THE BEST OF
NURSING HUMOR

Volume 2

THE BEST OF
NURSING HUMOR

A collection of
articles, essays,
and poetry
published in the
nursing literature

Volume 2

COMPILED AND EDITED BY

COLLEEN KENEFICK

ASSOCIATE LIBRARIAN, HEALTH SCIENCES CENTER LIBRARY
STATE UNIVERSITY OF NEW YORK AT STONY BROOK
STONY BROOK, NEW YORK

AMY Y. YOUNG

CATALOG LIBRARIAN, WISSER LIBRARY
NEW YORK INSTITUTE OF TECHNOLOGY
OLD WESTBURY, NEW YORK

HANLEY & BELFUS, INC.
PHILADELPHIA

Publisher: HANLEY & BELFUS, INC.
                  Medical Publishers
                  210 South 13th Street
                  Philadelphia, PA 19107
                  (215) 546-7293; 800-962-1892
                  FAX (215) 790-9330
                  Web site: http://www.hanleyandbelfus.com

The Best of Nursing Humor, Volume 2   ISBN 1-56053-272-6

Library of Congress Catalog Card Number 92-75985

Last digit is the print number: 9 8 7 6 5 4 3 2 1

For my loving husband,
Erwin London,
whose indulgence, patience, and grand style
never fail to amaze me.

CK

This book is dedicated to my son
Scott
for helping me keep in focus
the important issues in life.
To watch him grow is one of the
greatest blessings I have ever received.

AYY

CONTENTS

NOT YOUR AVERAGE DAY

LIVING LANGUAGE

THE DIFFERENCE BETWEEN YOU AND ME

ACCIDENTS HAPPEN

CHAOS AND COMPLIANCE

CONTENTS

LEARNING TO LEARN

ACADEMIC APTITUDE

CONTENTS

A PATIENT'S TALE

AT TIMES LIKE THIS

ACKNOWLEDGMENTS

This book is a product of the time, energy, ideas, and talents of many people. We are indebted to all those who played a role in its creation.

Most of all, our gratitude goes to the many authors who saw the humor and joy in the everyday and generously shared that by writing for others. Without their creativity, this book would not have been possible.

A project of this magnitude required extensive use of many academic and medical libraries in the New York metropolitan area. All of the librarians we have encountered graciously made their research material available.

Spencer Marsh, Miriam Swank, and other colleagues at the SUNY Stony Brook Health Sciences Center Library were enthusiastic supporters throughout the entire process.

Dr. Edward Guiliano, Clare Cohn, and other colleagues at New York Institute of Technology were most generous and unwavering in their support.

Special thanks are due to illustrator Phyllis J. Evans for expertly interpreting our fuzzy ideas into real drawings that capture the essence of each chapter.

Our appreciation to Linda Belfus and her staff for their tireless good humor, caring attention, and infinite patience in giving us the privilege of laughing our way into print.

INTRODUCTION TO VOLUME 1

A couple of years ago right before the end of fall semester, when the library was almost deserted, we overheard two nursing students complain about their classes and their interminable reading lists. We smiled at the familiar comments, but something struck a nerve when we heard one of them say "and none of it is even funny!"

Being medical librarians and having quirky senses of humor, we decided to find out for ourselves if there was any validity to that statement. Unable to locate material in a single volume on the topic of nursing humor, we began by searching Medline, CINAHL and the Nursing Studies Index. Most of the material in these indexes were articles about using humor as a coping mechanism or as a teaching tool. After a preliminary search, we were ready to agree that there really was nothing funny in the nursing literature.

Undaunted by the paucity of material, we decided to examine recent journals more carefully. An explosive growth in nursing journals occurred in the 1970s and, with this in mind, we decided to start with 1970 and end with June 1992. Eventually we spent untold hours scanning cover to cover 60 some journals published between 1970 and 1992. It became difficult to locate humorous pieces in most of the leading nursing journals published since the mid 1980s. Journals that had previously published humor or satire had eliminated those sections. Only North American and British journals were perused, with 33 journals eventually being represented in this collection. Our original intention was to select material only from nursing journals, but the search led us to pieces that were too good not to be included.

The following guidelines governed our selection process. All of the material had to be written by or about nurses. Every article had to say something about at least one aspect of the nursing profession and it had to make us laugh, chuckle, or at least smile. Humor comes in various styles, and since we both have very different senses of humor, we decided that we had to agree on the inclusion of each and every piece. We made no attempt to exclude material that may be viewed as sexist or controversial; rather the goal was to have a representative sample. Every effort was made to explore the rich diversity of nursing life. If more than one article covered the same subject, we included the funniest one or the one that we thought would have the broadest appeal. Some chapters are longer than others because more published material was found in those areas. Many of the articles selected deal with interrelationships and communication between colleagues, families, and patients, in keeping with the current emphasis on the humanistic side of medicine and nursing.

To authors and readers whose favorite material is not included, we apologize for the oversight. Please send us your cherished selections so that they can be reviewed for the next edition.

The articles are divided into nine chapters that chronicle the stages a typical nurse experiences during the course of a long career. Beginning with the trials and tribulations of nursing school, neophytes then discover the perils of job hunting. At this juncture, they also receive the first glimpse of "real-life" nursing. In the third chapter, the new nurse learns to cope with a plethora of diseases along with the nuts and bolts of treatment regimens. Learning to cooperate with physicians and using communication effectively are of paramount importance in a nurse's daily work. The sixth chapter details the world of academics and the mass media's perceptions of the nursing profession. With courage, humility, and compassion, the wonderful world of patient care is depicted. Exposing the realities of day-to-day nursing is the essence of chapter eight. In the final chapter, the fulfillment of pursuing this role over time is examined.

An extensive bibliography is included because many excellent articles were omitted. Most of these articles are of the same quality as those that were selected but did not fit into one of the nine chapters. Also, when both editors could not agree on the merits of a piece, it was excluded but listed in the bibliography. Unfortunately, many outstanding articles are included in the bibliography because copyright permission could not be obtained.

We hope that this volume will appeal to nurses, their families, and their associates in other health-care professions. Not every article will appeal to every reader, but everyone should find something entertaining within these pages. So sit back, put your feet up, relax, and enjoy.

Colleen Kenefick
Amy Y. Young

INTRODUCTION TO VOLUME 2

This is our second volume, and fortunately for the undertaking, we forgot the amount of work involved in the first volume and only remembered our joy with the end result. Organizing any book is a massive project, especially one that depends greatly upon the kindness of so many. Thus, we begin by acknowledging the talented authors who write humorous professional articles and their publishers for granting us permission to reprint them. We also took full advantage of the generous advice and comments given by readers of the first volume.

All new material was chosen for this volume, reflecting both the changing times and our maturing judgment. Selection criteria were the same as for the first volume since neither one of us has made the career move to become a nurse. Each article had to teach us something about nursing and at the same time fit our subjective definition of humor. Both editors had to agree on the inclusion of each piece, but in case of disagreement, a logical decision was made based on which one of us argued longer and louder on the merits of that particular piece.

Most humor articles and many editorials are either poorly indexed or not indexed at all. Very few selections were found by using indexes or by searching computerized databases. For this reason, we manually scanned 119 journal titles page by page from 1992 through 1997, with additional selective searches dating back to the early twentieth century. Although the majority of pieces selected are from the present decade, one of the earliest pieces is from 1917. For this volume, we extended the scope by seeking out humorous articles pertaining to nursing written by authors in other professions. The tone and inherent quality of expression, rather than the subject matter, were the most important criteria for selection. Fifty different journal titles are now represented in this collection.

This book is arranged into 12 chapters, recognizing that many activities occur simultaneously during a typical nurse's career. "Ideal Nurse" begins by examining prevailing attitudes and stereotypes of the perfect nursing image. Since every nurse must deal with some form of administration during his or her entire career, those "On the Top" are next exposed. In order to assist nurses in identifying and classifying unique characters they will inevitably encounter, "Field Guides to Rare Species" are included. "Not Your Average Day" recognizes that no day is average for those in the nursing profession. The next chapter, "Living Language," is composed of the infinite variations of language and word understanding. "The Difference Between You and Me" primarily dissects the relationship between nurses, doctors, and other health professionals. "When Accidents Happen" chronicles emergency room events that probably will not appear on your television screen anytime soon. Working with an amazing variety of patients, nurses learn to expect both "Chaos and Compliance." Since learning is now a lifelong process, "Learning to Learn" is no longer limited to nursing students. "Academic Aptitude" is written for those that toil in the ivory tower. In "A Patient's Tale," patients portray their adventures and misadventures while experiencing nursing care. The final chapter concludes by describing the infinite pleasures of current nursing practice "At Times Like This."

Over the last 10 years serious scholarly research into the use of humor as a complement to the treatment regimen has dramatically increased. Humor has been repeatedly demonstrated to have positive physiologic effects, reduce stress, facilitate communication, and to increase learning retention. Over the years, we have collected multidisciplinary materials that detail the use of humor as a therapeutic agent and have included them here in two bibliographies. The journal bibliography is divided into 14 broad subject areas that will assist further research into using humor appropriately in health care settings. With the one notable exception of Norman Cousin's landmark book, *Anatomy of an Illness as Perceived by the Patient* published in 1979, all books and journal articles included have been published since 1980.

Rapid changes have occurred in nursing and in nurses' perceptions of their chosen profession within the last five years. With the demands of managed care, increasingly sophisticated technology, and shorter patient stays, humor is needed more than ever. G. K. Chesterton once wrote that "Angels can fly because they take themselves lightly." While we are not advocating taking the business of nursing lightly, we are suggesting that we do not always take ourselves quite so seriously.

When nothing but a good laugh will improve the day, there will always be something in this volume to make you smile or laugh. Of course, each one of us will find our own personal favorites among the material assembled here. Our wish for you is to find some special articles within these pages to savor and share when you truly need a laughter break.

Colleen Kenefick
Amy Y. Young

IDEAL NURSE

The Almost Perfect Pledge

I will never again say to a patient, "This will only hurt a little."

I will provide all patients with zillions of possible treatment alternatives.

I will endeavor to learn from all my patients, even though it's nearly impossible.

I will abstain from revealing my co-workers' private lives in the elevator.

Above all, I will honor the ideals of Miss Nightingale.

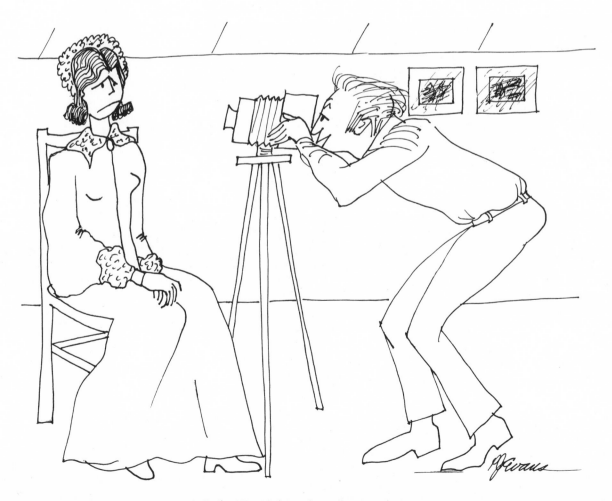

Smile, Miss Nightingale, and say "Crimea".

The Truth About Nurses: As Kids Tell It*

EVE R. WIRTH

Does anyone—other than nurses themselves—know the truth about nurses? Well, some kids think they do, or at least have inadvertently said what they think in humorous ways.

As a retired school teacher, I have collected some descriptions of nurses that were presented to me over the years by the 9-, 10-, and 11-year olds I have taught.

These boners were created via tests and reports: "A nurse is for helping folks when she is not needling folks." "I read that America is producing a large amount of nurses analy."

Then there are those children like Karl who manage to mangle metaphors: "I learned that nurses do a lot of hustling and bustling. They might be hustling and bustling in a hospital or a doctor's office. Who knows for sure. Why? Because it takes all of my learning to just learn that nurses do a lot of hustling and bustling."

My children tried to do their best on definitions on a quiz. RN is a "real nurse." LPN became a "long playing nurse." Then they were asked, "What kind of a degree does an RN have? One answer: "If she is normal—98.6, but if she is real hot it's around 105."

Perhaps they were right on target in this description of the real difference between male and female nurses: "A female nurse and a male nurse are eggactly the same, only the complete opposite in the you know where places."

Asked what they thought about nurses, my students had some fine opinions: "Studying to be an RN and ax-ally being one in real life on the job is a different colored horse story." And one of my favorites: "After hours nurses are just like real people. Once they take off their uniform, shoes, hat, stockings, and stuff and then they are ready to have fun."

In writing a report on nurses, one child even became quite emotional, although with more than 25 children in a classroom, there are always some extreme reactions. Here is some excess emotionalism in support of nursing that I cherish: "When I stop to think how great it is to have all those nice nurses working for us to get weller, I get a hot zooming all over my me. Then, just before the zooming stops, I get goose pimples that go pimply pimp on my left and right neck and a few in other places I can't say where."

Rebecca, a 10-year-old child, scribbled with her green pen: "All nurses are eggsited when they cure a sick person. And here is how they look when they did this: Their white cap goes up from their hair for gladness, their big eyeballs dance to the left of their nose and to the right of their nose, and then their nose goes in and out for thrills, and then their lips open wide and show their pearly tooth, and then if they have dimples like me, it goes in and out real fast, and then with a deep throat for happy tickles they are then ready to yell out loud, 'whoopee,' and that's the true story of how nurses look when they cure a sick person while they are working in a horsepit."

Another emotional reaction is Jill's: "After studying nurses, that they are a doctor's right arm and without her he would be crippled, I could have fainted on the school floor, if only I knew how to faint."

Tom wrote, "And here is something of an else I learned—a nurse is good if she always takes a doctor's odors real good."

How's this one for confusion?: "It takes high skill to be a great nurse. The smaller the hole, the higher the skill."

I pass, and so did all those wonderful students!

*Reprinted from Today's OR Nurse, ©1982; 4(7):72 with permission from Slack, Inc.

Are You Cut Out To Be a Nurse?*

Does your future lie in nursing? To find out simply complete our exclusive personality profile which sorts out the angels from the also-rans. Place a tick beside your preferred answer to each question.

1. You are running a bath for a patient. Do you:
   - (a) Use a bath thermometer to ensure that the water is exactly the right temperature?
   - (b) Use your elbow to test the temperature?
   - (c) Throw the patient in and take him out when he's nicely broiled?

2. The consultant surgeon asks for your hand in marriage. Do you:
   - (a) Throw your hat in the air with joy?
   - (b) Throw a right hook?
   - (c) Throw up?

3. The temperature is in the nineties. You are reprimanded for not wearing tights on the ward. Do you:
   - (a) Run the five miles home to retrieve your tights from the laundry basket?
   - (b) Apologise and promise to wear them tomorrow?
   - (c) Run into the sluice and paint your legs?

4. The hospital is short staffed and needs someone to do a night duty shift following day duty. Do you:
   - (a) Volunteer for the extra work—the hospital needs you?
   - (b) Keep quiet and hope no one asks you?
   - (c) Refuse because you are on a demo against staff cuts?

5. A patient tells you her life isn't worth living and she wishes she were dead. Do you:
   - (a) Tell her to enrol for pottery evening classes?
   - (b) Change her sterile dressing?
   - (c) Tot up her QALYs and write 'Not for Resus' on her Kardex?

6. You oversleep and are late in the ward. Sister sternly reprimands you. Do you:
   - (a) Sob in the sluice?
   - (b) Mutter in the linen cupboard?
   - (c) Thank her?

7. As a student you turn up for your shift to find no trained staff. The nursing officer asks you to take charge of the ward. Do you:
   - (a) Burst into tears?
   - (b) Go off sick?
   - (c) Agree and love every minute of the unaccustomed power?

8. You discover that one of the student nurses in your ward is the daughter of the general manager. Do you:
   - (a) Make sure she is given all the days off she wants?
   - (b) Treat her the same as the other students?
   - (c) Give her a hard time—who does she think she is anyway?

9. Your general manager complains that nobody likes him. Do you:
   - (a) Smile sweetly and say that you like him?
   - (b) Lie and say you don't know this?
   - (c) Throw him a stick of *Mum* rolette?

10. Out on the district you break down. Do you:
    - (a) Curse and ring the RAC?
    - (b) Look helpless and hope a man will come to your aid?
    - (c) Fix the bicycle puncture yourself?

11. The consultant surgeon suggests using a dressing you consider unsuitable. Do you:
    - (a) Smile sweetly and say, of course, he knows best?
    - (b) Smile sweetly and ignore his advice?
    - (c) Smile sweetly and apply the dressing to his mouth?

*Reprinted from Nursing Times, ©1987; 83(50):64–65 with permission from Macmillan Magazines.

12. Your health authority announces swingeing cuts in beds and services. Do you:
   (a) Not notice? You don't have time to read newspapers, listen to the radio, watch TV or count beds.
   (b) Write to *The Times?*
   (c) Take out private health insurance?

13. The government refuses to cough up this year's pay award. Do you:
   (a) Cancel your holiday and recycle your tights?
   (b) Get a job in America or in a bank?
   (c) Do agency work on your days off?

14. It's your round at the pub, but you are strapped for cash. Do you:
   (a) Decide you've got a headache and make a sudden departure?
   (b) Hold an impromptu whip round for Nursing Aid?
   (c) Order drinks all round—and one for the barman? After all, you only live once.

15. You are invited to appear on the TV show *The Price is Right*. Do you:
   (a) Spend the week before swotting up the answers thumbing through the *Argos* catalogue?
   (b) Refuse, saying the price is *not* right?
   (c) Place a notice in *The Times* announcing your forthcoming appearance?

16. You are asked to pose nude for *Penthouse* centrefold. Do you:
   (a) Agree, as long as it's for a £5 fee because you need some new tights?
   (b) Negotiate a £500 fee because you need a new job?
   (c) Refuse, pointing out that you are a man?

17. At a party an amorous male asks you what you do for a living. Do you:
   (a) Blush and admit that you are a nurse?
   (b) Change the subject?
   (c) Let him guess—grab his testicles and ask him to cough?

18. Which of the following songs do you prefer?
   (a) Stand by your man?
   (b) I will survive?
   (c) I'm leaving on a jet plane?

19. You decide you really ought to keep abreast of developments in nursing. Do you:
   (a) Read *Nursing Times*?
   (b) Watch *Casualty* on the TV?
   (c) Read another nursing journal?

20. You are appointed to Sister Plume's ward. Do you:
   (a) Get out your old copy of Florence Nightingale's *Notes on Nursing*?
   (b) Get out of her way.
   (c) Get out of nursing?

Real Nurses Don't Whine*

LEAH L. CURTIN, R.N.

Sometime ago, I found myself a captive at a no-frills conference of nurse theorists, researchers and graduate students. These worthies cared a lot about the theoretical foundations of nursing practice, but not at all about saunas or shopping. I hate to make generalizations, but there is an inverse correlation between smart-people and concern for creature comforts.

Abstraction to Distraction

Day after day the conference droned on from database to conceptual framework as speaker after speaker explicated in excruciating detail nursing phenomena in language only the initiated understood. We viewed pictures of slinkies and watched, in bemused bafflement, illustrations of theories that resembled nothing so much as thousand legged worms.

Night after night, I joined the group in the hotel's small seminar rooms to listen to lectures, to watch slides, and to make notes on what we were to cover the next day. No one suspected that, in college, responding to the question, "Define a biopsychosocial need," I had written, "chocolate."

This was not a crowd interested in such disingenuous frivolity. They were *purists* who had come to this seminar to *advance nursing science*. If they had known where I was coming from, they would have been shocked. They even talked *phenomenology* before breakfast!

I wouldn't have minded (too much, at any rate) wading through hours of mind-numbing jargon in the company of earnest scholars if there had been a Nieman-Marcus on the horizon. There was not. After landing at the airport, we had been transported by bus for two hours far into the countryside. Try as I might, I couldn't even find a Wal-Mart.

Listening to speeches read word for word from doctoral theses would have been bearable if, at least at the end I could have looked forward to a little bottle of wine and some munchies. Our hotel was situated in the precise center of a dry county.

There are few meetings held in parts of the world where you really have to fight to spend your money. You show me a nurses' convention and I'll show you a shopping mall. But, after three days, I gave up. I took my credit cards out of my bra and returned them to my wallet.

Meanwhile, the conference crawled along a treadmill to oblivion with stop-offs at boredom and monotony. I fantasized about sedating a speaker with a dart gun from the back row. In my day dreams I became the Queen of Hearts shouting "Off with their empirical heads." I knew I really was hallucinating when I became Meryl Streep between the sheets with Robert Redford.

Something snapped. The next day, I refused to come out of my room until the conference coordinator (I was supposed to give the closing address) pounded on my door and shouted, "Leah, stop *whining*. Real nurses can take a lot more than this."

"Venting" to "Vision"

"Oh yeah," I thought. "Real nurses shop . . . and they never, never talk theory before coffee in the morning."

Come to think of it, real nurses don't even know there is a controversy between phenomenalists and empiricists. Real nurses don't deal with phenomena, they take care of patients. They don't worry about empiricism and they don't split philosophical hairs.

They do worry about giving someone the wrong medication.

Real nurses use disposable needles. And carry at least 690 patients.

I was on a roll now! Real nurses do not need calculators. Real nurses do not fear doctors. Real nurses do not blame anonymous "others" for their problems and they do not go about mumbling that they feel "powerless." What real nurses do on their days off is sleep.

Real nurses do not spend hours illustrating a conceptual framework. They do not speak or write in polysyllabic circumlocutions.

*Used with permission from Nursing Management, ©1992; 23(12): 9–10.

Real nurses do not fret about transcultural experiences: they worry about paying off their *Visa* bills.

Contrary to popular belief, real nurses *do* read. They read spreadsheets, they read patient charts, they read clinical and pharmaceutical updates, they read anything written by Judith Krantz.

Real nurses are not overachievers: they really *are* that smart.

Real nurses are not congenitally late for work.

Real nurses aren't co-dependent: they can take care of themselves while they take care of others. They are not too busy to listen to a frightened family member.

Real nurses are not afraid to cry.

A real nurse is proud of the profession and never says "I'm just a nurse."

A real nurse learns how the system works—if only out of self-protection.

A real nurse doesn't think that "tough, rational, performance-oriented, competent and no-nonsense" are accolades which apply only to men.

A real nurse *will* go to an insanely boring six-hour lecture but only if she gets CEUs.

The One True Principle

For decades, nurses have looked to science for vision and answers. They have expected scholars to rationalize and justify and professionalize nursing practice. Why can't we develop a meta theory? How did nurses ever practice without supporting data? Why am I stuck working the night shift every Christmas when I have more seniority than 99 percent of the rest of the staff and I have perfect attendance and I always document accurately and completely on every patient chart?

Monads, diads, triads, deficits, magnetic energy fields—we search endlessly for understanding.

Quantum physics, the wellness continuum, the scientific method, nursing diagnosis, advocacy, co-dependence, the uncertainty principle, the wounded inner child—we try to resolve our place in the universe.

Rogers, Neuman, Roy, King, Orem, Peplau, Major

Margaret Houlihan—the greatest minds in nursing have peered into the chaos, looking for order.

Yet real nurses have always known the answer.

In their heart of hearts, they have known the one guiding principle that governs everything: *Patients will be sick 24-hours a day, 7 days a week, 365 days a year. Including weekends, nights and holidays.*

Fantasy to Reality

Close your eyes.

Picture a glorious mauve and peach office. The picture window frames a distant view of the ocean; deep carpets muffle any noise.

As you turn around, you see a nurse sitting behind a 12-foot mahogany desk. She is about 30. Her hair is pulled back in a chic chignon. She's wearing a $1200 Liz Claiborne suit, three-inch heels and sculpted nails. A telephone glued to her left ear, she is negotiating a contract for a seminar on the latest modifications of an adjusted-needs theory based upon intentionally-directed, energy-wave patterns as applied to self-help deficits among pregnant women in the final stages of labor on the third day after a full moon.

Open your eyes. *This is not a real nurse.*

Now, erase that picture from your mind.

Think about a hospital unit. It is Christmas Eve. Decorations hang limply on the walls. In the middle of this snowy night, a respirator wheezes oxygen in and out of a 24-year-old who almost succeeded in killing himself. Lights flash red and green on the monitors over the bed of an elderly woman in congestive heart failure.

How do you spot the real nurses?

They are the ones in rumpled lab coats, leaning over the side rails, trying to negotiate the only "contract" that really matters: person to person.

My reverie ended there. The Conference Coordinator was still pounding on my door. I girded my loins to face another day.

She is right you know.

Real nurses don't whine.

Nobody Ever Told Me:
A Humorous Look
at the Preparation
of Critical Care Nurses*

KATHLEEN G. HRIBAR, R.N., M.S.N., C.C.R.N.

"Nobody ever told me that in order to be a critical care nurse I had to . . ." I find myself saying this at least once a shift, generally while contorted on my knees, juggling syringes, IVs, and hemostats. In order to help future critical care nurses avoid these surprises in the job description, I propose several changes in their current mode of preparation. This article will point out some current inadequacies and discuss the curricular changes needed to prepare efficient practitioners. Deficits exist in today's educational preparation of critical care nurses in three major areas: physical fitness, language and communication skills, and sensory assessment skills.

Physical Fitness

While height cannot be physically altered, nursing schools should start screening this variable more carefully. The ideal height for critical care nurses is 6 ft or more—for reaching those convenient IVs that hang on the ceilings, readily accessible light switches behind and under beds, and trapeze bars built for Larry Byrd. For those less-than-ideal candidates, early remedial work in pole vaulting, high jumping, or mountaineering skills may compensate. Nurses should maintain their weight at approximately 90 lb (41.7 kg) or less for squeezing into tight bedsides, medication areas, and locker rooms.

Critical care nurses should develop their strength until they can bench press their own weight. This would add incentive for keeping well below that 90-lb mark on the scales. Speed should be evidenced by demonstration of a 4-minute mile. Finally, future critical care nurses must develop enough endurance to survive a 3-day weekend without food, sleep, or bathroom privileges. Dance marathons disguised as a means of funding various charitable organizations

(even one's own school of nursing) are excellent for the development and assessment of these abilities.

Thus, to be truly complete in the area of physical preparation for critical care nursing, schools should make the following inclusions in their mandatory curriculum: Jane Fonda Aerobics I, II, III, and IV, power lifting, military survival training, and marathon running. Schools might also make available optional classes in competitive darts (remedial), javelin throw (intermediate), and chainsaw juggling (advanced). Participation in intramural arm wrestling tournaments should be wholeheartedly encouraged, perhaps with extra credit points offered to the winners.

Language and Communication Skills

No present curriculum covers those specialized communication skills needed by the critical care nurse. Variable voice projection is necessary to communicate confidentially in an open-style unit. This is especially valuable to avoid shouting the more intimate steps in the clean-catch urine collection procedure and awakening the rest of the unit.

In order to interact with intubated patients, especially the confused, restrained patient who signs with head and shoulder motions only, nurses ought to develop telepathic communication skills. Hyperbole must be learned in order to minimize and maximize the impact of one's statements as needed. An example of such a hyperbolic derivation is:

1. You have a slightly abnormal heartbeat (*To the patient*)

2. He has a third-degree block (*To a coworker*)

3. How do I get a priest STAT? (*To the nursing supervisor*).

Finally, abbreviatology (the art and science of abbreviation) must be fully embraced. A critical care

*Reprinted with permission from Critical Care Nurse, ©1990; 10(2): 26–27.

nurse should be able to write two full pages (assessments, charting, etc) with five or fewer complete words, "A 45 yo WM with SOB, CP, and HTN" is one very brief example.

Nursing schools could readily develop formal coursework in both hyperbole and abbreviatology. They could be taught much like foreign languages, with recitations of hyperbolic derivations and conversational abbreviatology. Sign language courses are not recommended because of the obvious difficulty of teaching complex hand movements to the narcotized and/or restrained patient. Instead, schools might offer more universal skills such as hula dancing or hieroglyphics for independent study.

Educators should advise students to participate in cheerleading for the development of encouragement skills and voice projection. Those with more advanced language skills might choose to pursue ventriloquism to help their future patients ask those burning questions when the doctors are around.

Sensory Assessment Skills

Very specific sensory skills are required to fully assess the acutely ill patient while screening out the critical care unit environment. Both smell and hearing must be intensively developed in order to finely assess patients at the same time that constant background noise and various noxious aromas are tolerated, even ignored. Nurses must also fine tune their visual acuity for use in variable and generally undesirable circumstances. Assessing the color and circulatory status of cold Clara's feet at 3 AM is always a challenge.

Meeting these objectives is the job of all faculty involved in nursing education. Increased time in organic chemistry and biology lab courses may help the olfactory sense accommodate itself to constant bombardment by noxious stimuli while attempting to filter out the more significant odors like smoke, gas, and burning lab books. Continued academic emphasis on large lecture courses with poor articulators presenting will help develop those fine listening skills while learning to tune out the chorus of "what-did-she-says" in the background. Large lecture courses are also useful for developing fine visual acuity. Educators should be instructed to use only overheads and slides with volumes of fine print, especially slides of cellular organelles, Gram stains, and any electron-microscope-produced slides. Remember, the content is not important; instead, such coursework should emphasize and subsequently test the sensory skill developmental component.

Other Recommendations

Mechanical and electrical engineering courses would be helpful for operating complex machines, pumps, monitors, and computers. Architectural drawing would surely help in the construction of complex laddergrams required to analyze the elusive cardiac arrhythmia. Perhaps offering a major in nursing with a minor in engineering would prove to be a winning marketing strategy for making one nursing school a favorite.

A new avenue of study is the field of negotiation, including nuclear disarmament, hostage situations, and union negotiations. Any course in this specialty would prove useful in future dealings with patients, families, and coworkers who insist upon getting the only chocolate doughnut. Addition of these courses would be left to the discretion of the individual educational center.

All in all, we do a pretty good job of preparing critical care nurses. With some purposeful fine tuning and redirected emphasis, the present educational structure will prepare them to meet their daily challenges, master their profession, and truly enjoy being critical care nurses.

How to be a Crack ICU Nurse*

PAULINE DONNELLY, R.N., B.S.N., C.E.N.

The ICU nurse. Some say it means Icy Cold and Un-friendly. Intolerably Condescending and Uncivil, or maybe Impenetratingly Contemptuous and Uncompromising. Whatever your definition, these traits are not inborn. The following steps can get you started along the way to becoming a Crack ICU nurse.

First get rid of your nursing school smile. ICU nurses are a grim, serious lot. Their patients are CRITICALLY ILL!

Replace that smile with a chip on your shoulder. Thinly disguised contempt for other nurses is the rule and intimidation is the key to control these nurses. If a Med-Surg nurse has the audacity to transfer a patient to you, make her sweat by firing questions at her, like: "What's his crit? What's his K? Any ectopy?" Sneer when you say, "You didn't listen to his breath sounds? Did you try to palp a BP?" Yawn when she tries to redeem herself by reciting the color and consistency of his last five bowel movements.

Remember that ER nurses are your most dangerous enemies. They have the power to admit patients even when you have no beds. Supervisors bend over backwards to shuffle inpatients around for these EMERGENCY patients.

ER nurses are also difficult to intimidate because they have answers to all your questions. Astute observation can save the day, however. Glaring omissions can be pointed out, such as: "No-one signed this clothing sheet . . . wrote a laxative order . . . totalled this I&O sheet . . . labeled this IV bag." Don't get too carried away or they will punish you by delivering your patient while you're in report, leaving for lunch, or giving trach care.

Never forget that visiting hours are visiting hours. When visitors barge into your unit five minutes before the hour, firmly turn them back, reminding them that you need to complete your life-saving work if they expect to visit a live family member.

Use visiting hours for family teaching. Teach them not to touch anything without your permission. Teach them to rely on your judgment since the patient's doctors can't agree on anything. Finally, explain DRGs to them; this will motivate them when you teach them how to administer TPN in the home when their loved one is discharged.

Practice that Incredibly Cranky and Unaccommodating look in the mirror until it's perfect. No, that's not it. Try again. No, that's Immeasurably Cheerful and Uplifting—that's for the other floors. Now you've got it. Congratulations, and welcome to the world of ICU nursing!

*Reprinted from Journal of Nursing Jocularity, ©1991; 1(1):13 with permission from the author.

What Type of Nurse are You?*

CHRISTINE STEPHENS, R.N.

You're quick to label your nurse-colleagues, so you can tell who to stay away from and who you can depend on in a pinch. But do you know where you might stand in their eyes? Take this quiz to find out.

1. **How long have you been a nurse?**
   (a) 5 years or less.
   (b) 5 to 20 years.
   (c) 30 to 60 years.

2. **What effect do you have on your patients?**
   (a) Knowing you're on this shift evokes an irresistible urge to press the call light button every five minutes.
   (b) Knowing you're on this shift has reduced the call light pressing urge to within normal limits and only with reasonable requests.
   (c) Knowing you're on this shift has caused an intense fear of touching the call light button.

3. **Your hair style is:**
   (a) Ponytail.
   (b) Short bob.
   (c) Beehive.

4. **Your eye wear is:**
   (a) Not needed.
   (b) Contacts or fashionable frames.
   (c) Horn-rimmed bifocals.

5. **Your effect on your co-workers, doctors and supervisors is:**
   (a) Chuckling indifference.
   (b) Mutual respect.
   (c) Bladder incontinence, heart palpitations, "fight or flight" response, hives and/or hyperventilation.

6. **Your preferred uniform is:**
   (a) White pants, top with bunny or daisy print.
   (b) White pants, plain scrub top, or one with a professional or tastefully humorous print.
   (c) Stiff white uniform dress, cap, support hose and orthopedic shoes.

7. **You received your nursing training at:**
   (a) A respectable university.
   (b) A respectable university, plus inservices, conferences and continuing ed tests in nursing magazines.
   (c) Field training as a battlefield medic in the Korean War.

8. **You handle a medical emergency by:**
   (a) Breaking out in a cold sweat and calling for help.
   (b) Working confidently with the rest of the crash team.
   (c) Bulldozing the crash team aside while you administer to the patient by yourself.

9. **How do you handle demanding families?**
   (a) Find a good hiding place.
   (b) Calmly and competently answer their questions.
   (c) Give them your most evil stare and send them scurrying off in fear.

10. **How do you handle questions from supervisors and state inspectors?**
    (a) With a weak and tremulous voice.
    (b) With confident and knowledgeable answers.
    (c) With a malicious sneer.

Analysis

Count up the number of A, B and C answers you gave.

If you answered A to most of these questions, build your expertise through study and experience to gain enough nursing knowledge to function as a reasonably competent nurse.

If you answered B to most of these questions, you are a competent and experienced nurse, and a valuable asset to your employer.

If you answered C to most of these questions, you are a certified vintage nurse. Look around and see how nursing has changed.

*Reprinted with permission from Journal of Nursing Jocularity, ©1997; 7(1):14–15.

The Case of the Reluctant Role Model: From Health to Heresy*

LEAH L. CURTIN, R.N.

I'm not sure when it all began, but I can date some of its most pernicious manifestations back to the A.N.A. Convention in Houston, Texas. Houston in June is hot enough, but in 1980 Houston was having a heat wave: temperatures routinely reached 118°, the humidity ranged around 95 percent, and air-conditioned buildings were opened to the public to help prevent heat stroke. *And the nurses at the A.N.A. Convention, young and old alike, were expected to jog.*

Casting disbelieving eyes on my earnest colleagues and exhibiting all the self-sacrifice of the early martyrs, I offered to participate by staying in my air-conditioned hotel room and *praying for their survival.*

Unfortunately, my ruse did not fool those zealous advocates of self-improvement who insisted that I had a *duty* to be a health role model. Undaunted by my piteous cries of incapacity, they dragged me down to the streets of Houston. Only the most cunning behavior saved me from becoming nothing more than a greasy spot on the cement. When my colleagues rounded the first corner, I slyly slipped down a stairway leading to an air-conditioned underground shopping mall wherein I found a delightful little restaurant which happily served buttered croissants and steaming coffee at 6:00 AM. I finished just in time to splash some water on my hair and face, join my colleagues upon their return and assure one and all that I'd found the experience zestful indeed.

Since that time, matters have become desperate: no sooner do I order a double chocolate brownie with ice cream and hot fudge sauce than some 80 pound nurse comments, "I certainly wish that *I* could afford to eat *that* many calories." If I sit at a meeting with my legs comfortably crossed, inevitably someone informs me that it's bad for my circulation. And, while I grudgingly gave up cigarettes, colleagues who find it necessary to remind me—as I daintily sip my gin and tonic—that alcohol destroys brain cells are treading on thin ice. My duty to be a health model seemingly has no end.

Health research . . .

In self-defense I searched the literature: what all does one have to do to model a healthy life? I started with the Utah studies. Conducted in the 1960s, these studies confirmed what my mother taught me (and she didn't even have a government grant!): don't drink or smoke or carouse. While these findings were discouraging to someone of my inclinations, at least the subjects were human. Most of the other studies have been conducted using rats—singularly puny ones grown in laboratories for the express purpose of proving that almost everything is hazardous to your health.

If these studies are to be believed, to live a long and healthy life (and, incidentally, to be a health model) one must not drink alcohol and coffee or smoke cigarettes (or anything else for that matter), or eat much red meat or sausage or bacon or too much of anything else. One should work, but not too much or too little. One should marry (neither too young nor too old), have children (neither too many nor too few), go to bed and arise at about the same time each day, exercise regularly, remain geographically stable, and avoid noise, crowds and white bread and white sugar (both of which cause a gruesome death within hours of ingestion).

Moreover, the data indicate that one must eschew all food additives—a very difficult chore when most plants and animals are grown by multinational corporations which deliberately fill them with chemicals for the express purpose of poisoning their unsuspecting consumers. However, the government, ever watchful, requires them to reveal all chemicals and additives on the products' labels. The only problem is that the government doesn't require that they be translated into English. Consequently most labels are written in a foreign language decipherable only by chemists who have specialized in the field. As a general rule, consumers can figure that the more syllables per word, the more dangerous the additive. My research indicates that addi-

*Adapted with permission from Nursing Management, ©1986; 17(7): 7–8.

tives with more than six syllables cause instant death in laboratory rats.

Not that this means much: according to most studies, laboratory rats are getting sick on just about everything we eat—including diet colas. After extended study of the studies, I've concluded that today's laboratory rats are incapable of living in today's world (and no wonder, when you consider the sterile environments, controlled diets, and exercise regimens they're forced to follow!). I suggest that all future studies be conducted using New York City Sewer Rats, which undoubtedly have lifestyles far closer to most humans anyway.

. . . provides data—both offensive and defensive

By now it should be abundantly clear to all readers that my character has steadily deteriorated since that fateful day in Houston in 1980. I've become a fair imposter, a pretty good cheat, and a truly artistic liar. I don sweatsuit and sweatbands without any intention of sweating. I steal food from friends' plates on the premise that it's not fattening if I didn't order it. I've discovered that if I move the bathroom scale to a place where the floor slants a little, I can lose five pounds without struggling.

I have become convinced that calories really are dietetic measures of tastiness. Cheesecake, for example, has a great many calories, whereas turnips have practically none at all. Going on a diet has become something like opening a bank account: a calorie saved is a calorie earned. Thus I can wash down a whole bag of potato chips with a diet cola and still count up the calories I saved. I rationalize my failure as a health role model with lies: "If I just look at an eclair, I get fat" (so now I have to eat with my eyes closed); "I injured my foot last week in aerobic dancing class" (so now I can only stroll leisurely through Saks); "Really, I enjoy working long hours" (so now I can't even *complain* with credibility).

It all goes to show how persistent moralizing leads to corruption.

The nursing profession today is plagued with health zealots bent on improving others, particularly their colleagues. This had better stop before there are no honest nurses left, to say nothing of no collegial relationships.

Perfectly innocent nurses have been accosted by colleagues who do missionary work under the pretense of health teaching and who generously share their newly acquired techniques in the hope of making others as healthy as themselves. Their fervor is so great that they will spare nothing, not even the feelings of those whom they wish to save. If you protest that you do not want to change your lifestyle, they offer to help you develop enough insight to recognize the error of your ways. If you complain that you don't want to know your errors because you're perfectly happy the way you are, they reply, "You only think you're happy." Some wish to rid you of your excess poundage, others of your slovenly muscle tone, still others of your guilt about being chubby and unfit. If you protest that you feel no guilt, you are given a patronizing smile and assurances that they *understand* how you feel.

The pleasures of correcting others are seductive: the hidden passion aroused at the sight of another's failings; the suppressed feelings of superiority at someone else's weaknesses; the flush of generosity that accompanies a resolve to set the poor soul straight; the warm glow of satisfaction as one displays, for the benefit of others, one's superior knowledge and/or behavior. Are not these the reward of virtue? Can I, whose profession is nursing, whose calling is to promote the health and well-being of others, condemn this practice?

Yes. Unhesitatingly and completely.

A professional does not trade on personal relationships—or, heaven forbid, social ones—to demonstrate virtue. One engages in health teaching almost exclusively upon *request*. People seldom refuse help *when* they've asked for it and *if* it is offered in the right way. One does not seek out evildoers like a policeman setting a speed trap—waiting anxiously for an opportunity to pounce on offenders. Indeed, one *can* model healthful behaviors provided that one is not too obvious or arrogant or self-righteous. Otherwise, however well-intentioned your attempts to Set a Good Example for the less-disciplined, they will be repudiated.

The More Things Change*

GILLESPIE RICHARDS

"I'm glad you shared your concerns with me," the staff development instructor confided. "I hear you saying that this is stressful and I am certainly more comfortable when you verbalize these needs."

This form of language is an integral part of nursing education at the hospital where I recently began orientation as a staff nurse. After all, why be direct and just say "Yup!" when you can "hear where someone's coming from"?

My mentors know how to "talk nice" like this. These out-of-uniform, used-to-be nurses know how to account for objectives, goals, actions, expected outcomes—and yet make hair appointments. They all seem to be "into" aerobics, wear size three slacks, and talk about vital options such as skinned chicken breasts in wine sauce and "doing juices" on their coffee breaks.

Much to their credit, they *can* run a VCR. All things being equal, this is as essential as spotting a good wave form from a Swan. Sometimes I feel as though I've been left to watch films for the same reason I leave my two sons in front of the TV: so they—or, in this case, I—will not "awaken" before the tape runs out. I don't blame my instructors. They're supposed to explain the red tape, teach me the paperwork, and worry that I'll kill somebody while I'm still on orientation.

Being new is no fun. Being new and old is even worse. This hospital is full of clear-eyed, flat-stomached youth. They handle complex patients with ease and are up-to-date on all the machines we use to torture those patients. I report off to one wellness devotee who does tendon stretches against the hallway wall during the entire report. I wonder what she has in mind for patients on complete bedrest? My report is likely to start with the daughter's phone number and the wife's whereabouts. Her report consists of parameters, diameters, numbers, rates, and acronyms.

They wear a lot of memorabilia on their uniforms: pins, nameplates, flowers, "I care" buttons, "Love a nurse" buttons, their stethoscopes. I don't know how they get dressed in the morning. Or how they undo a uniform to wash it. I'm thrilled when I find clean nylons on my first rummage through my drawer.

And then, since these young nurses were "oriented" before me, they seem to enjoy practicing their caring on me. They ask me open-ended questions like, "Who are your significant others?" and "How are you adapting to this career change?" Once we've shared and verbalized a while, the real question comes out: "How old are you, anyway?" And when I say 38, their eyes glass over and their lips stick to their smiling gums and I can actually see them putting me in that special place one puts people who are *almost 40*.

I'm not really old, and I'm as healthy as a horse. Several times I've tried to come down with diseases to get some attention, or to get time off from my 24-hour on-call position known as "mother." Nothing ever showed on x-ray, though; my disgustingly healthy glow never dimmed. Occasionally it crosses my mind to call in sick because of hemorrhoids, bunions, corns, varicose veins, cellulite, gas—but I never have the nerve.

I am chastised, though, when I see some of the patients in this subacute care unit. They suffer from total body failure and have lines and tubes in every God-given orifice as well as in some newly constructed ones. A warning beep sounds, and I wonder if the fries are ready at McDonalds, yet I know that here it means someone on a vent is not breathing. Caring for 80-year-old patients, we see everything go, one thing after another. We seem unable to identify a polite time or place to stop giving care, so on we go.

The tearful wife of one elderly man asks me if he will ever get well, and I can't remember how to talk nice. I have no way to make "no" sound like "yes," so I just reach out my hand. He's a good learning experience, my ticket into acceptance by this young clan. Sometimes I see a big circle in life, tying together my youthful co-workers with this half-old nurse who can't get sick and with these very old patients who can't get well, no matter what we do.

And it's then I realize that I am already oriented.

*Reprinted with permission from American Journal of Nursing, ©1986; 86(8):982.

ON THE TOP

This is the era of managed care, but not necessarily caring management. Settling accounts and balancing books is of primary importance to management while attempting to meet the diverse needs of competing forces. Model managers know that when freed from justifying their existence, nurses will be more creative, inventive, and productive.

Nurses continue to perform at ever increasing skill levels, determined to provide their best despite myriad limitations. It is a daily struggle to remain optimistic, all the while observing the rapidly changing health care environment.

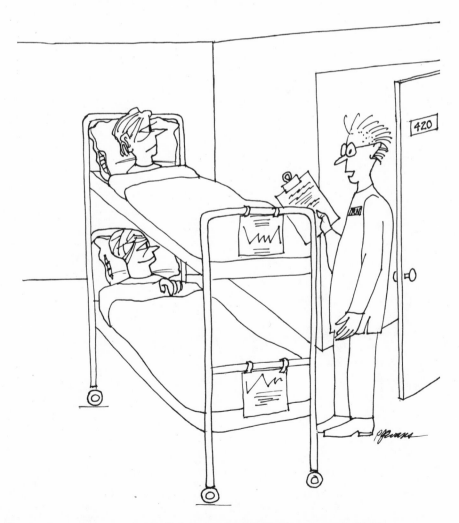

"Good news! Your HMO finally approved a ladder."

Meaningful Management*

An attempt to break down the "Them and Us" barrier

- Please stop shroud waving.
  Don't mention patients.

- There is no question of further cutbacks.
  They have already been decided.

- I think this will be an exciting challenge for you.
  You're being moved to manage the Pathology out-patient service.

- You have a completely free hand with this budget.
  It's overspent and the chief executive has noticed.

- I think we should call a meeting about this.
  The chocolate digestives I bought last week are getting stale.

- These figures need careful examination.
  Could someone please explain this budget print-out?

- I don't have the figures to hand.
  You're underspent but I don't want you to know.

- Of course, I take the broader view.
  I have no idea what you are talking about.

- We are forced to streamline the service.
  We must increase the number of managers.

- It is important that you ring me with any problems.
  I have just bought a new ansaphone.

- I like to keep in touch with the clinical side.
  I never miss 'Casualty' and 'Surgical Spirits'.

- My door is always open.
  I leave it like that when I am out of the office.

*Reprinted with permission from British Journal of Theatre Nursing, ©1994; 4(2):25.

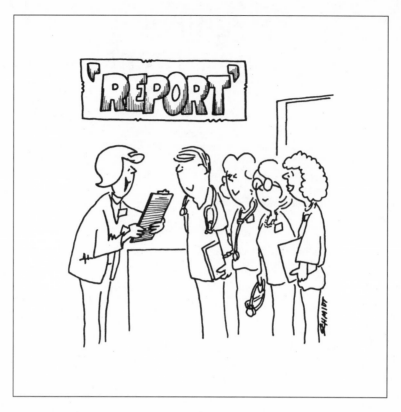

. . . 203 has four small pizzas and 206 just got a giant box of brownies . . .

Dear New Assistant Nurse Manager*

TOM HICKEY, R.N., M.D.

Welcome! Compared to me, I hope you are a better nurse and a better manager. I also hope you are as interested as I've been in inspiring the staff to look things up in one of the many current textbooks on the shelf behind them, instead of just asking whoever is sitting next to them to describe "The Right Way." I've never found a copy of "The Right Way" but keep hearing arguments between people who seem to have read different editions.

Key closing times: (Phones go dead 5 minutes earlier)

Cafeteria—6:00pm. (If you didn't get your supper by 6:00, plan on a clear liquid diet with maybe peanut butter and crackers.)

Kitchen—7:00pm. (To have dinner trays collected before they grow mold.)

Housekeeping—9:00pm. (When you need recently-vacated beds made up.)

*Used with permission from Nursing Management, ©1992; 23(10):90.

Maintenance—10:00pm. (To change a light bulb—on a good day.)

Your unit—Never. You have been carefully selected by the E.R., supervisors, doctors and other assistant nurse managers on the basis of your magical ability to find them one more bed on one minute's notice. Be prepared.

Avoiding disastrous tantrums at the bedside: Remember that a certain surgeon's patients are always "doing fine." Example: "Hello, doctor, Mr. Smith is 'doing fine.' He ate all his jello and his leg is nice and pink. However, we can't get a blood pressure on him and the E.R. doc is starting Dopamine. Otherwise he's 'doing fine.'"

The kiss of death: Passing on advice from one doctor to another. Example: a consultant tells you, "Just tell Bob he might want to switch to quinidine." If you fail to say instantly, "tell him yourself," you will spend the next three hours calling back and forth with messages like, "He said to ask you if you didn't see some article in last year's 'Annals of Medicine' about pro-arrhythmic effects of quinidine." (Will one of you guys *please* just give me an order?)

When things go crazy

1. Call the supervisor and calmly and concisely tell her the three or four major crises with which you are dealing. *Then* ask her if she can "spare someone to help out." You may get a nurse whose bad back prevents her from doing blood pressures, a unit-oriented nurse who can pick up a sick patient for the rest of the shift, or no help at all.

2. The phone may be ringing off the hook as dozens of "very close" relatives request individual detailed reports on a patient who went home last week. If this is keeping you from a crashing patient, you can tell the hospital operator that you are accepting no family phone calls for the next hour. Should they come to the hospital you can put a sign on the door saying "Special Procedure-No Admittance." Finally, when you take down the sign, be prepared to find that a forlorn hospital volunteer with a fistful of "get well" cards has been waiting patiently for an hour.

3. So far we have been lucky. Not one of our patients has died from going eight hours without a bath. (Actually, they didn't bathe several times a day back when they were working in their yards instead of having heart attacks.)

4. Prioritize. Sometimes the best you can do is keep all your patients alive until next shift. If you've been able to do that, be proud!

5. If you need: a helicopter, an ambulance, an unreachable doctor, a medication after the pharmacy closes, an emergency psychiatric consult for yourself or your staff—page the supervisor! Good luck!

Queen Busting

A Personality Profile of Hospital Royalty*
NANCY STEPHENS DONATELLI, M.S., R.N., C.E.N., C.N.A., JEFFREY B. JOHNSTON, M.P.A., R.N. AND ARLENE KIGER, M.S.N., R.N.

Do you remember the television show *Queen for a Day?* The program featured a chain of contestants, each one spreading her trials, tribulations and misfortunes as far as the TV signal would travel. After determining the most pathetic tale of the lot, the chosen "queen" would then reign over the activities for one special day.

Have you ever wondered where all those sad souls went after winning their title? Finally, after all of these years, we believe we have found the answer: many of them became nurses and continue their reign as queens in hospital units all across the country. All things considered, their behavior has changed only slightly over these many years. Why is this matter deadly serious? Queens destroy a unit's ability to work collaboratively, to grow professionally, and to offer the best in patient care. Therefore, if a unit is ever to offer true collegiality

*Adapted with permission from Nursing Management, ©1995; 24(1): 42–43.

and professional nursing care, queen busting is essential. Queen busting is not a sport reserved solely for management: queens hide some of their most "regal" behaviors when managers are around. Therefore, peers must take up the gauntlet of queen busting. Although this quest is not a sport for the timid or shy, it does reap enormous rewards. Often, busting a queen will relieve the enormous mental/emotional/physical load that comes from dealing with this personality. This, in itself, can make it seem as if extra staff has miraculously appeared!

In an effort to help you identify these stars of yesterday, the "Queen Profile" has been developed. Please take this profile test honestly and see if others on your unit, or even (horrors) you, qualify as a queen.

The queen (or king) profile

To complete the profile, circle all numbers that apply to you—or the person(s) of concern.

1. Frowns regularly, smiles rarely.
2. Is able to (and often does) quote verbatim from hospital personnel manuals.
3. Is quick to publicly criticize or identify which previous shift or nurse "didn't do it right!"
4. Has her/his own schedule calculated at least one year in advance, to maximize days off and vacation time. Also establishes long-range plans to effectively use future vacation time.
5. Hoards knowledge and/or expertise. Often is heard to say, "Just come to me and I'll tell you what to do," or "What? Don't you know that yet?" or "My way is best!"
6. Says, "We tried that before and it didn't work and won't work now because. . . ."
7. When asked to work with a group to identify and fix a problem, replies, "Nothing will change here, so why waste time talking about a fix?" If forced to attend a group meeting, these royal people:
   (a) Sit with arms folded across chest
   (b) Keep mouth zipped with a frown
   (c) Have outbursts of anger at management's inability to "fix it"
   (d) All of the above.
8. Often disappears from work areas for periods of time, leaving her/his patients for others to cover. Other times, says, "I'm going over to see [so and so] in [what-ever] department about a clinical problem," but isn't there if paged. Jokes about "making rounds" in various other units/departments.
9. Always hangs around the nurses station instead of patient rooms.
10. Is a "big-time" name dropper. Talks about how wonderful she/he is.
11. Makes no effort to attend educational classes and add to professional practice, even if learning is as close as the unit conference room.
12. If challenged/confronted/counseled, will sinisterly refer to an extensive private catalogue of "dirt" she/he has compiled on everyone else.
13. Will say, "Wait till you've been here a little longer. You'll see I'm right."
14. Always blames any event or mistake on someone or something else.
15. Hates *any* change.
16. Requires frequent and lavish praise.
17. Usually is not on duty when the unit has a "golden day" (smooth flow, collegial relations, great patient care, etc.).
18. Will always volunteer for anything that takes her/him away from direct patient care. Never tells other staff members, "I'll cover your patients so you can go."
19. Erupts in front of staff when some dramatic change is announced at a staff meeting.
20. Cuts people off mid-sentence or changes subject if it isn't her/his idea.
21. Bypasses nurse manager with "problems" and enlists the support of physicians/DON/VP.
22. Tells doctors/others that new nurses "are green and don't know any better."
23. Is angry/sullen if a "newer" nurse is in charge.
24. Feels free to unilaterally change unit patient assignments to get desired workload.
25. Sets peers up for failure by forgetting to cover call-offs or to tell nurses that doctors have called, and by not reporting doctor/patient complaints, etc.
26. Always talks about people behind their back, NEVER to their face!
27. Practices the "Three Bs":
   (a) Bickering
   (b) Backbiting
   (c) Bitching
28. Always "has to" go to lunch with the same people, at the same time, and sit at the same table.

Remembering
Home Care*

GERALDINE FIORIGLIO, R.N.

When the days go by and you wonder why
Just remember what you left behind.
As you relax in your garden and sit in the warm sun,
Think about your home care friends having all the fun.
Knocking on doors with no one to answer
Fighting the traffic, wondering "will it ever get better?"
Chasing after pumps that fail, catheters that leak,
Elusive veins and on-call each week.
No time for lunch or the money in your purse
Sharing one desk with every nurse.
Making this transition to "home health" or "home hell"?
All those new forms, 485, 487, what in heaven!
You can't forget those little ones, oh! What a pain yet a joy they've become.
The sad ones we've lost, the successes we've gained.
The need at times we have to complain, ventilate, or go insane.
And if you think we won't MISS YOU,
Then delusional thinking is coming through.

*Reprinted with permission from Home Healthcare Nurse, ©1997;
15(7):520. Edited from the original.

Dear Home Health CEO:*

IDA SANSOUZY

Dear Home Health CEO:

In this time of reengineering, down-sizing, right-sizing, and wrong-sizing, I have a suggestion for increasing productivity, adding to annual visits, and improving the morale and working conditions of all field nurses:

Requisition a recreational vehicle (RV), completely accessorized, for each field nurse. Here is an explanation of only a few of the advantages:

• An RV is a high-profile vehicle. It says, "Outta my way. I got patients to see." I can drive faster and see more patients in less time. The result: increased productivity.

• The demands for timely documentation continue to skyrocket. No longer would I be searching for a pen under the car seat nor honk the horn 5–10 times while sitting behind the wheel doing documentation. I would have access to a table, my laptop computer would be plugged in, and I'd be ready to begin documentation.

*Reprinted with permission from Home Healthcare Nurse, ©1997;
15(9):648.

• The cell phone and fax modem in the RV would allow me to communicate with physicians, case managers, and other caregivers quickly and efficiently. I could fax in an "add-on" order right away (such as one for a physical therapist). The physical therapist could potentially make a home visit the same day as a result of the speedy communication. That would add an extra visit to my daily stats and productivity indices. Over a budget year, what impact would that timely communication have as an advantage over our competition?

• When I'm too early for the next home visit, I can just pull the RV over, insert an educational video into the video cassette recorder, and learn about the nuances to managed care or a new reimbursable treatment. Time management to the hilt!

• To aid morale, the RV would allow me to take a break by meditating, using the RV's CD player, or taking a short nap, revitalizing my psyche and mental acuity.

• When the bladder calls, the facility is near. It's probably also clean and complete with the desired accoutrements. Less time is needed to complete daily bodily functions, let alone the time and stress now needed to find the location to do so.

• And, lastly, when hunger pangs are calling, there is a full-service kitchen behind the driver's seat. What's in the fridge? Do I use the microwave, stove top, or oven today? No more will I be a fast-food junkie. I'm on my way to a healthier lifestyle. I'll soon be a healthier employee, use less sick time, have improved productivity, and be a better risk for our self-insured health plan.

SO, when can I expect to move my trunk supplies?

Sincerely,

Ida Sansouzy
Your devoted field nurse

Formula for ED Staffing*

DEBBIE SUTHERLAND, R.N., M.S.N., F.N.P., C.F.R.N.

For the past several months, our emergency department has been undergoing redesign of our staffing patterns. This has been very stressful for our staff; change is often difficult. We were asked to contribute a staffing formula that was reasonable and would meet the department's needs. The night shift posted this formula for all to see. Perhaps other emergency departments enduring this process might benefit from the wonderful formula they created:

S = Staffing

P = Proximity to the full moon

R = Number of patients per hour

K = Number of helicopters able to fly

Z = Ambulances received in the past 24 hours

X = Temperature in Celsius

Y = Barometric pressure

Formula for ED Staffing

$$[(R-2) + (\Pi 3 \cdot \tfrac{4}{9})] \, \frac{Y + 3}{\tfrac{1}{52}} \cdot \frac{\sqrt{871} + 0.25}{(\tfrac{7}{15} - 3)} \div$$

$$\frac{[(X - \tfrac{1}{3})(Y + \tfrac{2}{3}) - \tfrac{3}{10}]}{\sqrt{7.1}} + \frac{\Pi 5^3}{\tfrac{5}{61}K} \div \frac{8}{17} +$$

$$\frac{R^2 - P^2 - X^2 \, Y^2}{\sqrt{Z^5}} - 1 + \frac{22{,}000}{0.75} = S$$

*Reproduced from Journal of Emergency Nursing, ©1996; 22(5):474 with permission from Mosby–Year Book, Inc.

Drills, Bills and Tulip Bulbs*

SISTER SUSIE

Hello there, Health Care Workers! You may remember that I had reservations about the computerisation of my Unit when it was first suggested. Well, you won't be surprised to learn that I was right to be worried!

Of course, the Head of the Directorate took no notice. He was so sure the computer would solve all our problems. The trouble is that he has been talking to the Outpatients Manager, who reduced the orthopaedic waiting list by 90 per cent in the first month after the system was installed.

Unfortunately, neither of them realised that this success was due to the system crashing after one week and losing most of the data. The consultant was a bit surprised to find his clinic empty on the Monday morning, but he used the spare time constructively by looking at the tenders to re-equip the orthopaedic theatre.

It looks as if Jowett & Sons, Painting, Decorating and Artexing, will win the contract. Do It All put in the lowest bid for the tender to supply new tools—or 'instruments', as they are learning to call them. But there is some question about the power capacity of the cordless drill, which might need to be recharged during a hip replacement. I understand a compromise is being worked out which may include a free set of patio furniture for the business manager.

Our own problems with the computer were more complicated. In fact, I wish the system had crashed. I can assure you no-one on my Unit would have rushed to resuscitate it. Except perhaps Nathan, who insists against all the evidence that it is not the computer's fault. I don't see how he manages to convince himself of that; we certainly never had the police here when we kept lists of patients in a big red book.

The problem started a few weeks ago, when a couple of gross of tulip bulbs from Amsterdam arrived at reception. Assuming there was another Royal visit or film crew due, the receptionists sent them to the estates department. There they were initially mistaken for exotic root vegetables ordered by the catering manager for the forthcoming Mexican lunch, and redirected to the catering department. Somebody did try to claim later that some of the bulbs were served to patients as the vegetarian option, but this was strenuously denied.

The bulk of the order was eventually returned to the estates department, who used them to brighten up the area where the staff social club used to be. It was only when the invoice arrived in the finance department that anyone questioned the order. The Public Relations Manager admitted that he might have ordered some bulbs on the off chance that someone important might visit during the flowering season. But he claimed that he would not have demanded that they be air-mailed urgently via Sydney, Australia.

The Business Manager, who frequently mistakes urgency for importance, and has been know to fax Post-it notes to himself to bolster his reputation as a mover and a shaker, denies all knowledge of the order. I think most people believe him. If he had ordered three gross of bulbs from Amsterdam, he would have arranged an executive seminar in the Amsterdam Hilton, and gone over to collect them himself.

Unfortunately, at this stage everyone assumed that someone else must have placed the order, probably as a last desperate attempt to empty the public relations budget before the end of the financial year. The invoice was paid, and by converting the rest of the budget into guilders, it was even possible to carry it over into the current financial year as 'foreign investments'.

Things were quiet for a week or so, but then other rumors started to circulate around the hospital.

A message had appeared on all the computer screens in the hospital reminding the Head of the Maternity Unit to renew her subscription to a pornographic magazine. Most of the admin staff seemed to have disappeared from the payroll data and were assumed to be working on a voluntary basis as the computer wouldn't print their payslips.

And, most excitingly of all, a huge sum of money had been electronically transferred to my unit budget by an unknown benefactor.

In spite of the disbelief of some of my colleagues, I was delighted—until last week, when the police arrived, and arrested Nathan!

*Reprinted with permission from Nursing Standard, ©1994; 8(39):44.

Detritus . . .
Reflections of a Practice Nurse*

ROSEMARY COOK, R.G.N.

Teamworking? Bah, humbug! We are being brainwashed by the teamworking gurus into thinking that if we don't do everything together on the count of three, then we have failed some secret test to which only they have the answer sheet. If ever there was a pointless invention, it must be the primary health care team.

We all know that there is more than one kind of nurse in the community, and that there are other people who are not nurses who also do things for patients. Why that means we have to be labelled a team, and need regular 'workshops' and 'facilitation', I have yet to discover.

I once read a really interesting piece about teamworking. It was about a Frenchman who had studied teams of agricultural workers. For some reason he did not study them shearing sheep or ploughing fields or milking cows; instead he watched them doing tug o'wars. What the researcher found was that people actually worked less well when they were in a team. On their own they would give it everything they'd got,

straining and sweating away, presumably grunting the Gallic equivalent of 'By'eck, I dunno if I can do it but I'll give it me best shot.' Once part of a team, however, the amount of effort exerted on the rope by each individual actually fell. Far from being inspired by the collective effort to even greater things, they mentally shrugged their shoulders and said of the chap next to them 'If'e wants to wants to pop 'is clogs, let 'im. Me, I take it easy.' And they did.

The trouble with really interesting bits of research like that is that you can never find them again when you want to show them to a teamworking guru at a workshop.

*Reprinted with permission from Practice Nurse, ©1996; 12(6):418.

Managed Care
Meets the Symphony*

"The president of a large managed health care facility also served on the board of his community's symphony orchestra. Finding that he could not go to one of the concerts, he gave his tickets to the company's director of health care cost containment. The next morning he asked the director how he had enjoyed the performance. Instead of the usual polite remarks, the director handed him a memo which read as follows:

The undersigned submits the following comments

and recommendations relative to the performance of Schubert's "Unfinished Symphony" by this city's symphony orchestra as observed under actual working conditions:

A. The attendance of the conductor is unnecessary for public performances. The orchestra has obviously practiced and has the prior authorization from the conductor to play the symphony at a predetermined level of quality. Considerable money could be saved merely by having the conductor critique the

*Reprinted with permission from Public Health Nursing, ©1996; 13(6):375–376. Edited from the original.

orchestra's performance during a retrospective peer review meeting.

B. For considerable periods, the four oboe players had nothing to do. Their numbers should be reduced, and their work spread over the whole orchestra, thus eliminating peaks and valleys of activity.

C. All 12 violins were playing identical notes with identical motions. This is unnecessary duplication: the staff of this section should be cut drastically with consequent savings. If a large volume of sound is required, this could be obtained through electronic amplification, which has reached very high levels of reproductive quality.

D. Much effort was expended playing 16th notes or semiquavers. This seems an excessive refinement,

as most of the listeners are unable to distinguish such rapid playing. It is recommended that all notes be rounded up to the nearest eighth. If this is done, it would also be possible to use trainees and lower grade musicians with no loss of quality.

E. No useful purpose would appear to be served by repeating with horns the same passage that has already been handled by the strings. If all such redundant passages were eliminated, as determined by the utilization review committee, the concert would have been reduced from two hours to about 20 minutes, resulting in substantial savings in salaries and overhead. In fact, if Schubert had addressed these concerns on a cost containment basis, he probably would have been able to finish this symphony!

I remain, Sir, your most humble and obedient servant."

The View Askew*

PAT VEITENTHAL, R.N.

For those of you who have not yet had firsthand experience in the joys of patient-focused care, here are some guidelines from someone who is currently in the eye of the PFC hurricane.

Hopefully—so you won't get caught off guard, like I was—these caveats will tell you when to duck, when to board up the windows, when to run, and when it's time to bury the dead.

You'll know PFC is coming when:
• For Christmas, administration gives you a ballpoint pen engraved with the hospital logo, instead of a 15-pound turkey.
• Your nurse-manager lets you work out your own schedule to conform, she says, to "your needs." Then she starts talking about how great it would be to have four days off—if only your department worked 12-hour shifts.
• You are asked to submit money-saving ideas to management, after which you're rewarded with a coffee mug on which is emblazoned—what else?—The hospital's logo.
• You start hearing phrases such as, "The ship is leaking; we've got to plug the hole."
• Outpatient areas are expanded, as speciality areas are shut down.

• Patients are discharged from the unit.
• Cash bonuses no longer exist—but administrative offices undergo complete remodeling.
• You see ancillary service people, who have been at your hospital for 20 years, crying in the bathroom.
• Licensed practical nurses are smiling a lot.
• In staff meetings, you often hear the words, "cross training."
• Supervisors disappear.
• Full-time positions that have been vacated are not replaced—but three PRN positions are filled.
• You start to see healthy eating tips listed on the "Job Board."
• The employee education office becomes the employee education closet.
• When a patient complains, "I can't find my nurse," it takes on a whole new meaning.

*Reprinted with permission by REVOLUTION—The Journal of Nurse Empowerment (1-800-331-6534), ©1995; 5(3):67.

FIELD GUIDES TO RARE SPECIES

The human animal is found everywhere in health care, from the hospital cafeteria to the intensive care unit. Although many species are beneficial, others are simply pests, causing havoc among families. When identifying species it is always best to disturb them as little as possible and to exercise extreme caution, because some can be vicious when threatened.

The diversity of individuals appears overwhelming, but by observing them in their natural habitat identification soon becomes possible. Each species or their near relatives exhibit unique behavior and folklore. This chapter will help you learn about their secret world.

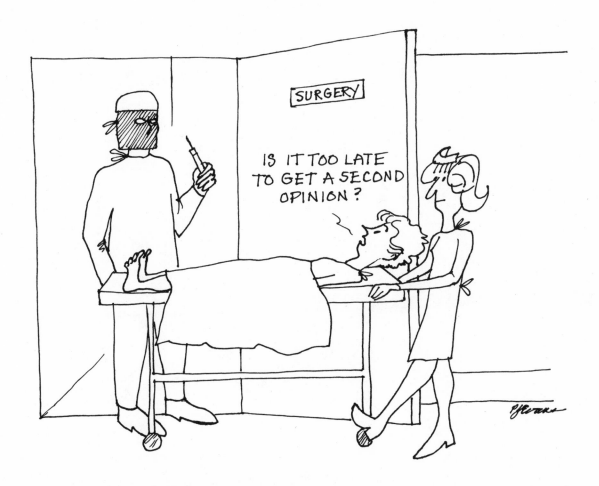

Bird Brained*

Even the most vitriolic opponent of NHS managers admits that, at times, they are necessary. Someone has to check up on nurses' ear-rings, harangue those returning from sick leave, and walk briskly through the wards from time to time. Someone has to come up with all those glossy booklets without which a modern health service could not possibly function.

But for the bedside nurse to survive the attentions of his or her own manager, it is important to be able to identify the particular species to which that manager belongs, observe principal characteristics (such as the mating call and boundary song) and behaviour patterns, and devise an adequate system for coping with his or her worst excesses.

The following descriptions cover the main species of health service manager. The most important characteristics frequently observed in the field are noted, together with suggestions on how to avoid alarming the subject, so causing it to fly off the handle.

Rare species

However, the nurse should remember, there is the chance of coming across a rare species, one who has gone off course from parts such as Europe or America, or from non-health service industries in this country. Such 'migrants' may choose to adopt their chanced-upon NHS setting, thus confusing the novice observer. They are perhaps most easily identified by their continuous alarm call: 'Downsize . . . downsize . . . downsize'.

The following species of manager are described in descending order of importance.

1. The Excellent Executive.

Almost invariably male, this manager rises rapidly to the top of the tree through a number of intervening perches on which he sits for a very short time. Each time he vacates one perch, after an interval of sometimes as much as two years, he leaves behind him much confusion among the sub-species. He has two degree-type markings on his letter headings, one of which is almost always in the shape of an MBA. His background in nursing has been rigorously erased, and neither marking nor behaviour reminiscent of bedside nursing will be observed out in the field.

His song is continuous and repetitious. Despite much field study by experts, however, its meaning remains unclear. He overcomes the songs from nearby lesser species by increasing his own volume and persistence. He frequently sheds innumerable leaves of paper, each containing a vocabulary that is as indecipherable as his song.

He is a good mimic. On hearing the song of the Powerful Politician, he is able to reproduce every word and phrase with uncanny accuracy. If he is asked to explain the meaning of his song, though, he flutters his wings irritably and repeats his call without variation.

The Executive is best handled by someone who is an equally good mimic. Try and learn by heart one or two of his favourite phrases, and repeat them when he flies past. Take several examples of his reports and mission statements into the field with you, so that you can be observed pouring over them and chirruping excitedly about their contents. You should find that your upward mobility becomes easier and you will soon be able to leave those boring old wards behind.

2. The Manic Megaphone.

Can be either male or female. This species is highly intelligent and brightly coloured, and the observer is left in no doubt at all about its presence within a particular habitat. Its song and call are both high pitched and loud, and reveal its whereabouts even when it cannot be spotted. Typically, its song consists of the oft-repeated trill of, 'Busy, busy, busy . . .'

Taking over nests

It has sometimes been confused with the cuckoo, because of its frequent practice of taking over the nests of lesser species. Having been set a task it cannot accomplish by itself, it habitually chooses a member of a lesser breed to carry out the work on its behalf. Once this has been done, however, and the item of work delivered, the Manic Megaphone turns on the other, tips it out of its nest, and takes all the credit itself. Despite this frequently observed pattern of behaviour, it is popular with other species of manager.

It responds well to loud cries of sympathy and support. Unshakeably convinced that it is the busiest species around, it seeks the reassurance of others that this is actually the case. Calls of admiration, such as, 'I don't know how you manage it' will be greeted by self-

*Reprinted with permission from Nursing Standard, ©1994; 9(6):39–40.

deprecating laughter and warm smiles. Beware, however, that you are not the next sub-species to be chosen to complete one of the Megaphone's unfinished tasks.

3. The Conference Collector.

A small, drably coloured species of manager that is rarely seen in its home territory. It frequently travels great distances to far-flung colonies and breeding grounds abroad, and so it is difficult for the observer to tell which is its preferred habitat.

On its return, it produces many leaves of paper, and the incomprehensible wording contained in these has led some observers to postulate that the Conference Collector is, in fact, an immature member of the Executive family. Others, however, assert that it is a distinct species. More research is required here.

Little advice needs to be given about the best way to handle this species, since it is so rarely encountered in the clinical situation.

4. The Silent Saviour.

Danger! On no account should you approach this species or in any way be seen associating with it! To be linked with the Silent Saviour is to give up any chance of promotion or career development for yourself.

This species is the favourite victim of the Manic Megaphone's attentions, because of its strong record in completing the latter's unfinished jobs and failing to grab the glory for doing so. Consequently, it remains comparatively low down the management tree, and roosts on the same perch for years, if not decades. Most managers claim they respect the Silent Saviour but are rarely seen in its company.

An interesting point to note is that all more senior managers approaching this species give out the same call: 'Can you just . . . , Can you just . . .' The Saviour is rarely heard making a call of its own.

5. The Desperate Dodo.

This species of manager is not yet as dead as the dodo, but is heading that way. It clings desperately to the lowest branch of the tree, and its greatest hope is that no one notices it there.

It is content simply to exist, and to draw its pay at the end of each month. It is frightened into ever-nearer extinction by the edicts that flutter down from the higher branches and, because it doesn't understand what they mean and doesn't know how to disguise that fact, it knows its days are numbered.

It is best left alone by the bedside nurse who should encounter no problems handling it. It has no identifiable calls, since its main strategy for survival is silence and subterfuge. It is in the late afternoons, when the sun sinks behind the management block, that its faint, shadowy form may be observed, scuttling furtively towards the car park. If spoken to, it has a tendency to jump in a startled fashion, or burst into tears.

As with all subjects, close study of the different management species will cause a greater fondness and respect for them. All creatures have a part to play in nature's grand design; even those such as wasps and managers do some good, even though it is not immediately obvious. As with wasps, though, you should avoid flapping angrily at persistent managers, as they can react unpleasantly.

The Reciprocal Natural Childbirth Index*

AL BERG

Introduction

The rate of cesarean section births has increased alarmingly in recent years,[1] so much so that some have suggested that the procedure be offered to every woman admitted in labor to a hospital.[2] We[3] think that's a bit much. We do believe, however, that the risks of vaginal birth in some women are so high that you might as well offer a cesarean section up front. In our experience the available biomedical risk scoring systems are not helpful. We have found that a system based on easily measured demographic and historical factors, administered at admission to the labor floor, predicts who needs a cesarean section extremely well. We call it the *Reciprocal Natural Childbirth Index*.

Methods

The *Reciprocal Natural Childbirth Index* (Table 1) is a simple additive risking instrument that can be administered in less than a minute. You can add up most of the score without even talking to the patient.

Results

We have used this index successfully for nearly a year. So far no one has scored less than 10, and the record score was 85. Of more than 100 women scoring 30 or greater, every single one ended up with a cesarean birth.

Discussion

We have found that a *Reciprocal Natural Childbirth Index* score of 30 or greater should earn the woman in labor immediate consideration for cesarean section. In fact, since you can get a score of 30 without even being in labor, someone with a high enough score could be offered a section at her convenience during regular working hours. We feel that implementing the index would save countless hours of needless labor, pain, and uncertainty.

Table 1. Reciprocal Natural Childbirth Index

Add points as indicated if the woman:

• goes into labor Friday afternoon	5
• has checked (or her husband has checked) cervical effacement and dilation at home	5
• arrives in a late-model Volvo station wagon	5
• has a hyphenated last name	5
• if the husband has one too	10
• is insured by a managed health care plan	5
• has more than four years of college	5
• if either parent is a physician	each, add 5
• if either parent is an attorney	each, add 10
• insists on calling all staff members by their first names	5
• brings her own naturopath to assist	5
• has a written birth plan	per page, add 5
• if printed on a word processor	per page, add 10
• spends more than half of labor in the shower	5
• brings her own Walkman®	5
• tapes are all New Age	each tape, add 5

Notes

1. Pick up any obstetrics journal.
2. *New England Journal of Medicine,* sometime in the last three years.
3. I couldn't get anyone to be a co-author on this, but I decided to use the editorial "we" anyhow.

Beastly Behavior*

LEAH L. CURTIN, R.N.

While visiting friends near the village of Lukachukai (located on the Navajo reservation), I met my first "house chicken." Reared from the egg onward with adult humans, *Chicken Cacciatore* was a bold bird indeed. Not for her the pitiful scratchings of the barnyard; rather she stole the choicest morsels from the plates of her human hosts. One day, however, "Catch"—for such was her sobriquet—got caught.

Beady eyes gleaming, saliva dripping from her beak (I had no idea before this that birds *could* salivate), she swept down upon a bit of meat and ran as quickly as her skinny legs could carry her toward the relative safety of the yard. She'd gone about 5 feet before her victim closed in behind her and gave her a swift kick in the rear. It lifted her 3 feet in the air before, with one tremendous squawk, she landed and spontaneously jettisoned a load of . . . er . . . "chicken droppings" on the spot.

Shocked by the entire proceedings, I mused (inadvertently out loud), "So that's what they mean when they say, 'I kicked the s#@* out of him.'" I was, of

*Used with permission from Nursing Management, ©1996; 27(4):7–8.

course, most embarrassed by my social gaffe. This earthy image, however, inspired me to reflect upon how often human behavior mimics animal behavior.

Speaking of chickens . . .

Endogenous to nursing circles, nurse chickens hold *bona fide* master's degrees in victimology. Crippled by poor self-esteem and an even poorer understanding of nursing's history, they undervalue themselves, their predecessors and their peers—and they blame just about everyone *but* themselves for problems created to no small extent by their own attitudes.

Given to squawking loudly in the privacy of the henhouse, they wimp out at the sight—or even the reported sighting—of a bully. Nurse-chickens make perfect rugs: they'll even pluck out their own feathers and weave them into welcome mats. Outwardly eager to please, they grumble and moan to one another—all the while laying plenty of eggs.

Nurses are *by no means* the *only* chickens in the health care henhouse; they're just the ones with whom I am most familiar by virtue of affinity and birthlines. I am aware of the many varieties and I mean no disrespect by my linguistic partiality.

In any case, with the prophets of old, I say, "Woe to the leaders of such flocks!" They must be wily enough to outwit the chicken hawks who'll scatter the birds at every opportunity. They also need the wisdom of an owl, the vision of a hawk, the courage of an eagle—and the skin of a rhinoceros to succeed.

Rx: Clearly, an ounce of prevention is worth a pound of cure. Recruitment into any of the health disciplines today should be limited to independent-minded—nay, even Libertarian—individuals who know that no one owes them anything. They must be educated scientifically and socialized into collaborative, multidisciplinary workforces committed to the supremacy of the empowered work-team.

For those already in the workforce, empowerment is the treatment of choice. Its implementation, however, raises many often-as-yet unanswered questions. For example, how do you convince a flock of birds who have always been rewarded for *following orders* to make their own decisions? Chickens who've learned through experience to cluck only after the rooster crows find it intimidating to "cluck" without the cue.

How do you teach hens who have *always* laid their eggs one-by-one in individual nests that the only right way to produce eggs today is as a team member whose synchronized patterns allow for timed delivery along critical pathways? That lone-hens (so to speak) are likely to get their eggs cracked? That ducks, geese and even emus lay eggs that are just as good—and maybe even better and cheaper—than their eggs?

How do you "empower" them when they *know* that people are eating fewer eggs today, and what with the downsizing of henhouses, they *are afraid* that they may be among those who end up as star attractions in the local KFC franchise?

How do you convince them that the old chopping block is now a launching pad? That wings grown stiff from lack of use *actually can* spread out and fly them to new destinations? That refusing to budge from their nests and laying more and more eggs actually is the *fastest way to the franchise?*

And, by the way . . .

Ostriches are becoming an endangered species. Prevalent in, but by no means confined to, the medical profession, they are easily spotted. Although very big birds indeed, they cope with changes by hiding their heads in the ground. The problem is that the ostriches rears are left *above* ground at a perfect level for faster-moving competitors to pluck out a tail feather or two—or to give them a hard kick in their gluteus maximi.

Unlike the chickens, they're weighty enough to remain in place. However, the earth muffles their cries of outrage, so all they get for their sputterings is beakfuls of dirt. To add to the ostriches' woes, their stubborn refusal to pull their heads from the ground leaves them vulnerable to future attacks from more and more aggressive predators.

Misfortunes, trials and tribulations abound for those who seek to change—or even partner with—the ostriches. Colleagues, entrepreneurs, governmental officials—frustrated with aborted attempts to educate or cajole them, have occasionally resorted to kicking their derrieres themselves before their more carnivorous competitors do them in. However, digging-in has always worked for the older ones, and only gale force winds of change will knock them off their feet. And great care must be exercised lest the younger ostriches, their gluteals still tender, pull their heads from the ground only to run in the wrong direction.

Rx: The patience of Job (and even he complained on occasion), the determination of Attila the Hun, the riches of Croesus—and perhaps the Sword of Damocles—are needed for success. It may be possible to save the younger ostriches through the use of heroic measures. If there is a reasonable hope for recovery, skilled leaders must draw their swords, dig the dirt from around the ostriches' heads, administer bank-to-bank transfers and bind them cheek-to-beak to the organization. Such methods should not be used on older ostriches or those in terminal condition: they've *chosen* physician-assisted suicide and more's the pity.

. . . And turkeys are making a comeback

No listing of birds in a contemporary commentary on health care would be complete without the turkeys. These ubiquitous birds leave their droppings littered throughout the health care system. Called by many names, these here-again-there-again-come-again-gone-again birds flock from one barnyard to the next, selling packaged weight-reduction programs to obese-but-hopeful clients and, of course, gobbling up grain all along the way.

Not without a place—they cut the fat by rendering it out (a.k.a. eliminating waste), by substituting low-calorie alternatives (*i.e.,* turkey-dogs for frankfurters, turkey-hams for the porcine variety, and frozen turkey rolls for the real thing), and by reducing appetites through selective programs of calculated anxiety—they're usually gone before the chickens come home to roost. Unlike the dishevelled caregivers they're called upon to help, they are distinguished by their sleek feathers, elegant wattles and indubitable aplomb: they know that they have the answers even before you ask the questions.

Rx: Anyone who has dealings with these turkeys had best know *precisely* what they need and how much they're willing to pay for it—negotiated up front and in writing. If you don't know, find out *before* you invite them in—and be sure to get a second opinion from a flock that knows it won't get the contract. Once they're inside the door, keep an eye on them—some are honest, but some are shifty and even shiftless (which could leave you shirtless!).

It also doesn't hurt to remind them that they're *visitors:* you own the henhouse and *you'll make all final decisions yourself.* Most turkeys do have something to offer—they've been bred for large chests and big thighs—just be sure they've got what you want. Otherwise you'll be the one on the platter rather than the one saying prayers of Thanksgiving at the feast.

A word about peacocks . . .

Members of this species strut about the place, displaying their tail feathers and demanding homage. Well-educated and well-groomed, they take few pains to hide their contempt for those they believe to be their hierarchical or social inferiors. Certainly the hard work and heartbreak of hands-on care is beneath them. They have forgotten, if they ever knew, that the mission of a hospital, clinic, home-care agency—and even a health network—is to deliver care to people. And the people who deliver it are the *revenue producers.*

Rx: It might do the peacocks a world of good to be reminded once in a while that *they are merely the middle men.* Few things are more sobering for the peacock than a run-in with a peahen—who can be a fierce adversary, especially when her chicks are in danger. And few things are more helpful than intelligent counsel from a wise mentor. Or more instructive than combat with a nearly successful competitor. Thus chastened, instructed and battle-hardened, the peacock just might grow up to be a fine leader.

A few good eggs . . .

This taxonomy is far from complete. We also have our share of vultures who, while never in short supply, seem to be breeding more rapidly today. And then there's the cuckoos who always have some weird gimmick to sell—and the pigeons who buy it. We also have plenty of parrots and cockatoos who can repeat only what they've heard. And the political magpies who chirp on forever about how we ought to fix the health care system—and, lest we forget, the ravens who tell us that we can't. Moreover, there is a lot of cross-breeding going on: thus, there are chicken-peacocks, turkey-ostriches—an infinite variety of combinations.

Space does not allow for even a cursory treatment of all the species and subspecies. However, a kind word must be said for the good eggs among us:
- the eagles who challenge us
- the owls who guide us
- the warblers who cheer us
- the doves who comfort us
- and the dauntless woodpeckers who search out and eat the pesky insects infesting our infrastructures (I think in more conventional circles they're called auditors and quality assurance specialists—and even whistleblowers). We also might want to thank the sparrows whose unsung work supports us all.

The Wonderful Variety of Pill-Takers*

CINDY LARUE, R.N.

Medication nurses soon find that every patient has a distinctive approach to taking pills. Here's how one veteran observer categorizes the different methods.

I have identified pill-taking patterns by the following broad patient categories:

Selective pickers: Patients in this category are those who repeatedly are given more than one pill at a time. Since they must select the sequence in which to take their medications, their choices automatically put them into one or another subgroup of decision-making technique: by color, size, shape, taste, etc.

Many take the biggest ones first; others start with the smallest. Sometimes it is the capsules that go first, or, perhaps, the tablets. Of course, the noncoated are hardest to swallow, so some patients want them gone first; others though, lead off with the coated ones, since they slip down so easily. Sometimes white pills disappear first, and the bright or multicolored ones are saved till last. But if the patient doesn't like bright colors, they go down first and the paler ones remain.

The variations, of course, are endless. Big red pills come before small yellow pills; but big yellow pills always come first. Some patients alter their selection methods by day of the week; others, with no particular rhyme or reason, switch techniques every day. It's a remarkably effective diversion for many patients.

Shot-glass downers: Their technique, simply, is "down the hatch." The patient takes the cup containing the pills (no matter how many are in it), tips his or her head back, and dumps the content of the cup into the mouth in one quick motion. Water follows quickly in the same manner. This is a very effective technique and gets the task done quickly.

Dry swallowers: These patients swallow their pills without additional liquid. Patients who do this are usually under 40, in my experience, and are rather unassuming. There are no comments or wasted movements. The patients merely put the pills in their mouths and—the pills disappear. At one time I was rather suspicious of these people and felt the pills were still lurking in their cheeks, but I have never been able to prove it.

Tongue flippers: This intricate procedure is usually done with one pill at a time. The pill is placed on the end of the tongue and then positioned on the roof of the mouth behind the front teeth. The water is then taken into the mouth, with the tongue remaining in position, and put at the back of the throat ready to swallow. The pill is then catapulted into the water with the tongue, and all is swallowed in one tremendous gulp (tongue flippers consider a drinking fountain to be a tremendous challenge).

Roulette swishers: To be a roulette swisher, one puts the pills and the water in the mouth at the same time, then rolls them around and around. At the appropriate time (only the swisher knows), the pills and water go down with a quick, precise backward jerk of the head. The roulette swisher is somewhat rare.

Gaggers: Some people naturally sputter and choke on anything they swallow, regardless of its size. Rarely is there a physiologic reason for this. The gagger always places the pill in the back of the throat with the thumb and index finger—naturally causing himself to gag! Sometimes it takes more than one glass of liquid to swallow pills, and, of course, water must be coughed and choked on too. Some gaggers insist upon swallowing their pills with something other than water, because water is "too thin." Other gaggers insist on water because anything else "makes me gag."

Chewers: This category includes patients who masticate their pills before swallowing them. These people prefer the bitter taste rather than risk "choking when swallowing whole tablets." Sometimes these patients simply break the pill into fours and then swallow it fourth by fourth. Occasionally, dissolving or mashing the pill in a carbonated drink or Jello will facilitate matters.

Gaggers and chewers are similar in that they both claim difficulty in swallowing. Here the difference

*Published in RN, copyright ©1976; 39(8):50–52, Medical Economics, Montvale, N.J. Reprinted by permission. Edited from the original.

ends. The gagger never attempts to chew, and a true chewer never gags.

Droppers: These patients cannot hang onto medications—a single pill or a cupful. These people are usually identified unexpectedly because 50% of the spills come without warning. And no matter how many pills are dropped, it is always a narcotic that is not found. It invariably turns out to be a white tablet dropped on the white sheets or a green one dropped on a green speckled floor. Too often, the pill is never found, and a narcotic waste slip must be filled out.

Commentators: The commentator may be among almost any of the previously identified groups. This patient greedily accepts the pills, sighs, shows them to all present, counts them, remarks about color and shape, gives a 10-minute oration on indications and side effects—whether factual or not—and, finally, swallows

them. Company always evokes a lecture. A nurse never seen before, any employee entering the room, be it a lab tech or housekeeping person—any new face is enough to evoke comment.

A commentator cannot always be taken lightly. Occasionally, he or she prevents a medication error. Since the commentator usually counts pills and observes colors, this patient can recognize when something is amiss.

Normals: Finally, we get to the 65% of the patient population who aid the nurse and facilitate medication-giving. Bless them! If possible, they stay near their rooms and don't busy themselves in the bathroom or on the phone as medicine time approaches. Many pour their own water and say "thank you." Strange as it may seem, the sickest patients often fall into this category.

The Therapeutic Value of Whimpering*

ROMA LARK, S.N.

As a nursing student in our small local hospital, I was struck by the different vocalizations that patients make in response to pain. I became curious as to whether these vocalizations would be good predictors of the length of stay in the hospital.

I was fortunate that our small hospital generated a statistically significant sample of patients with identical injuries: thirteen adult white males with traumatic above-the-knee amputations of the left leg combined with cholecystectomies. The reasons for the abundance of this somewhat unusual combination of injuries are twofold. As this is a logging community, the amputations resulted from chainsaw injuries. The cholecystectomies resulted from a research program undertaken by the chief (and only) surgeon, which I will address in a separate paper.

I assigned each of the patients to one of four categories: (1) Moaners, making noises like "Ohhhhhhhh"; (2) Screamers, a category that should be self-explanatory; (3) Whimperers, who make a noise like your dog when you step on it ("Mmm-Mmmmm"). The fourth category,

2 of the Stoics had actually died

Figure 1. Length of hospital stay by patient vocalizations

Stoics, really should be divided into two subcategories since two of the patients labeled Stoic weren't really being stoic but had expired.

As can be seen from Figure 1, the average length of stay in the hospital was 16 days for Whimperers, 19

*Reprinted with permission from Journal of Irreproducible Results, ©1993; 38(5):12.

days for Moaners, 20 days for Screamers, and 23 days for those Stoics who survived.

I attribute these results to the difference in care received by the various categories of patient.

Stoics obviously aren't going to get much care if they don't complain at least a little.

Screamers don't do so well because they just get more analgesia when they scream. ("Oh God, there goes 206 again. Give him another 10 grains of morphine, will you, I'm trying to finish a crossword here.")

As for Moaners, consider whether you would want to be around someone who is moaning all the time. We nurses have enough to put up with changing bedpans and dressings without listening to moaning.

Whimperers hit it just right. They make enough noise to let you know that something is wrong but not so much that you want to stay away.

Whimpering seems to be an excellent predictor of length of hospital stay and may also be a good strategy for getting yourself the most care from nurses, should you end up in a hospital.

Restaurant Review

COLLEEN KENEFICK
AMY Y. YOUNG

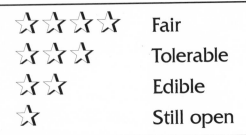

☆☆☆☆ Fair

☆☆☆ Tolerable

☆☆ Edible

☆ Still open

University Center Surgeons Table
13 Recovery Lane
911-SICK-RUS
Dress: Scrubs and gowns
Price range: Not affordable
Noise level: Earth shattering
Reservations: Required through insurance company

This cafeteria is conveniently located near the emergency department entrance. The sterile fluorescent lighting reflects off the polished white tile, giving the diners a ghostly pallor. Chef Bubba Knife impeccably balances flavor and flair in his unique hospital cuisine. To quote our venerable trustee, Dr. Crook's widow, "The egg salad is a direct route to heaven." Gusto and whimsy are the trademarks here, and all fat and sugar groups are well represented.

Don't shy away from the mystery meat stew, under-

cooked hot dogs, overcooked hamburgers, and faux french fries. For more timid diners, macaroni and cheese, stewed tomatoes, chicken hash, and steamed carrots are good choices. A single choice milk bar, dishwater coffee, and flat soda will complete every meal. For those still hungry for dessert, frozen apple pie or runny rice pudding are the top people-pleasers. A memorable meal in many ways.

☆☆☆

General Hospital Cafeteria
1 Hospital Drive
333-555-HELP
Dress: No code
Price Range: Pre-op dinner $10–$15
            Post-op dinner $15–$20
Noise Level: Slightly deafening

The General Hospital cafeteria (that old favorite), one of Central City's premier sites for meeting and dining, has been newly renovated. The eatery is now decorated in the nostalgic vein of the 1950s with exceptional lighting caressing the formica tables, heightening the food's visual appeal. The hospital administrator has not only hired the chef, but inspired him to create a novel menu. Chef Andre notes that since the hospital has been serving food in the same location since 1912, many of the favorites remain. "That food was good then, it's good now, and it will remain lively well into the next millennium. These recipes transcend time. My favorite meal is the remarkable gray meatloaf, mounded mashed potatoes topped with gelatinous brown gravy, and a side of wilted green beans."

Desserts are firmly steeped in tradition: blue jello floats on a bed of iceberg lettuce topped with a dollop of white soup. For those who crave elegant desserts, there is always golden cake accentuated by fluffy white frosting. Unforgettable!

Community Children's Hospital Cafe
Penny Lane
999-CODE-BLU
Dress: Clown costumes recommended
Price range: Prix fixe lunch $8
                      Special tastings $15
Noise level: Serene, with screaming, crying children
Reservations: Best made in person

Located next to the loading dock in the lower basement level, with a drop-dead view of the morgue. Follow the tunnels, and you'll know you've arrived by the aroma wafting from the sandwich vending machines. You can enjoy a return-to-life cocktail comprised of a medley of tiny shrimp, iceberg lettuce, cocktail sauce, and a liberal helping of hot sauce.

Kids of all ages will enjoy the catch-as-catch-can menu that may include: mushroom burgers, vegetarian platters, liverwurst sandwiches, stuffed cabbage, and fried fish. The kitchen's mashed potatoes lack both potatoes and creaminess, while the french fries are cooked in lard.

The kitchen ladies are very helpful when you can find one, making suggestions of the best chance of the day. The cafeteria clearly needs better views, but has the potential for delightful, fairly priced meals. Dining room appearance has improved significantly with the addition of a single silk flower on every table. Due to management's new lunch schedule and the long lines, you'll be able to choke down your own lunch or enjoy the specialties of the day in no time. It's a dining experience you'll like, but you'll want to like it more.

Deliver Us from Evil*

KAREN KELLY BOYCE, R.N.

In this shockingly frank field guide to nursing today, predators disguised as RNs stalk the hospital hallways in search of prey. The victims? That endangered species—the real nurse.

Real nurses may soon be as rare as bald eagles and humpback whales. Competing species within the nursing profession peck away at the truly qualified nurse until she either changes her colors and adopts a less caring attitude or flies away to more friendly environs.

During years spent behind the cover of tangled IV's and medication carts, I've observed four rather distinct species of nurses: the paper piler, the power addict, the wide-eye, and the realist. The way these four types interact creates the atmosphere in nursing today.

The Paper Piler

Identifying marks: The Paper Piler entered nursing for the pure sense of order, cleanliness, and organization it promised. She is thrilled by the word "professional." She is the only one who wears a cap when it is optional. Her shoes are always perfectly polished and look unworn.

Adaptive behavior: The paper piler can whip up a care plan in just three minutes that would astonish Florence Nightingale. She can chart with the clarity of a

*Published in RN, © 1982; 45(7):75–76, 78, Medical Economics, Montvale, N.J. Reprinted by permission. Edited from the original.

lawyer and reorganize the med books without blinking an eye. But she has one fatal flaw: She breaks out in a cold sweat of insecurity while trying to put a patient on a bedpan. And though she can dumfound you with a detailed explanation of 104's complex surgery, she cannot comprehend why 104 is crying, or what to do about it.

Flight pattern: The paper piler soon finds her niche. Through the sheer impressiveness of her store of knowledge, and her astonishing command of medical terminology, she quickly soars high above the ordinary flock of nurses. Secretly relieved, she finds herself far removed from patient care, and can often be spotted winging her way down any hospital corridor, her arms loaded with folders, schedules, and memos on improving efficiency

The Power Addict

Identifying marks: This species is drawn to nursing because of the "pain" of humanity—but not necessarily to relieve it. She may be an aide, an LPN, an RN, a lab technician, or dietary helper. I've often suspected that power addicts belong to a secret and powerful union that demands they be spread evenly throughout the hospital to maximize their influence. No matter what department, floor, or shift, there is always at least one Power Addict commanding the territory.

The power addict has a deep sense of insecurity and often a quite disturbed personality. Lacking the ability to control the personal aspects of her life, she cannot resist the urge to control and manipulate those weaker than herself. And who are more helpless than the captive sick on a hospital floor?

Adaptive behavior: The power addict rewards what she considers the "good" patient by quite literally leaving him alone. She punishes the "bad patients" (whom she calls hypochondriacs, junkies, and PIAs) by any means she can think of. If the patient has the nerve to disturb her during her break, she cures his "drug addiction" by making him wait two hours for his requested pain medication. If the aged woman on the far side of the hall rings for a bedpan, her reaction time is, again, slow. And if the old woman is then found to be "incontinent of urine," the power addict will let her know both by word and action that she is considered a lazy sloven. The next time that this woman has to urinate, she will probably fall in an attempt to walk to the bathroom. The power addict will then label her "confused" and consider the use of restraints. This nurse seems almost intoxicated with her ability to do harm.

Nor is the power addict satisfied by her dictatorship over the sick; she rejoices in her manipulation of the staff as well. It's easier for the charge nurse to send the new admission to another nurse than to endure the rantings and ravings of the power addict.

Flight pattern: It's easy to locate the power addict. If you can't see through her actions, just follow the sound of the loudest complaints. While hardly ever leaving her perch, or her sitting position, the power addict loudly reminds all within earshot (patients, visitors, coworkers) how "overworked" and "unappreciated" she is. Two other often-heard calls: "I'm on MY break," and "That's not MY patient."

The Wide-Eye

Identifying marks: Usually a Wide-Eye is a new graduate, but I have known more than a few who have clung to this stage for an extended time. A wide-eye enters nursing for all the "right" reasons. She radiates heartfelt sympathy. The words of her most respected instructors are branded on her breast. She has all the equipment she thinks she'll ever need: LOVE. She walks the hall wrapped in her delusion of "saving" the world, her uniform sprinkled with the stuff of sainthood. Her heart beats with the solemn belief that she can "make it better" just by wishing it so.

Adaptive behavior: The wide-eye opens the door to each patient's room with undaunted optimism. She has yet to hold a patient dying of brain cancer in her arms while he hurls curses and names at her. She has yet to wrap the body of a premature infant or sedate the mother who has just been told. She has yet to be punched by a psychiatric patient whom the physician claimed was "not violent," or to watch a young patient die of a blatantly "botched" surgery. She doesn't know that the paper piler is fretfully shuffling through the "incident" reports she fills out in all honesty, or that the power addict is just waiting for an opportunity to inflate her own ego by pointing out the wide-eye's errors loud and clear.

Flight pattern: Wide-eyes eventually molt their feathers if they stay in nursing for any length of time. With experience, they gain perspective and the refined emotional equipment that patients really need. If all goes well, a wide-eye eventually hatches into a realist.

The Realist

Identifying marks: The transition from wide-eye to Realist is usually so gradual that it's hard to pinpoint the moment or cause of change. One day the wide-eye wakes up knowing that she cannot "save" the world or do battle with the agonies of humanity. She simply does all she can to ease the agonies of her patients.

She has gone through that often ignored, but painful, process of learning her own limitations, and become a real nurse because of it.

Adaptive behavior: Blessed is the patient who has a realist for a nurse. She is the backbone of the nursing profession. Though overworked and underappreciated, she is too busy dealing with her patients' problems to worry about her own. She is often two steps ahead of her patients' needs, and she renders her experienced, excellent care with that extra smile and spirit that mean so much.

The realist recognizes her co-workers for what they really are. While she may not have names or categories for them, she knows them by sight. She is infuriated by the paper piler's forms, which take time from her patients. But she copes. She is impatient with the wide-eye, yet pities her, for she knows the painful process of self-realization she will go through. She sees the pain in the eyes of the power addict's patients, and she often finds herself in their rooms despite her own heavy patient load. She ignores the emotional games of the power addict. They do not impress her because she's there for the patient. The neglect and unnecessary pain inflicted by the power addict depress her, but she doesn't give up hope. She believes that "it is better to light one candle, than to curse the darkness." The flame of that candle burns in her heart.

Flight pattern: The realist knows the value of that flame, and through the years she protects this fragile fire. She hides it from the uncomprehending eyes of the paper piler and the open ridicule of the power addict. She reveals the flame only in her patient's room and often sees it reflected back. She notices that it flickers on occasion, but she closes her eyes and wills it alive. She is, therefore, totally lost and bewildered on that unexpected day when the flame dies.

It can happen overnight, when in pure frustration, she reports the behavior of a power addict to a paper piler and finds no one cares. Or she finds she cannot sustain her hope because she has too often watched the needs of her patient lost in the ever-grinding bureaucracy created by the paper piler. The disillusioned realist feels a weariness no vacation can relieve. She goes through all the stages of grief. First she is shocked, then angry, and finally resigned. For you see, there has been a death. A nurse has died.

Malice in Wonderland*

JUDITH VESSEY, PHD, R.N.C.
SUSAN GENNARO, DSN, R.N., F.A.A.N.

Dear Alice,

Congratulations! You have fallen into the wonderful world of research. There are treats to discover, drinks and cakes to sample, and marvelous people to come to know during your journey. However, a word of caution is in order. All is not as it first seems. Beware of malice in wonderland.† To avoid shedding tears, not to mention drowning in a pool of them, we offer this quick and easy guide of characters that need to be avoided.

The Harried White Rabbit. Usually this well-known scholar can be heard before being seen, running about uttering "I'm late, I'm late, for a very important date." (You can bet, as a research neophyte, that it isn't with you, despite your scheduled appointment.) Yet, you will be expected to perform library searches, collect data, or draft manuscripts or grant proposals on a moment's notice. This harried hare never has enough time to do a job well, but always finds enough time for you to do it over. Impertinent and impatient, this rabbit tends toward self-aggrandizement and sycophantism.

The Mad Hatter and the March Hare. "No room, no room," these two will shout should you approach them about joining their research party. Take the cue and

*Reprinted with permission from Nursing Research, ©1993; 42(2):67.
†With apologies to Lewis Carroll.

leave before it dawns on them that you might be a useful distraction. Should you mistakenly join them, your sojourn into the wonderland of research may grind to a halt. Time stands still for these two. Tenured and tired, they have little need to be productive. Basking in reminiscences of their past successes while sipping tea is enough for this pair in their golden years.

Queen of Hearts. Ever so stately, her royal highness commands respect by her mere presence. The Queen's methodological prowess, as well as her temper, are legend across the kingdom. Whether it's painting white roses red or "handling" difficult methodological problems using creative data analysis, her intimidated subjects do her bidding willingly. Who among them would dare question her majesty's decrees? Although not widely publicized, reports have surfaced that she also abused her animal subjects on the croquet field. However, her royal highness was successful in suppressing investigations to examine these potential violations of animal care protocols. Clearly, she has little regard for ethics but enough power to squelch objections. Cries of "Off with their heads" are enough to make anyone reconsider questioning her dictums.

Tweedle Dee and Tweedle Dum. This deadly duo can neither work *with* nor *without* each other. They take competitiveness to new heights, deliberately provoking each into doing battle. Although you may have an overwhelming desire to mediate their disputes, don't be caught between them when they duel. Remember,

Tweedle Dee and Tweedle Dum will never mortally wound each other, for their relationship is symbiotic. The same might not be true for your research career. If in doubt, just remember what happened to Humpty Dumpty, their last research associate.

Cheshire Cat. This friendly feline looks like the perfect mentor, appearing when you most need someone to listen to your concerns. Should you ask for assistance, direction is willingly provided. This kitty will purr about the quality of your work and promise to help your career. But beware. The help provided never seems to be quite accurate or complete enough. Yet, you may be convinced that your grant proposals will be funded and your manuscripts accepted more readily by agreeing to list this kitty as primary investigator or first author. At first you may be flattered by the attention. Later you realize that this cat is quick to claim the accolades of your joint successes for the mere mention of the Cheshire name. When difficulties arise in your relationship, as they surely will, it becomes apparent that this kitty's earlier helpful demeanor was merely an apparition.

So, dear Alice, please heed these words. As you travel down the path your research takes you, treasure the friends you'll make and savor the sweet taste of your successes. But do beware, and avoid any malice that may be lurking in wonderland. Although these notorious characters are few, should you mistakenly curry their favor, your dream of a successful research career will undoubtedly turn into a nightmare.

Hospiscope*

CAROLINE WEISS, R.N.

ARIES (March 21–April 20) Your normally strong and active personality needs to be pampered during this period of hospitalization. Develop a constant and vigorous grip on the call light. Keep alert by challenging all comers on your course of treatment and medications.

TAURUS (April 21–May 21) Your delicate sensitivities require attention. Request immediate transfer to a secluded corner room and have it redecorated to your

taste. As you are a late riser, you will need to cultivate the evening staff.

GEMINI (May 22–June 21) Your scintillating personality is an invitation to one and all. Your cleverness and charm endear you to your roommate who wishes you would limit visitors to a dozen at a time.

CANCER (June 22–July 23) As you tend to be easily distressed, try to get the hospital staff adjusted to your

*Reprinted with permission from American Journal of Nursing, ©1964; 64(10):115.

routine as soon as possible. Generally conservative, you occasionally send out for a pizza. Your astute advice on improving their hairdos is greatly appreciated by the nurses.

LEO (July 24–Aug. 23) Yours is a dramatic and colorful personality. Realize your leadership potential by organizing your fellow patients. Call a general strike unless something is done about the noise.

VIRGO (Aug. 24–Sept. 23) Efficient and neat, you are an ideal patient. You make your own bed and rinse out dishes after meals. Your analytical mind is being well utilized as you are preparing a new operations manual for the hospital.

LIBRA (Sept. 24–Oct. 23) Optimism and cheerfulness characterize your personality. You routinely order pheasant and champagne on your diet card. To maintain a careful balance in your life, you devote equal time to Westerns and mysteries on television.

SCORPIO (Oct. 24–Nov. 22) Yours is an outstanding personality—out standing in the hall when you should be in bed! Your mysterious nature is not fully under-

stood by the nurses who are mystified by how much you can stash in your bedside stand.

SAGITTARIUS (Nov. 23–Dec. 21) Yours is an independent and vivacious personality. Your love of travel will take you to x-ray, physical therapy, and the coffee shop. Your joviality has made you a legend among the orderlies who appreciate practical jokes.

CAPRICORN (Dec. 22–Jan. 20) Reticent and unassuming, you nevertheless show great sagacity in financial affairs. Now is a good time to buy stock in the hospital gift shop. Plan a cocktail party for the credit manager.

AQUARIUS (Jan. 21–Feb. 19) Your nature is both worldly and humanitarian. Your highly developed social consciousness has made you an authority on patients and staff. Set up a consulting service in the day room.

PISCES (Feb. 20–March 20) Your dreamy nature may make hospitalization difficult to endure. Consult the chief engineer about installing piped-in-stereo. Surround yourself with great literature (from the patients' library). Endear yourself by oil painting in bed.

Will Visiting Hours Ever End?*

JACK E. BYNUM, PHD
GENE ACUFF, PHD

Choose your favorite visitor from this rogues' gallery of all-too-familiar types.

They may arrive bearing gifts . . . or empty-handed, in groups of twos and threes . . . or in oceanic throngs that remind you of Peking during rush hour. They may be just what the doctor ordered . . . or the biggest barrier between your patient and recovery. They are, of course, the visitors, who hold as great a potential for good and for evil as any other part of hospital life.

This is not a guide *for* visitors, but *to* them; an analysis of the many varied ways they can drive you and

your patients into mental disarray or, at the very least, force you to put up the NO VISITORS sign. Not that it will do much good. There have been visitors since the day Adam lost his rib. Few things are in less danger of dying out.

The easiest category of visitor to recognize is the *Hale and Hearty* variety. Indeed, you can often spot this type at long range, sometimes even before he has finished parking his car at the hospital. He makes his

*Published in RN, © 1981; 44(4):50–51, Medical Economics, Montvale, N.J. Reprinted by permission.

entrance with all the subtlety of a cyclone. He beams goodwill, booming out his greetings through a smile that reveals more teeth than a Hollywood shark. The more terrible your patient feels, the louder and more euphoric this visitor's spiel becomes. Blinking through his postoperative stupor and nausea, your patient tries desperately to remember the name of this apparition who looks for all the world as if he were addressing a political convention.

The mental processes of the Hale and Hearty type are clear. Either he simply doesn't believe your patient is ill, or he thinks this kind of thirteen-times-life-size enthusiasm is just the thing to make him better.

You'll recognize the *Indulger* by what he carries. Making it a rule to visit only those on thousand-calorie, salt-free, sugar-free, fat-free diets, the Indulger never appears without a huge box of chocolates and butter cookies. Don't confuse the Indulger with members of a closely related species—the *Naturalists,* who bring bouquets of flowers and other pollen-laden hazards to the bedsides of the asthmatic or allergy-prone.

You only need to recognize the *Squatter* once: He never goes away. Arriving at the first permissible moment, and staying until forcibly evicted, the Squatter is one of your most difficult nursing challenges. Once he infests a room, no tactic or pesticide is effective against him. Your patient may feign sleep or coma, or, in desperation, acquire all the symptoms of a highly contagious disease. It won't help. Squatters are forever . . . forever observing your patient's every pain, every symptom, and every treatment. One theory holds that Squatters are frustrated medical students.

Occasionally, you will feel a sudden chill, a cold breeze blowing in the hospital hallway. A *Prophet of Doom* has just swept by, on his way to torment some unfortunate patient. This type of visitor is as sunny and fun-loving as Darth Vader. With a purely spurious but self-righteous authority, the Prophet of Doom conducts his own examination, not only of every square inch of the patient's anatomy but of every little piece of hospital equipment, as well. Everything he inspects is just another bad omen, another confirmation of his tragic prognosis. He sighs knowingly as he studies the mechanism for adjusting the bed. A true Prophet of Doom can, without saying a word, give your patient the impression that his doctor has just given him up as terminal.

The *Pryer* insists on a stitch-by-stitch account of your patient's entire medical history. He's the Woodward and Bernstein of medicine. Nothing escapes his inquisition. At times, it may be your responsibility to tell the Pryer that there just might be parts of the body that the patient does not feel like discussing in detail.

Finally, there are two varieties of visitors whom you must intercept with the utmost dispatch. There are those who might be called *Carriers*: the sick who visit the sick, coughing, sneezing, spreading cheer. And there are those *Disaster Fans* who are just plain dangerous, such as chain-smokers, equally impervious to polite pleas on wall posters and the presence of oxygen equipment.

And yet, in the final analysis, despite all outward differences, these various species of visitors are all brothers under the skin. For which of them, after inflicting a visit, will not respond to your patient's mumbled gratitude with the simple, yet profound question—"What are friends *for?*"

NOT YOUR
AVERAGE DAY

Day 1: I am special because I am a healing force.

Day 2: Dream of nursing as a joy, not a burden.

Day 3: No one is alone in the universe, except on the night shift.

Day 4: At the very center is pure stress.

Day 5: I forgive my supervisor for manipulating and controlling me.

Day 6: The universe is limitless, but my patience is not.

Day 7: Follow your bliss to the parking lot.

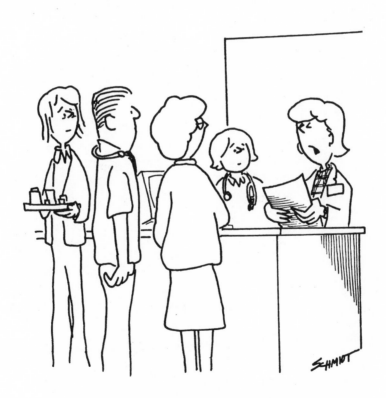

We're short-staffed, so here's the vacation schedule.
Betty, you go from 9 to 10:30, Tom goes from 11 to 1:15, Karen from 1:30 to 3 . . .

Home Care A to Z*

MARY ELLEN KILLEEN, A.C.S.W.

A is for Animals: aggressive, angry, anxious, angst-ridden, agitated animals. I have been dive-bombed by a loose bird, growled at by more dogs than there are in a large kennel, and had a nasty little feline use my winter coat as its litter box. The scarlet A goes to Abigail, a nervous twitch of a dog who mistook my thumb for lunch.

B is for Bathrooms. Finding the facilities while making your home visits can be the accomplishment of the day. Workers are divided on the issue of using clients' bathrooms. In some homes the drying panty hose and lingerie indicate visitors are not expected; other bathrooms look like they are just waiting to be included in a magazine photo display. If desperate, consult with the neighborhood postal person for suggestions. Remember, the cup of coffee at 8:00 AM leads to a search for a bathroom by noon.

C is for Car. A comfortable car with a great tape deck, air conditioning, space for pens and note paper, and a good supply of snacks in the glove compartment can make home care a joy. It doesn't hurt if the car is reliable and has good gas mileage, either. After a while your car becomes a home away from home and sometimes takes on a lived-in look: lived in with coffee cups, newspapers, extra clothes in case it rains or gets cold. One zealous nurse was really into her caring mission and worked three days straight; it seemed she had sufficient food and changes of clothes in her little red hatchback for the duration.

D is for Detour. You know the exact route from your office to Ms. Jones' house and then face the surprise of a big sign: Road Closed. Consider this one of the challenges of the job and a chance to be flexible. I once trusted the Highway Department's suggestions for an alternate route only to find a jokester had arranged the signs to lead nowhere. Now I trust my own sense of direction, check for homing pigeons, and after half an hour of flexible, challenging driving, call Ms. Jones for further direction. One is never lost, only detoured.

E is for Equipment. When you work away from your office and desk all day you learn to carry everything you need with you. As a social worker I have information on Social Security, applications for nursing homes and medical assistance, kids' books on dealing with illness, crayons and paper, and instructions on living wills. From time to time I also deliver tub benches or commodes. I draw the line on transporting enema gear. One of my colleagues was pulled over by a police officer after she assumed a light would stay yellow a little longer. When he saw the medical equipment in her back seat, he got in touch with his worry about his own aging parents and let this Angel of Mercy off with barely a verbal warning.

F is for Family and Friends. It is such a joy not only to hear about the important people in a patient's life but also to talk with them and sit right down for a cup of tea with Aunt Virginia. Homes are expansive enough to make room for many family members to talk about their reactions in a familiar setting. Some spouses who mouth only optimism in the house will share doubts and concerns while they walk you to your car. We see first hand what strengths and resources are in place for these families to face the challenges of illness. They may describe supports they have, but the description takes on real meaning when, during our visits, the phone keeps ringing with relatives checking in or neighbors are at the door with a cooked meal.

G is for Guard, the gut feeling that keeps you safe and free from harm. Some streets and homes are not as secure as they need to be. We in home care develop an intuitive or sixth sense that tips us off to something wrong. Always trust it and protect yourself.

H is for Home. It can range from a palatial spread to one room or a bed in a shelter. It can be an emotional and family-oriented place to which people return for visits and refreshment. With very sick people, it is spoken about poignantly as a destination and final place on the journey.

I is for Identification. Carry a photo ID to assure the client of your employment. It might not be a bad idea if clients also had ID badges. I did hear of an eager home care aide who briskly got down to the business of bathing the lady of the house, changing the bed linens, and finishing up her assigned jobs. She later was informed that, although it was a very refreshing bath, it had been administered to the wrong person and the lady next door was still waiting. Another nurse, on the sad job of pronouncing the death of a hospice patient, was startled when the putative deceased sat up in bed and inquired after the nurse's health (which at that moment became shaky). Her discovery of the error caused by patients with similar last names did little to alleviate the RN's fright, nor did she gain solace from her coworkers references to her as the Miracle Worker.

J is for Jump Rope. Jennifer, the young daughter of a client, was so sad when I visited her family for bereavement counseling. She showed me new birthday presents, which had done little to cheer her, and told me she didn't even know how to use her new jump rope. In no time I had taught her grandmother (in hand gestures that transcended our language barriers) and Jennifer how to go at it. It was healing for us all to hear laughter in that home.

K is for Key, most importantly a spare key to help you out when the other one is locked inside your car. Try not to lose your keys on the same day that your supervisor is making joint visits with you. Slight embarrassment may result.

L is for Lunch. Many home care staff make the mistake of skipping it, but a midday break refills the stomach and can refresh the spirit. Most of us drive by myriad offerings—Jamaican meat patties, places with salad bars and good soup, fast food joints. A peanut butter and jelly from home is not bad, either. There are wonderful places to sit and eat: in a restaurant, being served if it's been that kind of day; public parks; parking lots of McDonald's for great people watching; a cemetery for perfect quiet. My special break is eating peach yogurt and an apple, sitting on the bench near a small waterfall. I feel so calm, I can even handle a dog at my next visit.

M is for Maps. These are an absolute necessity. I trust the actual map rather than relying on the different directions my coworkers give. The poet draws a word picture: up a really pretty hill, past bright flowers in bloom, by an ochre-colored building and then go a while longer. . . . At least the engineer type is precise: drive 3.7 miles, turn right at the intersection, and left at the fourth set of lights.

N is for Nature. I love the chance to be outdoors for part of the work day. It is a bonus when a client suggests we sit on the porch or under a back yard tree. Driving to and from visits, I see the unfolding of the seasons, feel sunshine, notice changes in the weather, and have come to appreciate the raw power of ice, wind, and rain for making me a more confident driver.

O is for Office Staff. No one does home care without this group of angels back in the office, taking phone calls, tracking us down in the field with messages, telling us Mr. So-and-So just went to the hospital, sorting out billing questions. They also become telephone buddies with many of the patients. No picture of home care would be complete without their pieces of the puzzle.

P is for Participation in whatever the family is doing while we visit. I have helped with canning sauerkraut, jumped rope, answered the phone, and changed the baby's diaper. This willingness does not distract from the purpose of my visit, but somehow opens doors to the mutual work we share of getting through tough times.

Q is for Quarters. Dimes used to be enough for pay phones to call if you were running late. There is also the challenge in the city today of finding a phone booth or a working phone. The lack of them is discrimination against those of us not selling drugs.

R is for Recipes. Food is central to family life, and being offered samples and recipes is one of the delights of the job. In one typical week I was given instructions on cooking fichalings (a delicious concoction with spinach), baked stuffed lobster, no-cook applesauce, and kapusta (the only word of Polish I know but one that is sufficient).

S is for Suited. Home care helps define what work environment one is suited to. There is a freedom in being in the field and not in an office all day. I once considered—fleetingly—moving up the administrative ladder, but the thought of being inside at a desk without fresh air made me hyperventilate.

T is for Television, often competing for our clients' attention during a visit. One lady told me she never missed one particular soap in which all the characters suffered incredibly dramatic challenges. Watching it, she told me, confirmed that she wasn't all that bad off in what she had to deal with in real life.

U is for Umbrella. Remember the cardinal rule: if you bring it with you, the sun will shine.

V is for Volunteers, the group of generous people who consistently bring life, laughter, and hope to shut-ins. They build on the professional services and add lots of personal time and listening. V is also for Volunteer Director, who acts as a matchmaker for unions made in heaven.

W is for Whistling. My grandmother's admonition against this activity didn't cure me as well as one woman who looked as if an electric shock passed through her when I offered my latest musical rendition. She explained that my whistling almost shorted out her hearing aid. Now I always check for listening devices before I pucker up.

X is for Xenophobia, which is taboo, the antithesis to home care. Anyone with a fear of strangers will, and should, avoid this kind of work. One of the most positive job features for me is the daily exposure to a version of the United Nations and the chance to travel the world's cultures when I listen to clients' stories of their roots.

Y is for YAKs, not the animal variety (my reactions are clear on those), but the human type: Young Adult Kids, who live with or visit their ill parents. YAKs are on the threshold of adulthood and may evince contradictory reactions to sickness challenging the stability of parents and family life. I have seen YAKs provide the most tender and mature care possible and at other times regress to acting like the hurt children they are. Treat them gently and understand.

Z is for Zest, the trait that entices us to another day, another month, another year in the wonderful world of home care.

ENA Leadership Symposium: A Dream Come True*

VICKY BRADLEY, R.N., M.S., C.E.N.

Is there no end to this stress and strain? Are you still telling yourself that things will be better after this one next project is implemented, or that next week you are only going to work 40 hours instead of the usual 50 or 60? If the answer is yes, your denial system rivals that of the 50-year-old executive who presents with crushing chest pain, just positive it was something *he ate*. Your staff is not happy with administration (that's whose team they think you are on), and administration is not happy with staff (that's whose team they think you are on.) It is no wonder that nurses in middle management are cynical, stressed out, demoralized—and at times see no way out. As a result, the want ads are full of nurse-manager positions. When options like staff nursing, becoming pregnant, or going back to school

all look much more attractive than your current management position, you know that you are in crisis.

Managers will continue to face many challenges. One of these is to maintain a sense of humor while struggling with the many pressures of today's health care system. It is difficult to smile as you battle to cut costs, increase productivity, be competitive, be cost-effective, meet the needs of your customer, decrease turnover, implement CQI, decrease length of stay, remain clinically competent, design a new facility, and get ready for the Joint Commission on Accreditation of Healthcare Organizations. *Whew!* It is no wonder managers appear to have lost their sense of humor.

Let's see if you have lost *yours*. Try this "Mini Management Stress Test" based on five common scenarios:

*Reproduced from Journal of Emergency Nursing, ©1992; 18(4): 295–296 with permission from Mosby-Year Book, Inc. Edited from the original.

1. You find a plain white sealed envelope slipped under your door when you arrive in the morning. It contains which of the following?
   (a) A bonus check from your chief executive officer
   (b) An engraved invitation for a reception to recognize your staff's achievements
   (c) A resignation from a staff member

2. A distinguished-looking gentleman in a suit is waiting outside your office door. He is:
   (a) NBC's William Shatner, who wants you to co-host the next 911 television series
   (b) An experienced staff nurse who wants to work in your emergency department
   (c) The district attorney, who wants to subpoena five of your staff members to testify in a rape case

3. The hospital administrator called while you were out and left a message for you to call back as soon as possible. What is the call for?
   (a) To tell you about the $50,000 that was left to the hospital by a patient who received excellent care in your emergency department
   (b) To invite you and your staff to write a chapter for a management book based on your unit's achievements through the process of CQI
   (c) To share last night's ordeal of bringing a family member in for abdominal pain

4. Your night charge nurse asks to speak to you privately. Why?
   (a) To explain triumphantly how the Joint Commission on the Accreditation of Healthcare Organizations made a surprise visit and the department passed with flying colors
   (b) To explain how the night staff has developed a simple but brilliant plan to decrease length of stay
   (c) To tell you of the suspicion that a staff member is taking drugs

5. Your beeper goes off at midnight.
   (a) It is your staff, calling to say you won the lottery
   (b) It is your staff, calling to tell you they covered the night "hole" and you will not have to come in to work
   (c) It is your staff, calling to tell you the proverbial "bus" just unloaded and they desperately need an extra pair of hands

If you selected all *a*'s, you were dreaming. This commonly occurs with managers who are in crisis. Fantasizing is fun, sometimes therapeutic, and occasionally helpful for finding solutions we normally would not. If you are not having enough pleasant dreams, it is time for a well-deserved vacation. Tell William Shatner you are busy.

If you selected mostly *b*'s you had a great weekend. It is time to celebrate. All the CQI efforts of the ED team are paying off. You took some scary risks, implemented many changes, and your hair is grayer, but the payoff was worth it. Quick, while things are good, grab your friends or family and take a well-deserved vacation.

If you selected *c*'s most of the time, you are a member of the DSAC (Desperately Seeking a Change Club). Common characteristics of club members are as follows:

- You spend 95% of your time in meetings.
- You have a slight crick in your neck from holding the phone with it—"Look, Mom, no hands!"
- When in crisis, you eat chocolate.
- You feel guilty when you do not have all the answers.
- It is dark when you go to work; it is dark when you come home.
- Your answers to staff disgruntlement always start out with, "Things will be better after. . . ." (after the move, after the new nurses are off orientation, after the new medical director arrives, after. . . .).
- Your meetings with staff always end with, "Hang in there just a little bit longer."
- You are, that is you think you are, a little "touched" or you would not be in this job.
- You did not think this test was the *least* bit funny.
- You strike your heels together three times and say, "*There's no place like home, there's no place like home. . . .*"—but you are still in your office.

I Remember When. . .*

ANNA LEE FIELDER, R.N.

I REMEMBER WHEN . . .

- Windows in patient's rooms were left open in summer because there was no air conditioning.
- Patients received back rubs at bedtime.
- JCAH was someone's initials.
- Nurses stood up for doctors.
- Doctors didn't know you had a first name. You knew they did, but would not dare say it.
- You didn't know what a weekend was and worked 12-hour shifts, 5 days a week—and didn't ask why.
- Night nurses were served a meal.
- Coffee for nurses was free.
- There were no male nurses.
- There was no such thing as bonding with your newborn. You loved and wanted it or you didn't.
- Doctors were not worried about being sued.
- There were no ICUs.
- There was no QA.
- There was one performance rating. You performed or you were fired!
- The Director of Nurses talked with patients.
- There was no pantyhose.
- Nurses did not wear jewelry or slacks on duty.

- You polished your shoes before going to work, and you washed your shoe laces.
- You wore your cap and school pin every day.
- If you were called to the nursing office, it meant big trouble.
- Your head nurse was always addressed as "Mrs. or Miss."
- You reported to duty 15 minutes before the shift report.
- Doctors gave you a box of candy for Christmas.
- Nurses passed out nourishment at 10 AM and 8 PM.
- You smiled at patients.
- "AM care" was a bath, not a pan of water put on the bedside table.
- Patients were observed by nurses—not by machines.
- Little wires were not put on baby's scalps.
- Live-in was hired help.
- CPR was someone's initials.
- Nutrition was three meals a day.
- The patient had a name and was not referred to as a "cataract," "C-section," or "chole."
- *You laughed at yourself.*

. . . Sometimes, I wonder—has progress been made?

*Reprinted from Journal of Post Anesthesia Nursing, ©1989; 4(5):323 with permission from W. B. Saunders.

The Wayward Placenta*

GREG NELSON

There are times I get a little down about this way of life. Take the other night, for example.

I spent an hour in the pouring rain pretending to listen in earnest to a drunk couple explain why it wasn't their fault they drove through a mini mall at 80 mph. They created drive-through aisles in Bo Peep's Lingerie and Bubba's Tools and dragged most of the inventory out into a drainage ditch. It was impossible for them to be intoxicated, they explained, because they had eaten a large meal with their second bottle of tequila.

The driver had the only injury, a cut thumb from trying to pick up a broken beer bottle from his floorboard, and he kept grabbing my arm and belching his story in my face. Now, my newest uniform shirt is covered with mud, blood and I think some kind of lotion from Bo Peep's.

While waiting for the police, I reminded myself how much I love being a paramedic, although it took some convincing, even from me, as the rain ran down my collar and the drunk begged me to pull his car out of the ditch with the ambulance. Then he threw up on my shoes.

It all started because I wanted to be a hero. Oh, maybe not Batman or one of the Fantastic Four, but I did want to be the guy who came when "Help!" was called. All things considered, it's been a blast, but in reflecting on how I came to be a hero, I can't help wondering if Einstein was wrong and there *are* dice involved in the master plan. Standing there watching underwear and marital aids float by in the ditch, I chuckled quietly over how much fun I've had and what a strange route I'd taken to get here.

Sister Sunshine

In the late '70s I parted company with the United States Navy, having acquired a number of useful skills. I could fire automatic weapons, change clothes while floating in a swimming pool and give the appearance of intense labor while carrying a clipboard around. Above all, I learned how to mop. The Navy is very intense about its mopping. I even attended a three-hour lecture on the subject, complete with slides and a demo by a civilian expert. Really.

Despite having excelled at all my training and having received an honorable discharge, I was astounded to find no employers willing to pay me to either shoot things, carry a clipboard or change clothes in the water. There were, however, several corporations willing to take advantage of my government training in the area of linoleum hygiene (mopping floors). I sought— to no avail—a position of clipboard bearer, but all the prospects insisted I have some knowledge as to what goes on a clipboard, and there my studies fell short. Having exhausted nearly all of my $512 in government separation pay, I answered an ad for an Operating Room Assistant at a local hospital.

The Catholic nun who interviewed me, Sister Sunshine, had all the humor and charm of a drill instructor I knew in the Navy. I considered asking her if there was any relation, but she scared me too much to get past "Yes, ma'am," "No, ma'am" and "Sure, I'll become a Catholic."

Truth be told, I anticipated being turned down and, therefore, becoming eligible for unemployment checks, but to my dismay, they hired me. I got over being flattered after I learned it wasn't my natural charm but my mopping proficiency they sought. You see, despite its glorious tone, Operating Room Assistant means "The Big Guy Who Cleans Up That Disgusting Puddle." And I won't even mention the places I've had to shave people.

I was amazed at the never-ending ways I could be disgusted, and after a week, I was even considering re-enlistment. The worst thing I ever cleaned up after in the Navy was an occasional seagull.

A Disturbing Slosh

Well, just as I had reached my disgust threshold, I was summoned to the office of the Chief Operating Room Assistant, or as we called him COR ASS. COR lounged

*Reprinted with permission from JEMS: Journal of Emergency Medical Services, ©1996; 21(8):72–73.

behind his desk (it was an old Coke case), and said, because of my superior work ethic and the fact that other guy called in sick, I had been selected to attend a class that day. Thrilled at the prospect of being educated further in the linoleum hygiene sciences, I hurried to my assigned lecture hall. Imagine my disappointment when I learned the class was not in my area of expertise, but merely a CPR certification. At the end of the class the instructor handed me a card and said that should I hear the public address system announce a "CODE BLUE," I should report to the room number that follows and "help" until told to leave. Full to the brim with visions of Gage and DeSoto, Reed and Malloy, Lassie and Timmy, and a new feeling of self-importance, I waited eagerly for my chance at heroism.

There followed a frustrating week of good health among the hospital patrons, none of whom had the courtesy to suffer a cardiac arrest while I was on duty. Sometimes on my breaks I would follow some of the sicker-looking ones around just in case, well, you know. Then one Friday morning I was summoned to the desk in surgery, handed a large metal bowl with a towel draped over the top and given instructions to deliver it to the pathology lab located upstairs. Hearing a disturbing slosh, I inquired as to the contents and was informed it was a placenta in need of laboratory examination.

A few minutes later, I stood alone in the elevator listening to the easy-listening version of *Muskrat Love* when that fateful announcement came over the PA "CODE BLUE ROOM 207—CODE BLUE ROOM 207." The doors opened, and I shot out—determined to be the first hero to arrive. A split second too late, I recalled Newton's laws of motion because as the bowl and I went into motion, the placenta slid out from under the towel and landed with a resounding plop on the floor. (The placenta is undeniably one of the body's most useful organs but it's no great pleasure to look at, especially when it's oozing across cheap tile, dragging its cord behind.) All thoughts of CPR were wiped out as the placenta slid to a stop at the elevator door threshold. But even this horror was made minimal by the sights that followed. In rapid succession the elevator doors closed, and the half of the organ visible to me began a rapid journey upward, was severed at the elevator door ceiling and plopped down at my feet.

I said several prayers to various deities and pounded on the elevator button; it was at this point my day took a decided turn for the worse. As I bent over to retrieve the visible half of the organ, the doors opened and there stood the local Bishop, complete with purple sash and red face. Across from him stood the head honcho of the whole hospital. Fists on hips and heads bent slightly, they both looked down at the mangled organ then up to me and said in unison, "wh wh wh th th th he he he," well, you get the idea.

The PA system repeated the announcement, and I blurted out something to the effect that I needed to go. The regally dressed man of God looked at me, gestured to the mess at his feet and said in a thick Irish brogue, "Please feel free to take that with you." Never before—or since—have I moved so quickly to clean anything.

Red Face's Advice

The now-disconnected placenta in tow, I arrived at Room 207 and was hastily assigned to do compressions while a team crowded into the room and ministered to a middle-aged man. At the time, I understood nothing of what went on, except after about 10 minutes, he was pronounced alive and likely to survive.

I was floating down the hall, basking in the glow of my own self-worth when that same Sister Sunshine who hired me approached and gently said, "The Bishop would like to see you, my child." Then she did something that really terrified me. She smiled.

Minutes later as I sat in the head honcho's office and tried to remember just what I had disliked about the Navy, Bishop Red Face placed a gnarled hand on my shoulder and gave me some advice that has served me well in my career as a paramedic: "DO NOT PLACE YER BUTT IN MOTION WITHOUT ENGAGING YER BRAIN."

Touched that this seasoned old administrator would take the time to console me, I looked at him with mist in my eyes and stuttered. "Th-th thank you sir, I'll remember." "Good," he replied, "now turn in your scrubs, and get out of my hospital."

That day I left forever the profession of Linoleum Hygiene and got a job on a transfer ambulance that required only, of all things, that I be CPR trained. Over the years, I became an ECA, EMT and, finally, a paramedic. Through it all, the noble words spoken to me that day have served me well. I still occasionally place my butt in high gear without first considering the consequences and every once in a while, I get that same good feeling from that day in the hall before Sister Sunshine sent me to Red Face.

Yeah, most of the time I love being a paramedic, but sometimes, like the other night in the rain, all I can think of is, "Which store did all these batteries come from?"

A Work Stress Test*

GAIL WEISHAUS, R.N.

It is Stress!

I call stress the "toxic shock of the spirit." If you are not quite sure whether you are suffering from this chronic malady, perhaps the following test can enlighten you.

This Is a Test

Are you suffering from work-related stress? Take the following quiz, answering yes or no.

1. Have you ever taken a patient's vital signs and in a desperate need for paper, you wrote the results on your hand?

2. As a traveling nurse, does your car trunk or back seat look like a central supply closet?

3. Have you ever been so hungry, tired, and rushed that you drank a can of food supplement for lunch?

4. Did you ever get caught in the rain and ingeniously use a blue pad to protect yourself?

5. Have you ever thought of dumping Prozac into the city water supply?

6. When you hear that annoying beeper noise do you drive to a bridge to get out of your car and throw the beeper into the water?

7. As the beeper plummets into the water, you faintly hear it go off and without hesitation, jump in after it?

8. Do you ever find yourself admiring people's veins?

9. Are you starting to break away from using descriptive terms such as "clay-colored" or "coffee ground" and find yourself using more creative phrases such as "Burnt Sienna"?

10. When you hear the term *"Anna Phylaxis"* do you think it's one of your patients?

11. Do you believe that the office first aid kit should contain Valium for the staff?

12. Does your appointment book planner have every weekend marked "on" or "off" for next year?

If you answered yes to any of these questions, then you may be suffering from **STRESS!**

Of course these questions are all tongue and cheek, but there is a smattering of truth in this playful quiz, and it is this familiarity that should make us take a step back and laugh at ourselves.

When we feel stressed and ill at ease, or "dis-ease," as I prefer to call it, we need to balance these feelings and promote an internal feeling of well-being. How long does it take for you to recognize the symptoms of your stress, overload, burnout, or feelings of disease?

My recognition day came to me while I was working as a hospice nurse. I had several oncall emergencies during the week, and I remember starting out on this particular day, praying at a red light to find the time to complete my scheduled visits without any emergencies or interruptions.

As if the angels had delivered my message, I miraculously made all my visits without a single peep from my beeper. I smiled as I was driving back to the office thanking my guardian angel for allowing me time to complete my work.

As I entered the office, my angelic smile of accomplishment immediately disappeared from my face when an angry supervisor jumped out of her chair and proceeded to yell, "Where were you? I've been beeping you all day, and you haven't answered any of your beeps!"

I felt so enraged by her accusations that I immediately took my beeper and threw it on her desk. At that moment, I realized that I had just thrown down my remote control garage door opener. At first there was silence, and then the entire office erupted into laughter: everyone was laughing because I had been wearing my garage door opener instead of the beeper. I laughed with tears in my eyes at the humor in this situation.

Did I feel so stressed about completing my visits and finishing my office paperwork that I unconsciously grabbed anything even remotely feeling like a beeper and wore my garage door opener all day? I believe this was a sign that I had been working on empty and needed respite. This laughter was a cathartic for me and the rest of the staff. It proved to be a spontaneous tension popper that added a much needed break during an intense moment.

*Reprinted with permission from Home Healthcare Nurse, ©1997; 15(1):65–66. Edited from the original.

Test Yourself
. . . and Everybody Else*

KATHERINE MACKAY, R.N.

ENTERIC DISEASE

As a public health nurse, you have been following the S. family for salmonella control. This family includes the mother; seven children, aged 20 years to 10 months; three grandchildren aged 11 months, 5 years, and 3 years; and one all-American dog, age unknown. During the 9 months you have visited, the family has been enlarged by the arrival of one hamster and the birth of five puppies. Your nursing assessment is that Ms. S. is a congenial generous woman but somewhat limited in her ability to comprehend anything she cannot see.

You have completed your health teaching but continue to visit in order to supervise the collection of four consecutive negative stool specimens from each family member, four-legged as well as two-legged.

1. **Of the following comments, which would be most characteristic of a 10-year-old boy who has never turned in a specimen kit?**
    - (A) "The boogeyman jumped out of the bathroom and stole it."
    - (B) "I left it at school . . . I think."
    - (C) "Bobbie keeps hiding it on me."
    - (D) "What's a specimen kit?"

You have received negative stool culture results on all the S's except the 10-month-old baby. On a particularly wearing Friday, you find a lab slip face down on your desk.

2. **Your most appropriate action is to**
    - (A) set your bag on the lab slip and head for the coffee machine.
    - (B) hold your breath and turn the slip over.
    - (C) take the rest of the afternoon off.
    - (D) slide the slip under your blotter and make a note to look at it Monday.

The baby's lab report states "negative for salmonella—positive for shigella."

3. **The appropriate action for you to take is to**
    - (A) go to the staff lounge for coffee, taking along change for the candy machine.
    - (B) file the lab slip under S for Smith.
    - (C) start collecting booklets on shigella and specimen kits for the S. family.
    - (D) question the accuracy of the report and suggest a quality-control study in the lab.

4. **When you call Ms. S. to inquire about her youngest baby's health, her most likely response would be**
    - (A) "*She's* better, but my 11-month-old granddaughter is vomiting."
    - (B) "I didn't call you because I thought she was just cutting teeth."
    - (C) "Bobbie lost the card with your number on it, so I couldn't call."
    - (D) "The small kids have all been at my sister's for two weeks, so I could pack. We're all moving in with her so that I can watch her kids—she got a job as a cook at the university hospital."

5. **Probably your most therapeutic action now is to**
    - (A) take your accumulated overtime, starting immediately.
    - (B) start collecting specimen kits.
    - (C) ask your supervisor to lighten your caseload.
    - (D) attack your backlog of paper work.

Months pass, all S. stools are negative, and you are preparing to close their case when Ms. S. telephones.

6. **She is most likely to say which of the following?**
    - (A) "Thank you, nurse, for all your wonderful health teaching. I'm sure that by practicing good hygiene we will diminish our chances of contracting any more communicable diseases."
    - (B) "My sister and I are opening a fast-food luncheonette and want you to be our guest at the grand opening."
    - (C) "The babies are sick again, just like the last time."
    - (D) "Our dog had puppies again and we want you to have the first pick as soon as they stop having diarrhea."

*Reprinted with permission from American Journal of Nursing, ©1977; 77(2):342.

A Tribute to Home Care
(The Art of Home Care)*

PAULINE SHEEHAN, R.N.

The first major adjustment to home care is having to drive past garage sales. In 1 year, a registered nurse missed 67 garage sales and 11 half sales—half sales being that upon slowing down, one realizes that it isn't that enticing after all.

There is the Christmas shopping issue. Pre-Christmas traffic jams back one up through several traffic light changes. So, if you are particularly unlucky to work Saturdays between major malls, you experience the stress of Christmas shopping without doing any of your own shopping.

Then the weather warms up! The plant nurseries burst with more temptation.

A new marketing tip may be to ride the hospital elevator. For example, on the elevator someone noticed the home care badge and asked if the nurse would take care of their mother when she was discharged. "Talk to the hospital discharge planner," she responded.

Don't try to eat on the restaurant-lined streets between 11:30 AM and 12:30 PM. They are too busy.

Don't go to retirement centers during lunch hour.

Don't try to telephone physicians between 12 and 2 PM.

Make a few useful lists of services that are on the right side of streets: (1) clean bathrooms, (2) phones, (3) fast foods. If a place has all three, wowee!

More hints: Knock on the door louder than the hard of hearing person's television.

A word about finding the homes: The sun rises in the East and settles in the West, that is until you cross a bridge. East of the bridge, the sun rises in the North and sets in the South. The reason is that mountains have been known to move 90° when you drive across a bridge or around a mountain. It is not known how this occurs, but it is a fact. No one else but you knows this, so directions are off by 90°.

Don't let the mountain mobility factor alarm you, because by the next time you turn left, the mountain returns to its former place and you are still going north. It's not that big of a problem as long as you remember

that everyone else is wrong; you just have to make a 90° adjustment in their directions.

One set of directions read, "take the paved driveway between the two white houses and stop at the mobile home on the left." Nobody answered the door. After peeking in the window to discover it was a storage shed—a metal, mobile-home-like storage shed—the nurse glanced around at the houses with large glass patio doors facing open decks. Of course, out came the dogs, then the resident.

"Well, I'll be . . . there is a mobile home about a block farther!"

Parking: Be alert about where to park. Check for the apartment complex visitor parking, which will always be very far from the apartment that you visit. Don't feel sorry for yourself when you pass by the handicapped parking. The other nurses don't get to park there either. Avoid the 1-hour parking places, for that is when you will visit longer than 1 hour.

Your day will be a series of stops and starts. But remember, at every stop, lock up; at every start, buckle up.

Be polite and gracious. You are a guest in their home. They may hold a grudge if you run over their flower beds, fences, dogs, or children. And, never, never, never injure their caregiver.

Oh, inside the home! Once inside, you need to figure out who is the patient. One has to be wary about assuming who the patient is. The one who is on oxygen is not necessarily the patient, neither is the oldest one, the one with the most medication bottles, the one with the most physical ailments, nor even the one in the hospital bed—rather it may be the one playing cards in the kitchen. And to complicate this further, a different person may be the patient than the one at your last visit.

Comments about other assumptions: The one who looks older may not be the parent. The one who looks the same age may not be the spouse. Check the face sheet for the patient's age and gender. These facts can help you figure out who is the patient.

Once in a home, the apologies roll, "Sorry my house

*Reprinted with permission from Home Healthcare Nurse, ©1995; 13(1): 82–83.

is a mess." Yet, it's cleaner than how you left your own home that morning.

Other uses for the face sheet: jot down the name of their children, neighbor, dog, cat, or canary. You can peek at the names, and get credit for your good memory.

If you can't read the doctor's name on the face sheet, or you have never heard of that doctor, look at the prescription bottle. You may have to look at several, but usually you'll find one with the doctor's name—spelled correctly, to boot.

One wishes that one would always remember to check the ending mileage before going into the office.

The dream—running water; a wastebasket; a Mayo stand, which holds supplies or meals; and an overhead surgical lamp in every home.

Inservice Education for Northern Nurses

KAREN GRAHAM, R.N., B.N.

MURPHY'S LAWS FOR NORTHERN NURSES

- Fog will roll in and obscure the airstrip 10 minutes before the med-evac plane arrives.
- One med-evac engenders another.
- The med-evac plane will be gone past recall before the second emergency arrives at the health centre.
- In the midst of preparations for an emergency med-evac, you will need to see at least three sick children.
- White-out weather conditions cause premature labor.
- On Sunday afternoon at 4:00 p.m., the sound waves from the phrase "You've had a quiet weekend" will cause all hell to break loose within three hours.
- The need for a radio consultation with a physician causes solar flares.
- If the satellite telephone is out, the RCMP emergency radio is not being manned at the other end.
- All northern planes are on time—until such time as they don't appear.
- The merest wisp of a thought concerning sleep or going to bed at a reasonable hour will cause the emergency telephone to ring.
- If you have not had a delivery in months, two women in labor will arrive on your doorstep simultaneously and deliver within five minutes of each other.
- There is a high degree of correlation between a serious emergency occurring and the start of labor among prenatal women.
- A woman in premature labor who is "not doing much" will be in vigorous labor within 15 minutes after take-off. (You will have no delivery equipment because you "won't need it").
- The severity of an epidemic and the number of serious emergencies are directly correlated to the number of staff on holiday.
- A sick baby who has kept you up for three nights in a row will experience a miraculous recovery on the med-evac plane en route to the hospital, arrive back on the next plane and promptly get sick again.
- Med-evacing a plane-load of children with bronchiolitis at a reasonable hour of the day ensures that there will be at least two children per health centre crib and croupette by 22:00 hours.
- The number of children who arrive for their well child clinic appointment is directly related to the number of emergencies and the degree of chaos occurring on well child clinic day.
- The degree of difficulty in obtaining a blood specimen from an infant is directly related to the likelihood of the plane not arriving or being so late as to make the specimen worthless.
- Waiting until you hear that the plane has taken off will not avoid the consequences of the above law. The plane will either overfly or turn back or you will be unable to find the patient.

Reproduced with permission from *The Canadian Nurse/L'infirmière canadienne,* ©1994; 90(3):33–36. Edited from the original.

• Having received the news that the med-evac plane has "gone mechanical" and it will take at least four hours to fix, you send escort, family and assistants home to rest. Then the pilot will call, stating that the plane is fixed, the weather closing in and if he doesn't take off in 20 minutes he will be stuck for the next 12 hours.

• A long-awaited specialist will arrive when the patient with the appointment is out hunting and cannot be contacted.

• If there is a dental visit scheduled at the same time as a physician's visit, the audiologist will decide to come too, and then the senior nursing officer will decide to come for a week's assessment of the functioning of your health centre.

• If the staff of your health centre decide on ma-

jor spring cleaning and rearrangement of the facilities, the regional nursing officer will arrive with VIPs from headquarters or overseas visitors.

• If headquarters want a survey questionnaire returned to them by July 1, it will land on your desk on July 17.

• If you arrive new to the community, the sealift/barge order for yearly supplies was due in the regional office three days before your arrival (and no copy of the previous year's order can be found, nor is there an inventory of present supplies).

Axiom for northern nursing: A sense of humor is necessary for survival.

Corollary: Survival is necessary for a sense of humor.

Have You Mastered "Stresscalation"?*

RUTH DAILEY GRAINGER, PHD, A.R.N.P.

STRESSCALATION INSTRUCTION MANUAL

—Think negatively, particularly about yourself. Charity begins at home, you know.

—When something bad happens, think *only* about that. Don't let reality-oriented thoughts distract you from catastrophizing.

—When you are worrying (worries are movies in the mind), carry the worry to a certain level, then stop the movie, and never finish it. This will keep your worry/dread/anxiety at its optimum high level.

—When you are able to think negatively about an event, multiply its effect by seeing the event *over* and *over* in your mind. Thirty-seven is the optimum number of times to replay a negative event. If you replay it fewer times, you may not have the opportunity to escalate the stress of its pictures, sounds, feelings, and pessimism. If you play it more times, then you could actually get bored. Be careful of this.

—"What-if" should be your middle name.

—No self-respecting stresscalator would be satisfied with keeping stress to yourself. Share it with a friend.

—Live in the future. You should be concerned about the future because it is yet to be. Forget about *now*, for in just a moment, what is now will certainly be then, and it will no longer exist. *Now* is only a frivolity. You'll burn that bridge when you get to it!

—Promote BM behavior. (Bitch and Moan—the louder and longer, the better.)

—Play it safe. Don't take chances. You wouldn't want to be blamed, would you? What if you made a mistake? What if it didn't turn out right? What if . . . What if . . . (but that's your middle name).

—If you have a deadline, postpone as long as possible working on the project. It is so thrilling to go screeching in at the last moment, anxiety level flying, heart pumping, brain racing, feeling all fired up about it finally.

—When it is certain that you are *not* going to meet the deadline, the least you can do is panic. Scream a lot, moan, get angry at other people instead of your-

*Reprinted from American Journal of Nursing, ©1992; 92(9):16 with permission from the author. Edited from the original.

self, get everyone else in a tizzy, find someone to blame other than yourself, throw a tantrum. Scape-goating can be miraculously rewarding.

—Take every opportunity to have a pity party. Only invite friends who will feel as sorry for you as you do. Remember, he who dies with the most people feeling sorry for him wins.

—If interactions with a certain family member leave you disturbed and distressed, find time to talk with this individual even more often.

—The time to leave for an appointment is the exact time you should arrive.

—Ignore any advice that requires you to "postpone your actions" or "sleep on it." In the morning, you might not feel like you do now, and the opportunity may be lost.

—Answer every phone call, no matter when it comes in, what you are doing, what it takes you away from, who it is from, or what they want you to donate to! You wouldn't want to be curious, now would you?

—Deep down in your heart, you *know* that you could be *perfect* if you only tried a little harder. Really put the pressure on yourself to achieve perfection.

—Talk loud and fast. You'll get more words in edge-wise that way, and others will hear you better. If they seem to be confused or not following you, get angry at them for being stupid.

—Pay attention to the faults of others. You know that they aren't paying attention to their own (unless you advise them of these faults).

—It is unwise to say "no" to others for any reason. If someone wants you to do something that you don't want to do, surely their reasons for wanting you to do it are better than your reasons for *not* wanting to do it.

—When you are sick, pay adequate attention to all your symptoms, and frequently check to see that they are, in fact, worse. Report often to as many other people as you can find.

—Don't let go of slights, irritabilities, etc. Keep them close to your heart, massaging them, elaborating on them, cherishing them.

—Escalate the intensity of any situation. It's exciting, it upsets others, and you *do* get a lot of attention.

—Be sure that old family traditions are passed down to your children even if they "inherit" low self-esteem, depression, guilt, and abuse.

Now that you know more about how to stresscalate, the choice is up to you.

The "Hop Till You Drop" Theory of Nursing*

R. KANE

Some theories of nursing are willing to confront the marked gender structuring that still prevails in nursing, and some are not. The "hop till you drop" theory of nursing is one that recognizes and addresses this gender structuring. Most nurses are women. Most environments they work in are controlled by men. The "hop till you drop" theory of nursing is an acknowledgement that this fundamental and fundamentally true situation has meaning.

A variety of responses are available to women in contemporary society that enable them to live, day to day, with gender-structured situations predicated on the assumption of an innate inferiority of women, often expressed as an assumption of an innate superior-ity of men. The average-thinking person knows that there is something amiss in this world view, and may even surreptitiously wish to be free of these embar-rassing assumptions, but like McDonald's, Coca Cola, and poor and taxes, they seem to endure and intrude themselves into our lives.

Even when we know these views are dysfunctional, we continue to embrace and live them out, despite our best intentions and overwhelming evidence to the con-trary.

Some women attach themselves to powerful men with ample resources, and devote a substantive por-tion of their lives to shopping; hence the clever bumper sticker philosophy "shop till you drop." Some

*Reprinted with permission, Nursecom, Inc., from Nursing Forum, ©1992; 27(4):35–36. Edited from the original.

become passive, cute, darling, helpless, perhaps best captured as "fop till you drop." Some adopt a stance of domestic intensity, home-creating, and cleanliness, which one could call "mop till you drop," while others create elaborate styles of manipulation to achieve desired goals, using a "sop till you drop" approach. There are others.

The one of particular interest to nursing, however, is one that might best be called "hop till you drop." Adherents to this theory spend most of their careers working chaotically, assuming responsibility for their own jobs and those of one-half of their units, running chaotically from task to task, attempting finally, once and for all, to gain credibility. The seduction of this theory is an ongoing belief that if one just keeps working harder and harder, longer and longer, one will finally be acknowledged as a peer rather than as an inferior. Because this outcome never is achieved, the nurses who use this theory just keep hopping until they drop.

The theory enjoys considerable popularity because it veils an implicit hopefulness attractive to many nurses who inherently find despair unattractive, yet flounder in search of a basis for hope. They do not choose to be passive parasites, and in the process become activists, people committed to a cause, energetic producers. They are wonderful to have on staff, in leadership roles, as floaters. They can be counted upon in every situation. If they must stay up all night to complete the report, they will. They "know" the report is just one more brick in the building of credibility. The hope they manifest endures, touchingly.

The lurking danger in the theory, of course, is the amazing seduction such nurses offer the exploitative personality: now there's a real nurse. All the fuzzy and sentimental stereotypes of the all-giving mother float up on folks' fantasies, and the "hop till you drop" nurse assumes more and more responsibility, cajoled by such phrases as "no one does it better than you" and "we know we can count on you" and "you're my favorite nurse." No problem. The "hopper" gets "hopping" and adds yet one more task to an already overwhelming burden.

Nurse colleagues appreciate such "hoppers." Since some nurses elect a substantially more passive posture when confronted by persisting sexism, or choose outright to deny the existence of such sexism, the "hopper" becomes an invaluable resource. Athena-like, she charges into the foray for the many, carrying a banner of hope, resilience, and strength. Lesser colleagues, more prone to seeing life as an observer sport, watch the show, relieved of numerous onerous tasks and responsibilities. The "hopper" hops on.

The key delimitation of this theory is the short lifeline of the adherents. While invaluable in the short run, they either burn out prematurely, or eventually "drop." Many drop early, disillusioned. Some drop later, but with a lurking sense of betrayal in their hearts. None, tragically, change the system. Yet, one must acknowledge, they get a lot of work done in the interim. There are worse things than "hopping till you drop," and the adherent intuitively knows this truth. Until creative alternatives are available, however, "hoppers" will continue to select this theory as their paradigm of choice. At least it pays the bills.

Live and Let Die*

ROGER NAPTHINE

You might not think that Andreas Vesalius and I have anything in common.

Vesalius was after all, a famous early doctor of medicine—physician to the court of the Holy Roman Emperor Charles V.

Me? Well, I am a relatively obscure nurse.

But there is something we do have in common: we have both mistakenly pronounced as dead a person who was still alive.

In Vesalius' case, this was quite a tragic error. Believing a Spanish nobleman to be dead, Vesalius commenced an autopsy. When he opened the chest he discovered a heart still beating. Not surprisingly, the autopsy itself led to the nobleman's death. Vesalius was sentenced to death, but this was commuted to permanent exile. Vesalius died in a shipwreck while undertaking a penitential pilgrimage to the Holy Land.

My error was not so dramatic.

We had all been waiting for Mr. Castello to die. His death was obviously not far off—all the signs were there. His irregular respirations were becoming quieter, shallower and less frequent. I was checking his condition as often as I could throughout the evening shift and his continued, steady deterioration was quite apparent. But it was not so easy to get close to his bed as he was now surrounded by his family who wanted to be with him and who had taken over his care in these final hours.

When his family suddenly burst into loud cries of "He's dead! He's dead!", I was not at all surprised. However, I couldn't get into his room. I certainly couldn't get close enough to actually inspect the body, as the family had flung themselves over the bed, embracing him, kissing him one more time. They did not want to leave and it would have been cruel to ask them to go. I would allow them a few moments of privacy before I intruded.

I could however see his still body at the centre of all this loving but distraught attention. Mr. Castello was dead and I had to prepare for the tasks of post-mortem care, of the 'last rites'.

I thought I would save time by ringing his doctor to announce the death of Mr. Castello.

'Well, we expected that didn't we, Roger? There's no point in my coming in. I'll take care of the paperwork in the morning. Thanks.' He hung up.

But when eventually I had edged my way to Mr. Castello's bedside, I saw his chest move up and down—yes, it was the faintest trickle of a heartbeat. Mr. Castello was still alive although completely unresponsive.

As I'd not told his family that I thought he was dead, there was no loss of face in telling them quietly that yes, he was very, very weak but he was still alive. And yes, they were welcome to continue their bedside vigil.

Later that night Mr. Castello's feeble grasp on life finally loosened. He died very quietly.

Whether his doctor even noticed the discrepancy in times between his being told of Mr. Castello's death and the time written on the formal report, I've never found out. He never mentioned it to me.

But I knew. And eventually so did other nurses. Word of my over-enthusiastic 'diagnosis' soon spread around the hospital grapevine.

Are you surprised then to learn that after this I became somewhat cautious in my declarations on patients' deaths?

Well, I'm somewhat relieved to know I'm not the only one who can get it wrong.

One of the great, persisting fears of our culture is that of being buried alive.

And of course, you can't be buried alive unless someone—the attending doctor, for instance—is mistaken in pronouncing you dead.

Although brain-dead people are legally regarded as dead, their life-like appearance and the presence of artificially maintained warmth and perfusion of tissues makes it possible for nurses to regard them as 'living dead.' During the process of organ retrieval, their status changes to that of an organ donor. This status is preserved even when the kidneys and liver are being removed. But when the heart and lungs are removed, then the person is irretrievably dead. No amount of wishful thinking will now restore the person to life—the patient is now 'dead dead'.

This belief that some states of being dead are more definitive than others, echoes the old belief that per-

*Reprinted with permission from Australian Nursing Journal, ©1994; 2(2):32–33. Edited from the original.

haps we aren't really, absolutely dead until something quite final is done to our body.

So, do I still feel foolish about my premature announcement of Mr. Castello's death?

Yes. Not because I was wrong, for I am obviously not alone in that. I feel foolish because I hadn't checked the patient before concluding that he was dead.

And that was poor nursing practice.

The Last to Go*

It is commonly known in the nursing field that the seriously ill patient can still hear. The sense of hearing is the "last to go." Accounts of patients awakening from coma states and reciting conversations of loved ones or caregivers confirms this belief. This experience confirms that patients do hear and can respond to the nurse in special circumstances.

Mr. J. was an elderly man admitted with a cerebrovascular accident. He had been in the hospital for two days when I was assigned to his care. The previous nurse had reported that Mr. J. was weak, in a fetal position, and did not speak clearly, only groaned when moved or disturbed and he was known to be deaf. My

initial assessment found Mr. J. to be exactly as the nurse had reported.

During the shift, I was to apply an antifungal cream to Mr. J's perineum and gluteal fold. As I neared his bedside, I touched him and explained what I was about to do. "Mr. J., I have some ointment to put on your bottom—can you roll over and show me your bottom?" I began raising the sheet when he very clearly stated, "I'll show you mine, if you show me yours."

Needless to say, I was very surprised! (These were also the only clearly spoken words he said that evening.) Hearing may not be "the last to go" afterall—it may be the sex drive!

*Reprinted with permission from Kansas Nurse, ©1994; 69(3):6.

LIVING LANGUAGE

Iris Ciliaris was working a dreaded shift to the left for the Greater Trochanter Systema serving all incisured peplos. It was a quiescent nocturia when all helix broke loose.

A triose of patients renin, verbomania with excitant, as casualties of St. Anthony's fire. The first one through the threshold was a Dandy-Walker with caput femoris. Iris saw the Seconal patient, and in a minuthesis knew he had shotty lymph nodes. Nexus was Marie-Foix suffering from burning foot syndrome.

Aftercare of these patients, Iris met the couple Duo Denum at Mercier's bar. While listening to Peri Stalsis on the stereotaxis, they ordered gingivo tonics with limen.

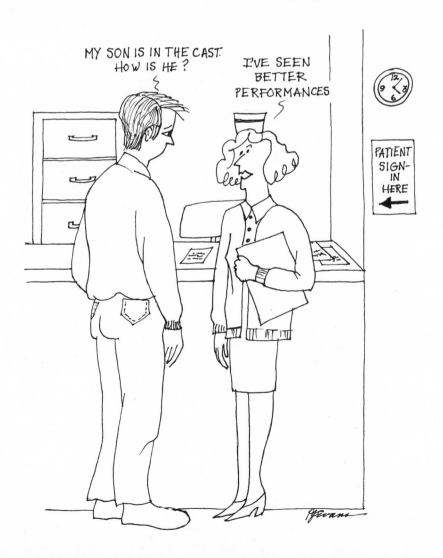

How to Read Nursing Employment Ads*

ANITA BUSH, R.N., C.C.R.N.

As the worldwide nursing shortage makes recruiters more competitive and our remuneration more equitable, it's easy to become misled by the slick advertising some institutions have adopted. In order to help you avoid feeling misled, here are the real-life definitions of the most common ploys used to attract nurses.

WHAT THE AD SAYS . . .	WHAT IT REALLY MEANS . . .
"Competitive pay"	Pay is as low as we can get away with and still have our body count be reasonable.
"Salary"	Hourly wages based on time clocks or time sheets.
"Challenging environment"	A lot of really sick patients, short-staffed, little support from managers and administrators, a high-density of "difficult" physicians and bitchy nurses.
"Excellent benefits"	Minimum legal requirement, one or two low-cost perks and eventually you will get to take a vacation . . . maybe a couple of days next year.
"Diversity"	You're required to float to cover units you don't feel competent to work in, and don't say you're not comfortable there. "A nurse is a nurse is a nurse."
"Tuition reimbursement"	We have a written policy, but your schedule will be so bizarre that you'll never be able to complete a course so don't even bother enrolling in one.
"Committed to professional development"	You're expected to serve on many committees and task forces, to participate in your manager's projects but we're so short-staffed right now you'll have to do them on your off-duty time. And no we really can't pay you any extra for this work you do for us, but since we need all this for our accreditation, if you don't do it, we'll have to write that in your performance evaluation.
"Free housing"	We had to close some beds since we couldn't staff them so you can stay right here in-house where we will call you anytime of day or night to come to work.
"Clinical ladders"	12-foot ceilings from which everyone hangs the IV's, i.e. very old building.
"Research opportunities"	We want you to discover how to do 12-hours of work in the 8-hours they pay you. Also they want you to figure out how to care for 50% sicker patients with 33% fewer staff. No statistical knowledge needed.
"Job security"	If you're licensed and breathing you can work 'til you die.
"Inter-facility transfer opportunities"	We have seasonal peaks and troughs so they'll float you 2000 miles away.

*Reprinted from Journal of Nursing Jocularity, ©1991; 1(1):14–15 with permission from the author.

WHAT THE AD SAYS . . .	WHAT IT REALLY MEANS . . .
"Per diem"	What's that?
"Free parking"	Some places still charge you money to come to work.
"Medical coverage that includes chronic kidney care"	That's part of a new union contract since staff rarely get a chance to go to the bathroom.
"Salary-in-lieu-of-benefits"	Silly goose! Who said you could have both?
"In-house continuing education"	We can't schedule you for 2–3 days off together just because you want to attend a workshop. Even though the class is required for your job, we'll still charge you money to attend.

Words to the Wise*

H. ALLETHAIRE CULLEN, R.N.C., M.S.N., F.N.P., C.E.N.

I understand that for most layfolk ours is a foreign language. Why else would we say "cyanotic" instead of "blue," "aggressive" instead of "nasty," and "dyspneic" instead of "in big trouble?" Why indeed? Why would physicians refer to "cardiac tamponade," while nurses refer to the same condition as "decreased cardiac output related to restrictive factors?" And why, oh, why, would we say, "This will be just a little pinch," when what layfolk would say is, "Like riding a bull at Gilley's for 3 hours?"

It's an interesting concept. Doc-talk. Nurse-talk. Lab-talk. Business office-talk. I now present the natural sequela to the aforementioned: patient-talk. It is *real*: each of my examples is genuine. But it is odd.

You probably were not confused the first time someone told you that a patient was having "the shock." You, of course, recognize that as a lay term for a cerebrovascular accident (CVA). You, of course, are brighter than I. I became aware of the phrase "the shock" in triage. An elderly woman rushed in and said that her husband was in the car, "having the shock."

I need to digress for a moment, so you will understand my confusion. Here in Rhode Island, natives usually preface sentence objects with "the." One does not have loose stools; one has "the diarrhea" (or more often "the diarrheas"). For a headache, one takes "the

Tie-nolls." You do not come to Kent County Hospital; you go to "the Kent" or "the Miriam", or even "the R'Di-land". (Of course, natives have also been known to say, "Next time you cut through my yard, go around," and if you stand next to someone, you are said to be "side by each." In point of fact, an especially cheerful team on the 3 PM to 11 PM shift is known for singing, "So we'll travel along/singing a song,/side by each." But now I truly digress. . . .)

So when the woman said her husband was having "the shock," I, thinking like an emergency nurse (always chancy at triage; better to think like a patient), said, as I followed her to the parking lot, "Is he bleeding somewhere?"

"No, no, no!"

"Did he fall? Has he a fever? An infection?" (I was running out of types of shock here.)

"No, no! It's the shock! The shock!" (Shades of Tatoo: "The plane! The plane!")

What it was, of course, was a stroke. A CVA. And we ministered to the patient, and he did well.

My brain did not.

Shortly thereafter, a young man came in complaining of an earache. It was pretty bad, he told me, and his brother had had one not quite as bad, but bad enough so that his eardrum was stretched and bulging.

*Reproduced from Journal of Emergency Nursing, ©1993; 19(2): 171–172 with permission from Mosby-Year Book, Inc.

His name for it: "o-tightness medium." (I tried not to grin. Had his brother's earache been worse, it might have been "o-tightness large.")

Some time later, a woman inadvertently explained the entire Mideast crisis to me. She was extremely uncomfortable and had been short-tempered with her children. She knew she could restore family harmony, she said sincerely, if we could just give her something for her Sinai infection. (Henry Kissinger, please take note.) And while I am reflecting on that part of the anatomy, one of my colleagues tells of the woman who assured her that she had clogs coming out of her sinus cabinets. (So that's where Imelda Marcos was storing them!)

Since then, I've learned to accept (with equanimity, if not a giggle) patients with pinky eye, Midas valve prolapse, sugar diabetes, and hyena hernias. I had a man (a very embarrassed gent, I hasten to add) tell me he had female anatomy. Clutching his bottle of sublingual nitroglycerin, he told me, "I have vagina." Sometimes you can give the best patient care by doing a little patient teaching. There are no words to describe the relief on this man's face when I taught him the word "angina."

Patients tell me that they have stayed overnight in the "extensive care unit." They have had daily "heartograms" when admitted there. Patients also get put on bedrest and heparin therapy when they are admitted with "flea bites."

Then there was the woman who came to the triage booth for a confidential chat. "I need to know if you take care of this kind of thing," she said, "I'm from out of town. It's my husband."

"What's wrong with your husband?"

"He's Oriental."

I assured her that we cared for all patients in need, no matter what their race, creed, gender, insurance status, etc., etc., etc.

"Yes, yes," she said impatiently. "But can you help my husband?"

"We'll certainly do our best. Can you explain what's wrong?"

"I told you. He's Oriental."

Visions of Orwellian personhood changes flashed in my mind. "You want to change the fact that he's Oriental?"

"It came on him so suddenly."

"He didn't used to be Oriental?"

"No, he was perfectly normal."

I was about to give her a lesson in race relations when it suddenly dawned on me. "How long has he been confused?" I asked.

"Just since he got up this morning," she said, without missing a beat.

"So this *disorientation* has never happened before?"

"On, no," she replied, and I am pleased to say that we got her husband the care he needed, promptly, with no more social psychology from the triage nurse, thank you very much.

Of course, patients are not the only ones who have trouble with the language we use. I remember a sweet receptionist who consistently charted the chief complaint as, "Patient states having trouble removing his bowels."

Still and all, there are patients, the dear hearts, who tell us that they take a water pill called "latex." How many of us have had elderly gentlemen tell us that they have "prostrate problems?" (Yes, I understand the reference, but the perverse part of my brain always wants to suggest that if such a gentleman would only get off his face, his problems would be over.)

There came a day when a teenager told me he thought there was something wrong with his salvation glands. I almost asked if his lymphatic system was having a revival.

As a Rhode Islander, however, I must confess that my favorite story has to do with the gentleman who came in with an intractable cough. Bear in mind that everyone in Rhode Island has a boat, or a relative with a boat, or plans to get a boat, and that most of us have within our circle of friends at least one commercial fisherman, and you will understand that I was not at all surprised to hear this man tell me that he had barnacle pneumonia. He was a quahogger; he was probably right. What did surprise me was the emergency doc who spent the rest of his shift singing under his breath, "Shiver me timbers and blow me down! I'm Bronchial Bill the Sailor."

It is the moments like these that make me sure I will stay an emergency nurse forever.

Help!*

SAMUEL N. GRIEF, M.D.

Time is of the essence in the modern family physician's office. With everything we're responsible for, it's no wonder that doctors have come up with an abbreviated language of medical acronyms to save time (and some major tongue twisting) when conversing with colleagues. With the advent of managed care, these acronyms have become a dime a dozen. I'm beginning to feel overwhelmed.

Don't get me wrong. Without acronyms, medical professionals the world over would be battling a terrible outbreak of writer's cramp. The sheer length of some medical terms makes the word antidisestablishmentarianism look short. However, I think things are getting a little out of hand.

Over the last decade or so, we have witnessed a dizzying array of new technology—all, of course, with their unique acronyms. Each department of medicine seems to have its own list, contributing to the growing lexicon. At x-ray, we hear about CT, PET, MRI, IVP, KUB, DSA, and CXR. At the laboratory, terms such as CBC, SMA, ABG, LFT, TFT, BUN, HDL, LDL, TSH, FBS, and RBS are regularly bandied about. Cardiologists talk about CAD, ECG, MI, PTCA, CABG, LBBB, ETT, MUGA, and more. Pulmonologists are wont to mention COPD, RAD, PFT, PPD, TB, PPH, FVC, PEF, IPF, and, everybody's favorite, SOB! You get the picture.

Here in New Hampshire, managed care has become a major force in the health care industry. Unfortunately, along with it has come a new bunch of medical-bureaucratic terms that are usually referred to by their acronyms. And let's not forget all those insurance companies with their long names. For example, Harvard Community Health Plan was called HCHP. Just when I was getting used to that, Harvard got capitalistic and merged with Pilgrim Health Care to form Harvard Pilgrim Health Care, or HPHC. U.S. Health Care is an easy one (USHC). Healthsource is even easier (HS). Private Health Care System is pretty straightforward: PHCS. Traveler's insurance, however, is known as MetP. At least Prudential Care Plus is logically called PCP. Not so good, though, when in the same sentence you are using a catchphrase of the medical system: primary care provider, or PCP!

To make matters worse, at my family practice we refer to our doctors and nurse practitioners by their initials, usually including their middle one. This is meant to avoid any confusion, especially with the call schedule. The use of medical providers' initials has become so widespread that some staff know me by my initials, not by name:

"Where is SNG?"

Recently, the medical staff have begun taking liberties with my initials:

"SNiG, can I ask you a question?"

"Hi, SNiGgy!"

You get the point.

So, one day I went across the hall to speak with my colleague PPF regarding a patient. PPF wasn't there that day, but DTD was covering for him. Unfortunately, she was busy helping SJC and ML solve a medical problem on one of their mutual patients with IDDM and CRF. Off I went looking for a corridor consult from RRD instead, but he apparently had been AWOL the entire day. Frustrated, I returned to my patient with a possible torn ACL, whose ROM was limited. I decided to send him for an MRI and an orthopedic evaluation ASAP.

My next patient had a long history of BAD and OCD. She claimed that her lithium and her antianxiety agent were contributing to her recent flare-up of IBS. She also wanted me to do something for her CTS. I ordered an EMG, prescribed an NSAID, and sent her to an OT/PT for her wrist and an RD for dietary help with her bowels.

Later, a patient with SOBOE came to see me. His ROS was negative, but his father had had multiple CVAs, PVD, and ASHD. The patient was a 50-year-old man with HTN, BPH, and IBD. The exam was normal but his ECG wasn't. Over at the hospital, his CKs were elevated so he underwent a cardiac catheterization PDQ, which showed multivessel CAD. A CABG was successfully performed the next day.

Finally, in walked my last patient of the day. Mr. B's health insurance card showed that he had HS POS. But I knew that this patient really had HS HMO. Mr. B was here to show me his recurring skin rash and request a referral to see the dermatologist (Dr. C) in Boston. I told Mr. B that Dr. C was not in his health plan. Mr. B became irate, telling me that he had checked earlier in the day and Dr. C was a member of his PPO. I informed him that Dr. C was not in my PHO nor my IPA. If he wanted to see Dr. C, he would have to switch MCOs. Mr. B went on to tell me that as a VP of a large corporation, he wanted to be treated like a VIP. He insisted on seeing the medical director. Off he went.

Acronyms certainly do speed up the handling of patients over the course of the day. There's a price to pay, though, for all these shortcuts. The list of acronyms commonly used in my family practice is not only enormous, it's growing faster than the national debt. It's hard to keep on top of them all. Daily acronyms like DPT and MMR are easy enough. Most of us can handle the simple diagnoses of UTI and PID. However, when two or more abbreviations are being used for the same condition, things can get pretty fouled up, sometimes leading to a SNAFU. For example, one recent patient of mine received a diagnosis of LBP (low-back pain) and went to get some physical therapy. When the therapist saw the referral, she thought I had sent over a patient with low blood pressure! Some patients with DUB are upset because they think that I wrote DUMB on the superbill. COLD is sometimes mistaken for just a regular URI when the practitioner really means chronic obstructive lung disease. It's enough to give you GAS (generalized abbreviation syndrome).

To all those readers who long for the days when acronyms were rare and the spoken word was cherished, the next time a patient walks in with temporomandibular joint syndrome, bright red blood per rectum, gastroesophageal reflux disease, eustachian tube dysfunction, or seasonal affective disorder, don't forget to speak slowly and carefully. Above all, remember that "less is more." Now I'm off to see my next patient, who is MAD (maximally aggravated at doctors) because I am certified by the BOARD (blatant overuse of abbreviations repetitively by doctors).

Humor is Good Medicine*

GEORGE M. BOHIGIAN, M.D.

Medical Dictionary Terms

Enema	Not a friend
Fibula	Small lie
Rectum	Dang near killed 'em
Seizure	Roman emperor

*Reprinted from Missouri Medicine 1992; 89(9):679–680, copyright © 1992 The Missouri State Medical Association. Edited from the original.

Humor is Good Medicine, Volume 2*

JOHN C. HAGAN, III, M.D.

Medical Dictionary Terms

Bacteria	Back door to a cafeteria
Bowel	Letters like A, E, I, O, U
Cataract	Rich person's car
CAT scan	Search for a kitty
Cauterize	Made eye contact with her
D & C	Where Washington is
Condom	Death sentence
Genital	Non-Jewish
Impotent	Distinguished, well-known
Labor pain	Hurt at work
Nasal	End of a hose
Nephrotic	Overly anxious
Olfactory	Aging infrastructure
Recovery room	Place to upholster
Rheumatic	Amorous
Semen	Ship's crew
Terminal illness	Getting sick at the airport
Tibia	Country in Africa
Vein	Conceited

*Reprinted from Missouri Medicine 1992; 89(11):781, copyright © 1992
The Missouri State Medical Association. Edited from the original.

The Adventures of A. Little Tush, MD, Detective Doctor, Forensic Physician, PC

Episode 1. When Tush Comes to Shove, or Medicine and Pleasure Don't Mix*

WALTER S. WIGHTMAN, M.D.

So, I'm in my office. Art's Medical Building. The ventral side of town, if you catch my mesial drift. It's the time of day when a curbside consult with some medicinal EtOH is just what the doctor ordered. In other words, I'm nursing a Brompton's cocktail back to wellness and looking forward to a chaser of whiskey and rifampin, that is. No such luck. In a voice that could wake the expired, my nurse, Ann Esthetist, insufflates the intercom:

"A patient here to see you. Are you still practicing?"

"Until I get it right, my little narc, Ann. Send the worried wellnik in."

Whoa, baby. Look what's just ambulated into my exam room. I mean, this dame is no Edna Everage. A limbic system nonpareil—that is, she has legs from her Unna boots all the way up to her hips. She's so hot, she's febrile. Me, I play it so cool, I've got rigors. I mean, I'm really shivering. Well, tremoring, essentially, though not intentionally. She can see I'm a fasiculus of nerves.

"Don't worry, Doc," she says, "I'm like an edentulous computer. I don't byte."

Then, she winks at me. So, I give her a little winky back, and my heart skips a beat. After a short interval, she starts up again.

"Dr. Tosh?"

"That's Dr. Tush. With a *u*."

"Well, if you aren't with-a-me, you're against-a-me."

Don't I wish. But I don't risk my license for nobody. She articulates once more, temperomandibularisly, giving me something else to chew on.

"Dr. Tush, I need your help with . . . ahem . . ."

"I'm a doctor, not a dressmaker, sister."

"And I'm not a nun. But I need you to sew up a case for me."

Her and two or three bazillion other patients in the city naked, I mean, naked city. And the jamokes with the toughest problems all seem to find their way to the shingle hanging outside my door. (Ann says I should just get a regular sign, seeing as how ninety-nine percent of the clients think I'm a roofer wearing a white coat.)

"So, tell me about, ahem, your situation, Miss . . .?"

"That's Mademoiselle, uh . . . Turcica."

That name. Always leaves me with an empty feeling. But I had to put my pituitary dysfunction aside and act like a professional. So, I pretended to take a phone call and ignored her for five minutes while I flipped through a chart before I let her tell her story. She went on for what seemed like minutes. I didn't even get a chance to interrupt after the obligatory 18 seconds.

Tells me her entire family figures in the caper. From ol' Pap Smear to Gran Uloma and even Uncal Gyrus. But the chief complainant in the whole sordid history is Ante Partum, a pleasant 41-year-old white woman who looks younger than her stated age. Seems poor Ante finds herself in the family way with an estimated date of confinement handled by Federal Express. That is, she's ready to deliver anywhere, anytime—and, if she's like most gravidas I know—overnight. The fetal kicker is, nobody's got a clue cell as to who's on the male end of this Luer lock.

A quick whiff test tells me there's a fishy odor about l'affaire Partum. But chances are I won't need a chi-square test to tell me who the parasexual perpetrator is. It's more than probable that the offending agent is that well-beyond-standard deviant, that arch aortic dissector—Professor Maury Artery, medical director of the Sherlock Homes for Old Doctors Named Watson.

When I tipped Turcica to my suspicions, her pilars erected in fear.

"Oh, my L-L-Lord," she stammers.

And people wonder why doctors get God complexes?

"What should I do, Dr. Tush?"

Who do I look like, Albert Schweitzer or somebody?

"Take two aspirin-free pain relievers and *don't* call

*Reprinted from The Journal of Family Practice, ©1995; 45(1):13–14. Reprinted by permission of Appleton & Lange and the author.

me in the morning. I'm going to be up late, making a little house call on a certain professor friend of ours."

So Tush is on the trail. But it's always nice to put a little differential in your diagnosis. That means calling in some specialists from out of town.

"Annie, he makes my skin crawl, but get on the cutaneous horn and contact Dermatitis the dermatologist. Next, ask Ariasis to worm his parasitical little butt over here, pronto. Then, pressure Ulcer, that so-called vascular surgeon, to honor us with his presence. He's pretty handy with a scalpel. Just make sure he wears gloves this time. And, oh yeah, notify all the otolaryngology people at the newspaper, as well as at the TV and radio stations—the entire otitis media. Artery's a sucker for publicity."

The consultants and I lure Artery out of hiatus with promises of a free cholesterol screening and lunch on the pharmaceutical rep. We catch him like a man about to have a prostate exam—with his pants down. I obtain Tush's version of informed consent.

"I'm gonna clamp down on you, Artery. And all the bypass graft in the world won't spring you on this one. Consider yourself under cardiac arrest."

Artery pulses paradoxically, then says in a strangulated voice:

"What do you take me for? Some incipient hernia just out of Holthouse? You can't incarcerate me. I'll rupture first."

Then he starts laughing uproariously, which I consider strange under the circumstances, since I could never get a risus out of him before.

Next thing I know, the Turcica broad shows up with Ante right behind. (What we in the profession know as the Anteposterior position.)

Out of the Borrel blue, Partum pipes up:

"I have an admission to make."

"Ridiculous," I says, "you don't even have hospital privileges."

"No, no, Tush. I mean, Artery isn't the fecundator," she says.

"Then how . . .?"

"I went to Vincent Vitro's Casa del Pregnancy."

"You don't mean . . .?"

"Yes, it was a Vin Vitro fertilization."

Talk about your culture shock. Even the Professor was speechless. But it was just an aphasia he was going through, for I soon had to endure yet another Arterial line:

"Well, well, my good Dr. Tush. It looks like you've laid a rather large egg. Your case just went right down the Fallopian tubes."

Since then, Turcica and everybody else treat me like I've got the Boobonic Plague. But I keep busy; Tush is not one to sit around on his rear end. And don't you worry, I'm the Arnold Schwarzenegger of physician detectives. I'm like a bad case of athlete's foot. I'll be back.

When DOS is Not DOS

A Commentary on Computer Technology and Nursing Terminology

MARILYN M. TEETER, R.N., M.S.N.
DAVID WELLMAN, M.B.A.

Is it DOS or is it DOS? Is it CD or is it CD? Is it ROM or is it ROM? Is it CONFUSING? Yes, it is. And only a nurse trying to learn to use the computer can understand why.

Today, many in the field of nursing are becoming more aware of the need to become computer literate.

The contemporary trend in hospital care is toward computerization and nursing educators are emphasizing computer use in the classroom. Indeed, the National Council Licensure Examination is now computerized. While we applaud this evolution, it is not

*Reprinted with permission from Computers in Nursing, ©1995; 13(6): 301–302. Edited from the original.

without its problems, many of which are unique to nursing. To nurses, especially those who complain of limited math skills, the computer represents a major obstacle to their practice, and is not seen as a tool to enhance their skills and ease their burdens.

Learning any new and complex skill is challenging, but under certain unique conditions the undertaking of acquiring computer knowledge is even more challenging. It is the view of computer instructors that anyone can acquire computer skills. This view tends to focus only on the mechanics of the training process, while largely ignoring intangibles. Relevant intangibles for some nurses include technophobia and confusing, conflicting terminology. Consequently, many in nursing have found that the claims of computer specialists are a bit optimistic.

The computer field has long been criticized for maintaining a vocabulary that is entirely too technical for meeting the needs of the user interested solely in basic applications. Nonetheless, manufacturers persist in labeling ON and OFF switches with binary notations of 1 or 0 and designating devices for attaching a mouse or printer as COM1 and LPT1. While this alone is difficult for the learner, there is another twist to the problem of mastering the terminology for the nurse. This twist can be labeled *confusion of dual meanings* as evidenced by the fact that DOS is not DOS to nurses. The Appendix contains a brief list of the principal computer terms that vex and confuse the nurse. The list clearly illustrates the disparity between the common use of a term as known by the experienced computer specialist, and the meaning to the nurse.

Dual Meaning

Terms	Computer Meaning	Nursing Application
ADA	Programming language for Department of Defense	American Diabetes Association
AI	Artificial intelligence	Artificial insemination
BPS	Bits per second	Biophysical profile score
CAD	Computer-aided design	Coronary artery disease
CD	Compact disk	Constant drainage
DIF	Data interchange form	A differential blood test to identify types of white blood cells
DOS	Disk operating system	Day of surgery
DRAM	Dynamic random access memory	A unit of liquid measurement
DTP	Desktop publishing	A type of immunization for diphtheria, tetanus, pertussis
Echo	A batch command to display message	Shortened form of echocardiogram
EMS	Expanded memory system	Emergency medical system
FM	Frequency modulation	Fetal monitoring
Input/output		Terms referring to the monitoring of fluids as they are taken in and lost from the body
IV	The last column in a LOTUS spreadsheet	Intravenous
K	Kilobyte—1024 bytes	Potassium
Loop	A set of program instructions	A form of an intrauterine birth control device
M	Megabyte	Meter
MAP	As in memory map	Mean arterial pressure
MD	Command to create a subdirectory	Muscular dystrophy or initials after a physician's name meaning Doctor of Medicine
MS	Microsoft or millisecond	Multiple sclerosis or medical-surgical
Node	Connection point in a local network that handles messages	Small rounded mass
NS	Nanosecond	Normal saline
OEM	Original equipment manufacturer	Optical electron microscope
OS	Operating system	Left eye
PC	Personal computer	After meals
PICA	A unit of measurement equal to 1/16 of an inch	A craving to eat a nonfood substance

Terms	Computer Meaning	Nursing Application
Pitch	A horizontal measurement of no. of characters per linear inch	The quality of a tone
PRN	Default printer	When required
PROM	Programmable read-only memory	Premature rupture of membranes or passive range of motion
RD	Command to delete an empty subdirectory from a disk	Registered dietician
ROM	Read only memory	Range of motion or rupture of membranes
RLL	Run length limited	Right lower lobe
SIG	Special interest group	Write on label
Terminal	Input-output device	Nearing the end

Hospital Hazards*

ROGER P. SMITH, M.D.

Hospitals are not good for your health. As a society, we have become more aware of our environment, and a greater emphasis has been placed on environmental hazards in the workplace. The Occupational Safety and Health Administration (OSHA—the folks who brought us horseshoe-shaped toilet seats) has been preaching safety for many years. Only recently have people viewed OSHA's work as anything other than the federal equivalent of underwear that rides up. However, OSHA's diligence has identified many previously unknown risks to those of us who must labor in the vineyard of disease. Now we find that those hallowed hospital halls are actually dangerous to our health. To assist colleagues who may not have had the benefit of an on-site inspection, the following is a list of syndromes, conditions, and complaints indigenous to hospital staff. Proceed with caution.

Beeperlinthitis—A vertigo-like state induced by rapid back and forth movement of the head made in an attempt to hear and interpret sounds coming from a pocket pager.

Borborygamortis—Hunger pains that occur at 2 AM and threaten to kill you.

Housestaff knees—A pre-patellar bursitis resulting from periodic and forceful genuflection at the feet of attending physicians.

Hallowedtoesis—Attending physician's feet.

Chart cart farts—The expulsion (sometimes explosive) of gastrointestinal gas due to the intense Valsalva maneuver required to move a chart rack with only one functional wheel. Usually result in only minor injuries, but have led to a need for Environmental Protection Agency waivers in some metropolitan centers.

Dysadmenorrhea—Painful administration.

Schizophrenic—A learned ability to use the diaphragm to both inhale and continue presenting a case at the same time. Found most commonly in interns. A leading cause of **inspirational aspiration**, in which your best thoughts are choked off.

Radiolunacy—An acute psychotic state induced by ineffective attempts to obtain copies of imaging studies from the clutches of the radiology clerk.

Chaparoaming—The glazed look in the eye and sense of wanderlust that occur while looking for an attendant to assist with a pelvic examination.

*Reprinted with permission from The American College of Obstetricians and Gynecologists (Obstetrics and Gynecology, © 1992; 80(1):138–139).

Dermatographia pigmentosa (Japonica)—A semipermanent discoloration of the hands induced by using writing devices bearing brand names (usually of antibiotics).

Acute otis-itis media—Traumatic inflammation of the middle or index finger arising from repeated rapid (and ineffectual) pushing of the elevator call button.

Acquired or contagious vertigo—That uneasy feeling engendered by dealing with dizzy members of the health care team.

CTDTs—Intense facial twitching accompanied by palmar cramping occurring when informed that computed tomography is not available and that an actual pelvic examination must be performed.

Glove and shocking paresthesia—The tingling sensation experienced in the hand immediately following the performance of a pelvic examination necessitated by CTDTs.

Primal stream—The primitive, but very real, sense of relief offered by finding a rest room after a very long surgical case.

Delirium tremendous—The semistuporous state seen acutely during 2 AM telephone calls (seen chronically in interns).

Dyspepsia—A panic state and form of caffeine withdrawal seen when the labor-delivery room vending machine is out of your favorite cola product.

Allergic lionitis—The plaintive bellowing sound heard when a sneeze sends hot coffee toward your lap. An excessively large spill may lead to irritation and pain in the gluteal region, known as **hot cross buns**.

Even a trip to the rest room is filled with danger:

Acute roll reversal—The abrasion of the thumb and first finger that results when the previous occupant places a roll of toilet paper backwards on the holder and leaves the end pasted down.

Gender deassignment—An uneasy sense of foreboding and guilt that occurs when using a "unisex" bathroom.

Acute pile-itis—We've all used the paper. Enough said.

Probing Reports*

ROSEMARY COOK, R.G.N.

There is no doubt that the general public is fascinated by all things medical. The media obligingly provide regular doses of medical dramas, medical documentaries and reconstructions of medical emergencies. There are doctors and nurses in all the best books, whether murder mysteries, detective stories or romances; and any human interest story in any newspaper is infinitely more alluring if the headline contains the words 'doc', 'nurse' or 'heart swap'. And now to further pander to this appetite for a taste of the Hippocratic high life, there is a new car from Ford called 'The Probe'.

What the public wants

This is not the work of some over-stressed automotive engineer whose son has just qualified as a doctor at the third attempt. Advertisers are employed to ascertain what the car-buying public actually wants, and they have to come up with names to fit the mood of the moment.

These are people supposedly in tune with the nation. They have a finger on the pulse of our subconscious desires. They spend huge sums of money on their market research, and know the country en masse better than they know their own mothers.

Arguably, they understand people better than the Health Education Authority, which is trying to persuade everyone to wear dark-coloured, long-sleeved tee-shirts in summer to protect them from those dangerous ultraviolet rays. They are probably better informed than the people who introduced the female condom to a disbelieving public.

*Reprinted with permission from Nursing Standard, ©1994; 8(52):43.

If the advertisers suggested The Probe as the right name for a new car, then it is obviously a Probe that the public wants. But who do they want to drive around in something named after a surgical instrument? Are they going to drive home from the dealers, rush into the house and exhort the family to come outside and admire their new Probe? When the chaps at work ask what sort of car they are going to buy this year, are they really going to announce proudly, 'A Probe'? When they ask the doorman at the smart hotel to bring the car around to the door for them, can they look him in the eye and say, 'Mine's the Probe'?

Alright, maybe they can. Maybe it's just that some of us have been a bit too close to the medical profession all these years and tend to associate probes with the places they go and the gooey stuff that tends to come out stuck on the end of them.

So, what will be next in the range? Perhaps they could trade up from their old Probe to a Scalpel even. Or perhaps a Ventilator. Or a Sigmoidoscope. 'I'm just popping into town, darling.' 'Are you taking the Probe?' 'No, I'll take the Siggy.'

Having come up with the name they think the public wants, the advertisers seem to be rather less sure of a storyline to go with it. The posters show only the car and the immortal words 'The Probe'.

So far there has been no sign of a proper television campaign, with characters and scenery and follow-up episodes. No doubt when it comes it will be the story of the tangled love affair of a doctor and a nurse. She will throw away her fur coat and jewellery, but decide to keep the car. He will go skiing with another woman, only to be spotted by her when she drives by in the car.

She will travel to America with a friend and toss the keys to the on-call room over the side of a bridge.

He will finally decide to give up medicine so that he can afford even bigger and better Probes, and will drive away watched enviously from the windows of the hospital by a lot of other doctors in white coats.

TV mini-series

After that, public opinion will demand that it is turned into a TV mini-series, and the characters will make guest appearances on chat shows, denying the existence of any relationship in real life. Meanwhile, TV listings magazines will run competitions to win a weekend stay in the hospital where the adverts were filmed.

Alternatively, they may just sack the advertisers and rename the car.

Medical Malapropisms (or a Stitch in Time Gathers No Moss)*

STEPHEN W. DAVIS, M.D.
TINA M. KENYON, A.C.S.W.

Several members of our Department of Family Medicine have been recording malapropisms and other unusual terminology that we hear in our daily activities. The classic medical examples of these are, of course, "sick-as-hell anemia" for sickle cell anemia, "smiling mighty Jesus" for spinal meningitis, "fireballs in the eucharist" for fibroids in the uterus, and, in our area of Rhode Island, the "Barrington enema." Our collection includes statements made by patients and, surprisingly,

by colleagues, as well as things we think that we may have heard but are not quite sure.

Our collection includes several of the common medical malapropisms, such as the "prostrate exam," "old timers' disease" (Alzheimer's), and "infant milk formula" (Enfamil formula), but we have organized the remainder of the collection into several categories.

The first category is "misuse of common phrases." Members of our department are involved with individ-

*Reprinted from The Journal of Family Practice, ©1995; 40(2):119–120.
Reprinted by permission of Appleton & Lange and the author.

ual and family counseling, and these sessions are ripe with examples. Perhaps the heightened level of anxiety in a counseling session leads to these slightly different expressions. Among the comments we have noted are:

- "He takes things out of content."
- "I took a walk to break up the monopoly."
- "When he said that, I was livered."
- "I have to have the notary republic sign this after-david."
- "I know that I need to buckle under and get going with my life."
- "Yes, but there is a stigmatism attached to that in society."
- "We'll burn that bridge when we get there."
- "I became an escape goat."
- "My husband and I had a falling down last night."
- "I'm not sure because I heard it second wind."
- "I think that I'm going to get an over-the-table job for the summer."
- "He should get right to the point and stop beating the bush around."
- "He drinks once in a great moon."

A variation of this category is the mixing up of terms from the popular culture:

- "I have too many mood swings—I feel just like Heckyl and Jeckyl." (Dr. Jekyll and Mr. Hyde?)
- "My husband had better watch those sexist remarks or he could end up just like those guys in the Tailgate scandal" (Tailhook and Watergate).
- She did not want to talk to us because she wanted to take a "catwink" (catnap and 40 winks).
- "My husband quit smoking cold duck." There are interesting interpretations here: is she referring to his "cold turkey" approach to smoking cessation or is she subconsciously referring to his favorite alcoholic beverage?

The other major category is the misspeaking of medical terminology. These certainly can include multisyllabic medical terms, but they also can include common phrases that get turned around:

- "My son's nose is always constipated."
- "My son was diagnosed with total body pneumonia at the hospital."
- The patient was asked "How are your spirits?" and he answered, "I don't have any spirits."
- "I have decapitating neck pain."

Medical terms, of course, can also lead to malapropisms:

- "I had a pack smear" (Pap).
- "I want the happiness shot" (hepatitis).
- "My headache was cured as soon as they swooped me into that MIA" (MRI).
- "I'm calling for the results of my throat sculpture" (culture).
- The mother said that her daughter had "noxemia, a skin rash" (eczema).
- "My son needs a scripture for hepatitis" (prescription for the hepatitis shot).
- "I had my breast monogram test" (mammogram).
- "The patient needs a stress test but without the threadmill" (treadmill).

Sometimes the phrases are classic, and in some ways they make more sense than the original expression. One of our patients reported that she had had a "Valium stress test." Another reported that her son had "mind-grain headaches."

A medical office form requesting information on a patient's method of birth control was returned with "none needed—partner was nutrilized." Several patients have expressed a concern that their problems are caused by "blood clog." One of our favorites, which certainly makes more sense than the appropriate medical term, was expressed by an overdue pregnant woman who said that she was "ready to be reduced" (rather than induced). The last phrase in this category was uttered by a colleague, which makes one begin to wonder whether there may be too much editorializing occurring in the listeners' minds: one referred to a child as the "splitting image" of his mother.

Medical Malapropisms: The Sequin (Sequel)*

TINA M. KENYON, A.C.S.W.
STEPHEN W. DAVIS, M.D.

- A female patient was having trouble seeing, so she made an appointment to get her *Cadillacs* done. (cataracts)

- While speaking to the triage nurse about a genital rash, the patient said, "I just want you to know that I'm married and we're *monotonous*." (monogamous)

- "My mother's going through *mentalpause*." (menopause)

- "I had a bad tooth that had to be *distracted*." (extracted)

- "Look at that sunset—it has all the colors of the *rectum*." (spectrum)

- A pregnant patient called to say that she was having *erotic contractions* (they were irregular too).

- "Yes, Doctor, I'm taking my *latex* every day." (Lasix)

- "I've been using my *glaucomameter* like you told me." (glucometer)

- "I feel awful—I'm just a *barrel* of nerves today." (bundle)

- An older man, several days after surgery, said he was suffering from *postpartum* blues. (postsurgical)

- "I'm still taking *frolic* acid." (folic)

- "I haven't had a Pap *scare* in a long time." (smear)

The following quips, among others, were sent in from the *Journal's* readers:

- A patient filled a prescription for Lasix. The instructions said to take for "*watery tension*." (water retention)

- "I was vomiting every half hour on the hour."

- "My discharge started last week, but I only noticed it today."

- "The pain was so bad, I got a bottle of Jack Daniels and drank myself into *Bolivia*." (oblivion)

- "We decided not to have an autopsy because he was already dead."

- "What can you do about my *very coarse* veins?" (varicose)

- "My son got kicked in his *tentacles*." (testicles)

- "I have a terrible itch in my *generals*." (genitals)

- "Will I need a *resurrectomy*?" (hysterectomy)

- "I've been to three doctors, but no one has helped me with my *virginitis*." (vaginitis)

- "I get sinus infections because I have a *deviant* septum." (deviated)

- "I have a bone to *beg* with Dr. Jones." (pick).

- "My father died of a cerebral *hemorrhoid*." (hemorrhage)

- "Does this medicine come as a rectal *depository*?" (suppository)

- "I'm having *contraptions* and I need my *epidermal*!" (contractions, epidural)

- A hospital operator announced the beginning of "Morbidity and *Morality* Rounds." (mortality)

- I recently had an interesting experience. The mother of one of my patients got alarmed when I prepped her son's arm and asked the nurse for some 4–0 nylon (heard as Formula 409). She said, "You're not going to clean the wound with that, are you?"

- "My doctor just diagnosed me with *prestigious* anemia." (pernicious)

- Family history revealed that the patient's father, who was a Navy man, died from "*sea roaches* of the liver." (cirrhosis)

- At a hospital in California, a patient was well known to the family medicine service. He was admitted in full arrest, resuscitated successfully, and returned to the floor after a period on a ventilator. After he was transferred out of the ICU, he exclaimed, "I remember clearly that the last time I was here I told everyone, DO NOT *INCUBATE*! Now I wake up to find out that there I was—*INCUBATED*!" (intubated)

Documentation, dictation, and transcription offer their own misinterpretations as well:

- In a discharge summary, "no papilledema" came out "no papal edema." In another, "perennial asthma" came out as "perineal asthma."

*Reprinted from The Journal of Family Practice, ©1995; 41(2):193–194.
Reprinted by permission of Appleton & Lange and the author.

- Here's a quote from a resident's dictation about a man with bilateral AK amputations: "His ankle jerk reflexes were symmetrically absent."
- A medical student's note stated, "The patient claims she got pregnant in Boston, which is impossible."
- The patient is scheduled to have a work-related injury.
- He had heterosexual exposure to a woman.
- It is unclear whether she is having sexual activity at the moment.
- She presents to urgent care with the inability to wait until tomorrow.
- Family history is positive for a mother who is a pessimist.
- A Welch-Allyn sigmoidoscope was transcribed as "well-challenged sigmoidoscope."

How to Speak EMS*

BRAD FARRIS, EMT-P

*What's in a name? That which we call a rose
By any other name would smell as sweet.*

—*William Shakespeare*

When is a Code Blue not a Code Blue? When it's a Code 7, of course. Your EMS team may not use Code Blue or Code 7 often, but in other parts of the country or other parts of the world, they're used every day. The EMS field has its own language, and although much of that language is similar from one place to another, there are some pretty remarkable geographic differences.

We are all familiar with the primary EMS vehicle, but we use a few different terms to refer to it. Probably the most common of these terms is "rig," more than likely borrowed from the over-the-road transport industry, where it is used to refer to a truck, usually an "18-wheeler." In the EMS field, a "rig" may also be a transporting ambulance, a fire engine, a rescue truck or almost any other vehicle.

Near New York City, it is common to hear the term "bus" used to refer to an ambulance. This is probably because at one time, many of the ambulances used in the New York City area were built by Grumman, the manufacturer of most of the city's passenger buses. Interestingly, you may also hear the term "bus" in the San Francisco Bay area, particularly in the East Bay. Near St. Louis, "wagon" is more commonly used. It's hard to say with certainty, but "wagon" is probably derived from "meat wagon," an archaic term that bears a derogatory connotation. In Los Angeles, Fire Department ambulances are referred to as "RAs," short for Rescue Ambulance. In the Midwest, the term "car" is used. A medic will say, "Which car are you working?" This is a holdover from the days when ambulances really were cars—like Cadillacs, Pontiacs and even Buicks. Of course, in many areas ambulances are called "Medic Units" and if the lettering on the back doors is just right when the doors are open, the lettering will just say "dic unit."

The names given to different types of calls may vary geographically as well. In the Pacific Northwest, a call for a person who is believed to be deceased may be dispatched as a "Possible Unattended." Unattended, in this case, refers to a person who expired with no medical personnel "in attendance." In other parts of the country, the more straightforward "Possible Dead Body" or "Possible DB" is more common.

The United Kingdom has developed a whole system of color codes to categorize responses. "Green" means available for work, while "Red" indicates that the unit is engaged on an emergency call, and "White" signifies a nonurgent call. "Blue" indicates that a critical patient is being transported to the hospital, where he or she will be delivered to the "A&E." (No, it's not a cable TV network. In the United Kingdom, A&E is short for "Accident and Emergency," the hospital emergency room.) The color Purple signifies a possibly deceased person,

*Reprinted with permission from JEMS: Journal of Emergency Medical Services, ©1996; 21(11):62–64. Edited from the original.

while "Purple Plus" refers to a person who is definitely deceased. Not surprisingly, the next stop for a "Purple Plus" will likely be the "Purple Annex," or the mortuary. The United Kingdom also gives us a couple of other interesting terms, including "RTA" for Road Transit Accident, and "barrow" or "trolly" for gurney. The distinctive two-tone air horns used in the UK, along with the standard flashing blue lights, have given rise to the term "Blues & Twos" to signify the use of lights and siren.

Color codes are used in some parts of the United States, as well. In western Washington, colors are used, among other things, as response codes. For example, "Code Red" is an emergency response with lights and siren, "Code Yellow" is a response without lights and siren, and "Code Green" is a cancellation. "Code Blue" indicates an urgent request for immediate police department assistance, and "Code Black" is a call for the coroner.

Many areas implement a system of "10 codes" inherited from police department radio codes. These are usually fairly consistent within a given area, but vary widely from place to place. Although "10-8" is nearly always translated as "in service," it doesn't always mean what you might expect. In many places, being "in service" implies that you are in quarters and available for calls. In some places, however, a unit that is "in service" is responding to a call, and in others "in service" indicates that the unit is available by radio.

Even similar codes can mean completely different things in different parts of the country or to different types of services. "Code 1," for example, can refer to a nonemergency interfacility transfer, an emergency call handled with lights and siren, or to a dead body, depending on where you are. "Code Blue" may refer to a cardiopulmonary arrest or to an urgent request for the police department. Another code used to request immediate PD backup, "Code 7," is used in many areas as a code to indicate that the unit is taking a meal break. In the Pacific Northwest, "Code 4" may indicate that CPR is in progress, while in many other areas of the country, the same code is used to inform the dispatcher that no further assistance is required.

Sometimes, jargon is used to refer to particular types of patients. Patients with COPD may be categorized as "pink puffers" or "blue bloaters." Someone who is very sick and getting sicker may be said to be "circling the drain" or CTD. Someone who calls for service often (say, every single day) might be called a "frequent flyer." In some places, a patient with agonal respirations is said to be "doing the guppy."

In the medical world, almost everything has an acronym, and EMTs and paramedics have, for my money, one of the most interesting collections. DRT is used in some areas for "expired" (Dead Right There). The ubiquitous "DFO" often used by patients and EMS types alike refers to a syncopal episode (Done Fell Out). Some other common acronyms are LOL (Little Old Lady), DAH (Dead as Heck) and FDGB (Fall Down Go Boom). One of my personal favorites is NUD (Nigh Unto Death).

EMS jargon is a rich and varied language. Like all languages, it has many geographical dialects and it is constantly changing. If you can speak "EMS" fluently in your area, maybe it's time to branch out and learn the dialect of some other area.

Statistical Software Definitions to Assist the Student in Understanding Available Commands*

SHIRLEY R. RAWLINS, R.N., C.S., D.S.N.

Diskette—a female disc.

A Drive—the operating mode of a compulsive software student.

B Drive—the operating mode of the "laid-back" software student.

C Prompt (alias Cognitive Prompt)—a command given to the student by the computer to indicate a need for thinking.

SPSS—a four-letter word the student may choose to type into the computer which is followed by the computer's retaliation by giving the student a C PROMPT; a derivative of this command is SPSSX which is a *really* bad word.

Hypothesis—a vague idea the student may have about something that might occur; for example,

H_o: number of attempts at running a program = number of successes in running a program.

H_a: number of attempts $\neq$ number of successes (Note: repeated tests of this hypothesis have indicated a tendency to reject the H_o).

Review—an option for the student who wants to count his/her mistakes; can be used to support the H_a given above.

Help—an option for the student who is desperate and considering jumping from the learning resource center balcony.

Home—a place seldom seen by a software student (except possibly after 7 P.M. when the learning resource center is closed).

Reverse Scoring—a method of entering data such that it is printed out backwards (Note: this is not a difficult procedure; the computer knows to do this automatically for a beginning software student).

Plot—a scheme derived by a coalition of computers to thwart students.

Variables—things that vary; in fact, they vary so much that they look different each time the student calls up his/her program.

Frequencies—A term indicating how many hours per week a software student finds himself/herself sitting in front of a computer screen (Note: Expected Frequencies is how often the instructor *expects* the student to practice on the computer; Frequencies is not equal to Expected Frequencies).

Barchart—a printout with lines, not unlike the floor design of the local after-hours hangout.

Crosstabs—an angry option; if selected by a student, this mode will put data into cells and square the student's Chi's.

***t*-Test** (alias Tolerance Test)—an option that may be chosen by a student with a lot of patience; the student must choose between being paired or grouped, and this choice may vary depending on the time of day.

Descriptives—a command that provides character references for the student who is not sure if he/she is in error, mean, deviant, variant, or just plain skewed.

Mean—a value label sometimes assigned to the instructor who assigns software homework (and then grades it!).

Standard Deviation—the expected mental deviation of

*Reprinted with permission from Computers in Nursing, ©1992; 10(5): 189–190. Edited from the original.

the software student from the norm as compared with the total university population.

Oneway—an option that means what it says; the computer quits if you do not enter commands correctly.

p **Value** (alias Possibility Value)—term on a computer printout; this symbol indicates there *possibly may* or there *possibly may not* be something significant in the numbers; the student's task is to then consult a classmate about what it all means. . . .

Regression—the level of operation for the typical software student; may be characterized by thumbsucking and/or assumption of a fetal position underneath the IBM PC's.

Transformation—the process a software student undergoes as his/her hair turns white and permanent brow wrinkles appear.

Software—a value label assigned by students to the patient, positive, supportive instructors who teach computer use to the student who is computer illiterate!

Finding the Right Word*

PHILIP BURNARD, PHD, MSC, R.G.N., R.M.N.

Nursing has got more complicated. This is due, partly, to the language involved. As nurse education has moved into the higher education sector, it has developed a suitably difficult language to go with it. Now it is time for a simple guide.

The following definitions are offered as an aid to anyone trying to get to grips with today's jargon.

You may find that things are not as complicated as you first thought . . .

Reflection: Doing something and thinking about it after.
Research: Asking questions, going out looking for answers, not finding them and suggesting that more needs to be done.
Experiential learning: Doing something, thinking about it, changing your mind and doing something else.
Assertiveness: Being appropriately rude to people.
Caring: Being nice to people, while maintaining eye contact.
Counselling: Having a chat—particularly after something awful has happened.
Counsellor: One who hangs about after something awful has happened.
Psychotherapy: More complicated chatting.
Group dynamics: Things that go on in groups—usually of an intriguing nature.

Student-centred learning: Doing most of the work yourself, scowling as you do it.
Adult learning: Doing all of the work yourself, smiling, weakly, as you do it.
Audit: Finding out what it's about and counting it.
Total Quality Management: Getting it right first time and being very smug about it.
Mission Statement: An outrageous porky about your aims as an organisation.
Self-assessment: Deciding on how you're doing, then lying through your teeth.
Quality assurance: Keeping up with the times. Staying glossy.
Mentoring: Keeping an eye on someone, whether you or they like it or not.
Supervision: Being kept an eye on, whether you like it or not.
The process of nursing: Coming on, doing things, caring madly, going off.

There are more, of course, but this list is just a start.

Few things are really that difficult. It's just that some people prefer us to think they are. Sometimes, of course, things really are more difficult than they appear. But that need not worry us here. We have enough to worry about already.

Happy nursing.

*Reprinted with permission from Nursing Standard, © 1995; 9(49):46.

THE DIFFERENCE BETWEEN YOU AND ME

Humor is often used as a strategy to maintain close working relationships between doctors and nurses. Used appropriately, humor reduces tensions that are an inevitable part of working with very sick patients and their families.

Historically, physicians have been viewed as the only experts in health matters and therefore more knowledgeable and competent than nurses. The give and take of laughter helps equalize the standing between status levels. A liberal dose of humor will break down formidable barriers, promote healthy interpersonal relationships among colleagues, and contribute greatly to serenity.

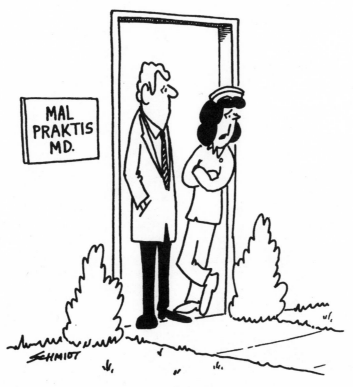

I don't think things will get better until you change your name . . .

What is a Doctor?*

PAT COTTER

From within the blue and green surgical garb, dark suit and tie, or various wild assortments of sport clothing, emerges a delightful creature called a doctor. Doctors come in assorted sizes, weights, shapes, and forms; but all doctors have the same creed; to admit patients, perform surgery, write stat orders, change dressings, and question nurses (all this during report, at precisely 3:00 P.M., just before class, or at mealtime) and to protest with noise, an efficient weapon, when they find an order not carried out that very minute, that very hour, or sometimes even that very day.

Doctors are found everywhere; joking in surgery, singing in the halls, having coffee in the doctor's lounge, writing at the nurses' station, gabbing in the patients' room, relaxing on the golf course but never, ever in the office when a patient is in pain, vomiting, coming in or trying to go out.

Doctors are fascinating: patients idolize them, wives learn to live without them, RN's ignore them, aides avoid them, students help them, and insurance protects them.

A doctor is Truth when discovering neglected orders, Wisdom with an "I might have known it" look, and Beauty with a compliment. A doctor displays sympathy in a medication error, kindness in teaching, and Hope for the future when a pre-clinical contaminates his entire sterile field.

When you are the busiest, a doctor is underfoot, gone with a chart, dictating, writing more and more orders, or calling for lab reports. When you have the time to make a good impression, you stammer, report on the wrong patient, throw away a specimen, or go with him to find a distended abdomen, a clogged Foley, an untidy room, or an ambulating cardiac.

A doctor is a composite: he has the power of a narcotic, the energy of a stimulant, the resistance of an antibiotic, the intestinal fortitude of an antiemetic, and the strength of all the pharmaceuticals combined. He is a minim of anger, a cc. of impatience, a dram of temper, and a whole ounce of understanding.

A doctor likes a conscientious nurse, a patient wife, a mind-reader, half-days at the office, one night of uninterrupted sleep, sharp scissors, dry dressings, a helping hand, a happy patient, and a charted morning temperature. He is not much for an inaccurate intake and output, midnight deliveries, shortened vacations, strict routine, paper work, history and physicals, hospital rounds, and Medicare.

Nobody else is so early to rise, or so late to the golf course. Nobody else can arrange to visit 26 hospital patients, remove four gall bladders, keep regular office hours, and handle emergencies at any hour of any day and still have time to follow every athletic event, deer hunt, and entertain, socialize, relax, and sleep. Nobody else could fill one pocket with a pen from the nurses' desk, a hemostat from the dressing tray, and the scissors from a student nurse so expertly that the object isn't missed for two full hours afterwards. Nobody else could go to school for a total of 20 years and still not learn to write.

Yes, a doctor is a magical creature. To a young girl in a starched blue uniform with a crisp white apron, black shoes, an innocent face, and an eager manner, a doctor is a Knight in Shining Armour, a Prince Charming, and a *real* Kildare. A doctor is her teacher, counselor, director and friend. She looks to him to answer innumerable questions, explain procedures, draw pictures, and share every bit of his knowledge in the brevity of one hurried minute.

The student watches this Prince Charming with respect, and from him she learns what no textbook can teach, for she gains experience, confidence, and trust. The doctor teaches her not only to work capably with a physical condition, but also to work with PEOPLE, to make people wholly well, in mind, spirit, and body.

Yes, the doctor is the eternal friend of the student nurse. We work with you, gripe about you, try to help you, but, most of all, appreciate you for your understanding, teaching, and guidance.

*Reprinted with permission, AORN Journal, (3 Jul/Aug 1965), pp 127, 130. Copyright ©AORN, Inc., 2170 S. Parker Road, Suite 300, Denver, CO 80231.

To Russia, With Love*

ROBIN WALTER, R.N., B.S.N.

Travel abroad with this nurse and her fellow clowns as they touch the hearts of strangers using the international language—laughter.

There are some things in life you do because you *ought to,* others because you *want to,* and then there are those things you do because *the deposit is nonrefundable.*

It was for this last reason—because I couldn't get out of it—that I wound up traveling to Russia as part of a humor-and-healing tour group only weeks after the country's fiery brush with civil war. Add to that a few news reports of diphtheria and cholera outbreaks in Russia, and you've got all the reasons you need to cancel getting up in the morning, let alone taking a trip abroad.

A yearly event organized by a family practitioner in rural West Virginia since 1985, the tour is open to anyone interested in experiencing the therapeutic power of humor. Participants are of all ages and from all walks of life. Our group, the largest so far, had 30 members and included two nurses, four physicians, and one radiology technician.

The travel agent assured me that everything was "under control." Had she forgotten that our group would be entering the country dressed as clowns? I felt like I was consenting to self-colonoscopy or a home biopsy—the kind of thing where you can never be sure of the outcome.

Preparing for the trip was tough. Oh, deciding what to pack was easy—clown shoes, a rubber chicken, "real" toilet paper. It was the phone calls from family and friends that made me nuts. Their questions—more like statements of fact, really—ranged from "Do you know what's happening over there?" to "Don't you hear what the press is saying?" to "Are you crazy?!"

My husband, hoping to avert long-term single parenthood, simply asked, "Can't you go as something a little more low-profile than a clown?" That's like asking if spouses can take call! Of *course* I was going as a clown. After all, it was the recommendation of our tour leader, an exemplary MD of the sort we all dream about (he has an anaphylactic reaction to profit and thinks there's a place for homeopathy in the ICU). Ever the optimist, he assured us while we were somewhere over Greenland that clowning and clearing Russian customs weren't mutually exclusive, and then drifted off to sleep, his mind seemingly at ease. I was skeptical, but 11 years of nursing have taught me to let sleeping docs lie.

From flying halfway around the world with a bunch of clowns, I learned at least two things: that the sound of a deflating whoopie cushion on a crowded international flight will cause the oxygen masks to automatically drop from their overhead compartments; and that the true test of maturity is how a person reacts to seeing a clown board the baggage carousel at the Moscow airport and be "claimed" as luggage by other clowns.

Our guides were charming Russian women who spoke perfect English—as long as it wasn't into the tour bus microphone. Then all you could understand were just two words—a number and "century." By the end of the trip, I had it pretty well figured out: The food was late 17th-century (unprocessed and unrecognizable—except for cabbage); the water was definitely 20th-century (bottled, with or without gas); and the bathrooms were any century B.C.

But we'd come to Russia to clown, not to complain, and clown we did—in Red Square, in front of the Kremlin, in and around the museums of St. Petersburg. Our antics were always met with enthusiasm, participation, and joy.

But nowhere was the experience more rewarding than in the children's hospitals we visited. We went to burn units, cancer centers, orthopedic hospitals, nephrology and urology wards, and children's psychiatric facilities. Nowhere was a patient's door closed to us, no area declared off-limits.

I tried not to notice the lack of equipment, the needles soaking in a pan of bleach, the stained gauze

*Reprinted with permission from American Journal of Nursing, ©1994; 94(6):44–45.

hanging to dry in the lab. Instead, I focused on the smile of a bedridden 10-year-old burn patient as he watched his mother laughing, with her face painted as a clown. I learned later that, with pain medications in such short supply, the two had shared mostly tears in the weeks since his accident.

I blew soap and bubble gum bubbles with my Russian colleagues, performed "feets" of magic with orthopedic patients, and pulled chocolate coins from the ears of the unsuspecting. I never wanted it to stop. But stop it did, abruptly and without warning, in a surgical hospital in Moscow.

Eleven clowns, an interpreter, and a Russian surgeon jammed into the 4´ × 6´ elevator. Jokingly, I remarked, "Do you think Soviet elevators have a weight limit?" Everyone laughed, and, as if on cue, the elevator jerked to a stop somewhere between the second and third floors.

The surgeon confidently moved toward the control panel and pressed the third-floor button. Nothing happened. He pressed the second-floor button. Again, nothing. He began to bang the control panel anxiously with his fists. The clowns instinctively huddled in the back of the elevator.

The surgeon stood motionless—his green scrubs draped and drawstringed, his mask dangling at his throat—staring at the sealed elevator doors as if they were scar tissue. Then he started yelling. Our interpreter refused to translate most of his brainstorming sessions with the second- and third-floor staff. But she did let us in on a few of the suggestions echoing up and down the elevator shaft:

"Would you like us to try greasing the line?"

"Try getting everyone together and ramming the door."

"Should we send for the Special Forces?"

After about a half hour, everyone was getting edgy. Three of us needed to go to the bathroom. Our surgeon, now bathed in sweat, reached for a cigarette. At this, the clowns went wild, lunging at him with hands waving in disapproval. Reluctantly, he stuffed his cigarette back in its pack.

Within the next few, anxious moments, we knew the Special Forces had arrived: The lights went out. So did one of the clowns. Some meditated, others prayed, and one clown, clutching his penknife, announced, "That's it! Five more minutes and I'm going through the roof!"

There was a heavy sigh from the corner of the elevator. A small voice mused, "And my mother was worried I'd be cold. . . ." Giggles gave rise to laughter, and the elevator again took its cue. The lights came back on and we ascended to the third floor.

From the barricaded, heavily guarded streets of Red Square to the open hospital wards, I discovered the universal power of humor. Soldiers in full military regalia danced with us, old women clapped their hands, children sang, people in pain smiled. Perhaps it didn't make the earth move, but it certainly had an impact on elevators.

With fond memories to guide me, I've decided to write a self-help book about my experiences in Russia. I'll title it *A Cross-Cultural Guide to Caring and Civil Disobedience.* You should be able to order it through any local bookstore, but the deposit will be nonrefundable. *Dasvidanya!* ('Bye!)

THE DIFFERENCE BETWEEN YOU AND ME

The Itch You Can't Scratch*

ROSEMARY COOK, R.G.N.

If anybody else asks me how my headlice clinic is going, I shall hand in my notice. I can cope with the receptionists leaning the other way, like corn in a breeze, when I approach the desk. Their diplomas did not prepare them for the possibility of a lot of human parasites using me as a stepping stone to their immaculate heads. As for the district nurse's cartoon of a line of nits queuing up outside my room, it was actually quite funny for the first day or two. I did move it though from the notice-board to the kitchen, so as to avoid giving the patients the impression that we are taking the current crisis lightly.

It's the doctors I can't cope with. In a surgery not usually renowned for its use of protocols and procedures, they have issued an edict—in writing, no less—to the effect that they don't want their surgeries clogged up by families with itchy heads, demanding individual examination. Since families with itchy heads persist in turning up at the surgery asking to be examined, they are all being diverted to me.

The doctors think that this is all very funny. They have christened my morning surgery 'The headlice clinic' and are prone to ring up in the middle of it to ask if I can fit in a blood test for one of their patients 'in between nits'. They find the subject of headlice hilarious. This is because they do not have children yet, and so have no sobering experience to draw on. Or it is because they had their children long ago, when having headlice was worse than having a criminal record and the memories are so traumatic that they have repressed them.

Our patients don't find it amusing. They usually arrive in states of deep shame and shock, insisting that their child has never had them before and that he or she must have caught them from the horrid little monster they sit next to at school. I console them with interesting snippets, such as the fact that headlice prefer clean hair. By the way, how do we know this—has anybody asked them? I also tell them that my children have had headlice too. Usually, my attempts at reassurance are so successful that their confidence is quite restored. They then turn on medical science and denounce the profession for not having found a way of preventing something so simple. Some of them get really demanding and want to know why there is such a problem with headlice this year. Here I am floundering. Is it the weather? Is it related to the fact that there have been a lot of ladybirds about this year? Could it be anything to do with the plague of wasps? Goodness knows.

The gnarled old countrymen who are wheeled out on nature programmes to predict the weather by counting the stripes on caterpillars, or other such methods, never say anything about headlice. I've never known one to break open a cowpat, sniff the inside and say: 'Ay, there'll be plenty of itchin' this Autumn.'

I have developed a method of dealing with this deficiency. It does not seem sensible to rely too much on the disarming effect of the truth by explaining to patients that we—that is, me and medical science—don't know the answer to their question. On the other hand, I am wary of over-using trite phrases about 'research' and 'clinical trials.'

There are some areas of research that I feel I should know about, such as wound care or the effects of the pill. But to imply I am completely au fait with the latest thinking on the life cycle of minor human parasites would be going a bit too far. I just smile knowingly, in a way that implies extensive knowledge about, and an interest in the subject. But I also smile wearily, suggesting that I have many more patients to see, which prevents me from sharing my expertise in any great detail. It is a subtle combination, which I practice for hours in front of a mirror.

So we are dealing with our headlice epidemic. I am doing the work and the doctors are signing the prescriptions. The practice manager has riffled through the Red Book to see if there is anything we can claim. I have explained that headlice don't figure in the banding system alongside coronary heart disease, but her grasp of anatomy and physiology is tenuous at best and she is still hopeful. I am just waiting for one of our afflicted families to make a complaint about the length of the queues for the headlice clinic. Then I shall send them in to see her. Since she hasn't quite got 'infested' and 'infectious' sorted out in her mind, she will probably conduct the entire interview from behind the filing cabinet. It is time I had some fun out of this crisis.

*Reprinted with permission from Practice Nurse, ©1995; 10(5):358.

THE DIFFERENCE BETWEEN YOU AND ME

The Bare Bones
of Teaching*

MARCUS GUNN

There is lots of encouragement these days for GPs to get out of the surgery and take their health messages into their community. And we are always being reminded that the term 'doctor' comes from the Greek for 'teacher'. So, like most GPs, I am happy to do a little community education: the occasional chat at the Senior Citizens' Club about healthy exercise, an interview in the local throwaway about melanoma protection, even a rare broadcast on community radio. And having a medical student in the practice is one of my great delights.

But nothing had prepared me for today's educational outing: taking my skeleton along to my son's primary school.

Getting there was bad enough. A fully articulated skeleton is almost impossible to fold up and stuff in the boot so there was nothing for it but to sit it up in the passenger seat, belted in and leering sightlessly out the windscreen. I think I was caught by every red light on the way to the school and thus developed a nice line in nonchalant shrugs each time another car pulled up alongside. One worthy chap took a look and exclaimed, 'Hey, mate! You've got a skeleton there!' I thanked him with a universal gesture.

I'm proud of my skeleton. It has lurked in my surgery cupboard for years, frightening new receptionists and making itself useful for patient education. It is, in fact, a great improvement on the box of bones I bought in my first year at medical school. The vendor was a hugely wise and rather shifty third year student who proudly showed me all the pieces, most of which turned out to be broken. The clavicle was in one piece, however, and he slyly rolled it between his fingers saying, 'This is the os penis. It slides out to make your old fella go hard.'

I didn't believe him. Really. Not for long.

Getting into the primary school was not too difficult. The gardener leant on his rake as I staggered past with my bony cargo but wisely he kept his thoughts to himself. The prep classroom hubbub subsided into awed astonishment as we entered through the back door.

The teacher, who is perceived by 5 year old Tom as being immeasurably old but is really about 16, clapped her hands brightly and gathered the class around her. 'Now, children, Tom Gunn's dad is here to tell us all about what is inside each and every one of us'.

'Good afternoon, children.' I began portentously, clutching my skeleton. 'Who can tell me what is inside every one of us?'

A curly-haired cherub stabbed her hand into the air. 'Poo!' she said brightly. She had already decided that I had more inside me than anybody else in the room. This assumption put her in the same mind as many medical students I have taught.

It took a good five minutes for the class to recover from this daring display of Wildean wit, despite the teacher frowning severely and me laying about myself with the skeleton's femur. When the children finally dragged themselves up off the floor, they watched me with eager eyes in case I served up another lob to their class clown.

Things improved from there, with twenty shining faces watching as I named the major bones (including a careful explanation of the clavicle and its role in, and only within, the shoulder girdle) and moved on to talking about what happens when something breaks.

'What do we call a doctor who spends most of the time fixing broken bones?' I asked. A little boy put his hand up. 'Daddy', he replied, proudly. Oh, great, I was showing the local orthopaedic surgeon's kid a skeleton. He probably cut his teeth on one.

The skeleton was rapidly losing its novelty value, not to mention several important parts as the children grew bolder, so I turned my attention to the teaching aids supplied by the teacher. In pride of place was one of those life size anatomical models with organs you can lift out. The children had learnt earlier about the brain, heart, lungs and stomach so I decided to point each of these out. The anterior rib cage lifted off easily enough, allowing the organs within to slide into a multicoloured pile on the floor. It's amazing how similar kidneys, spleens and stomachs all look when they are piled up on the carpet. The teacher watched sus-

*Reprinted with permission from Australian Family Physician, ©1996; 25(7):1174–1175.

THE DIFFERENCE BETWEEN YOU AND ME

piciously as I struggled to cram them all back in the body cavity. She didn't seemed pleased by my assurance that there were usually a few bits left over in real life, too. Tom came to help and had everything squared away within seconds. It looks like those Transformers toys were a good investment after all.

Having completely confused the children, my work was done. They clapped enthusiastically, Tom glowed with pride (bless him!) and I hoisted the skeleton over my shoulder ready to depart. We stepped out into the playground just as the bell rang, only to be swamped by torrents of children pouring out of every door, screaming with delight at the sight of a strange man with an awesome skeleton in the playground. I staggered out to the car under my ghastly burden, followed by a chanting crowd of urchins. The scene was like something out of a Frankenstein movie, with Igor being tormented by the townsfolk.

As I drove back to the safety of my surgery (with my coat over the skeleton's head), I pondered how it could be so much more difficult to educate a group of small children than to consult with adult patients one at a time. Maybe the difference is, although your patients might think you are full of it, they don't say so.

While I Got You on the Line*

KIM SHAFTNER, M.D.

"Hudson's Hardware. Can I help you?"

"Hello, may I speak with Lee?"

"Doc, is that you? This is Milt! I sure am glad you're back from vacation."

"Oh, hello, Milt. Actually, I'm still *on* vacation. Is Lee in?"

"Well, you won't believe this, Doc, but the very day you left, I had to go to the hospital. I've been on a leave of abscess for the past few days, and now I'm sitting here recapitulating at the store.

"Lemme tell you all about it while I got you on the line. I was just sittin' in my old easy chair watchin' Oper Winfree, when I got this awful pain in my belly—it went clean up into my goozle. I got up and took some Tylons and then some Pepso Bizmaul and didn't get nary a bit better. Then I went to bleedin' from my intestinals and dang if I wasn't feelin' pretty rotten.

"Well, Hester got herself all riled up and called the rescue squab. They up and hauled me off to the hospital and come to find out you was on vacation. That Dr. Meehan came and saw me and decided he had to keep me. He didn't know if I had a gaspin' ulcer or a high anal hernia, or if my pinnix was actin' up. He got this right serious look on his face and started talkin' abut floratory surgery.

"Well, to make a story short, they found out that I just had some gastroindoritis. They put that snake up my backside and found a rectal fisher and some chronic pollens but not much else."

"Milt, it's good to hear that you're better. Is Lee around?"

"You know, after I woke up from that cornoscopy stuff, I started weaseling in my chest. They thought it might be barnacle asthma or maybe emphysemo on account of my smokin' and all. Dr. Meehan came in and got that real serious look again and said something about a preliminary embolism and blood clocks. They did a lung scam and a cardogram, and one of them muggin' tests. Heck, they even put me on that Fredmill! I think they was looking for some heart filibrations, but they finally found out that I had brownchitis.

"So Doc Meehan has me on a gland diet and some Argumentin, and I'm doing a little better. I kinda like Dr. Meehan in spite of that serious look and all. I mentioned I might like him to be my doctor. He said that you was just as fine a doctor as I needed and figured I oughta stay with you for the time being."

"Milt, is Lee working today? I have a problem with my mower and I really need to speak with him."

"Doc, he quit last week. Nice talkin' to you though."

*Reprinted from The Journal of Family Practice, ©1997; 44(1):103. Reprinted by permission of Appleton & Lange and the author.

How to Drive Doctors Crazy and Ease Them Into Malpractice Suits*†

JANICE L. DENNIS, R.N.‡

Some of our nursing colleagues seem to think they can best serve humanity by making life miserable for those who "get wealthy on other people's ills," better known as good ol' Docs. A course is offered in basic techniques, called SD, or Subterfuge Doctors. This includes on-the-job training in the hospital, where the experience of day-to-day confrontation presents new challenges in subterfuge. For those nurses who have not taken the course, here are a few of the essentials.

When laboratory results are reported to you, give them only to the attending physician. Then, when the consultant calls, you can say, "I already told the attending, after all he is the patient's Doc." Or, alternatively, call only the consultant with the laboratory data so Doc will not know what is going on with his patient.

When faced with illegible physician handwriting, ask another physician to interpret the order and then, after giving the wrong dose or medication, say, "Doc So-and-so interpreted the order and I followed what he said it should be. (In choosing a physician to read the illegible writing, be sure to choose the one who causes the most static among the staff.) The other alternative is to say to the family, "I really would like to give Grandpa something for the pain, but Doc didn't write the order so I can decipher it, and he is on the 19th hole at the country club and has left orders not to call him."

When Doc writes "g," use either the metric or apothecary system, whichever will be the incorrect dosage (grams if it should be grains and grains if it should be grams). When the prosecuting attorney asks why you gave the wrong dose, you can say you were just following Doc's orders.

If a patient makes a turn for the worse at 5:30 AM, be sure to call the attending and all the consultants. At that hour it is difficult for them to get back to sleep. Also, during the night shift, be sure and shine your flashlight into the patients' eyes on 2 AM rounds. This will ensure that the patient will ask for another sleep-ing pill and you will have to call for an order for a second sleeper, further assuring Doc's good sleep.

When a surgical develops a staph infection, be sure to put the new surgical in the same room. This will guarantee a continuous postop infection that will keep the infection control committee busy. It will also assure a longer, more expensive hospital stay.

Put patients who need to be restrained in the rooms farthest from the nursing station. You can be sure of a negligence suit when they fall out of bed. Also, always place call lights where patients cannot reach them. (An efficient nursing station does not have many call lights to answer.)

If there is more than one physician caring for a patient, go ahead and follow all orders without asking questions. This way you can tell the family, "Grandma is not getting better because the left hand does not know what the right hand is doing," usually enough ammunition so that someone in the family will go to a lawyer.

When a patient turns critical and needs life-support machines, tell the family you would like to help but that you need Doc's orders and his answering service is busy. Never mind that minutes are crucial for the patient.

As Doc is leaving the floor, call after him, "By the way, Mrs So-and-so's blood sugar is 512 gm and she didn't look too good when I saw her an hour or so ago."

When a patient tells you she is going home on Tuesday, look concerned and tell her, "Dr Doe's patient had the same thing and she went home two days ago." This will start the patient pondering what is wrong with the medical care she is receiving.

When prepping a patient, shave the entire body. This will protect you if the surgeon has ordered the wrong prep. It will also make the patient itch while the skin rejuvenates and the hair grows back. The patient is then likely to remember only how intense the itch-

*Reprinted with permission from Postgraduate Medicine, ©1983; 73 (6):303–304. Edited from the original.
†Editor's note: This article was written in response to "How to Drive Nurses Crazy and Ease Them Out of Nursing" by Harvey N. Mandell, M.D., Postgraduate Medicine, 1983; 73(3):26–27, 30.
‡ADW, And Doctor's Wife.

THE DIFFERENCE BETWEEN YOU AND ME

ing was and not how well the operation went and to not recommend the doctor.

Always call Doc's office when he starts office hours and again just before he leaves. Also, always leave messages at all hospital switchboards for him to call back. This will keep you covered in case you do need him when he returns your call, and your time will not be wasted looking for him.

Always add cascara to the coffee you make on the unit. When Doc helps himself and does not pay, you can say he had it coming.

Obtain the wrong dressing tray from central supply. This will ensure that the surgeon will have to stand and wait in the patient's room with the operative site exposed.

Before Doc makes rounds, be sure all the patients he will want flat are rolled up in bed and all the ones he will want up are flat. Do not make rounds with him to properly position the beds. He needs to do this exercise because it will increase the strength in the arm he uses for his tennis serve.

Be sure that surgical instruments are dull and blunted. This will make surgery more exciting. When the blaming starts, reach in your pocket and turn on your tape recorder.

When the Doc who always steals your lunch will be on duty, be sure to prepare your sandwich with mayonnaise and let it stand out of the refrigerator, preferably in the sunshine.

Finally, if the family tells you what good care Doc took of Grandpa, raise your eyebrows and say, "Wait until you get his bill!"

Dear Mark . . .*

MARK RADCLIFFE, R.M.N.

This week I have raided the postbag and, in an effort to be useful for once, I am going to try to answer some of your problems.

Q: You know those little tube-like things with white ear nipples at one end and a baby drum at the other? What are they then? All my mates have got one. Can I have one? Signed Doctor Descriptive.
A: Dear Doctor. That'll be a stethoscope! Yes, you can have one but please remember that they are important listening tools and should not be used for flicking colleagues.

Q: I have been seeing this man for six months. I am a nurse and he is . . . well it doesn't matter what he is, suffice it to say he is not a doctor. Anyway, he wants us to start kissing with tongues.

I am not sure if I am ready for that kind of commitment. Apart from anything else this tongue business strikes me as terribly unhygienic. I certainly do not want anyone without a medical degree licking the inside of my mouth.

However, he is a very nice man and there aren't any cute doctors around the hospital at the moment. What should I do? Signed Stella Steristrip.
A: Dear Stella, I am surprised some of your more worldly colleagues have not offered you advice on this matter. A lot of people kiss, often quite randomly. Ask your friends at work to supply you with some aluminum foil. Next time you go on a date with this nondoctor, line your mouth with it before you leave the house. It may make speaking and eating a tad difficult, but it will enable you to kiss with confidence.

Q: My girlfriend does not speak to me. I have not seen her for four months and the last I heard she had moved house and become engaged to some bloke from Stevenage.

The last date we had went rather well, I thought: she was outside the chip shop with her friends and I went past on the bus.

Do you think I should write her a letter telling her the relationship is over or should I carry on in the hope that things can be the way they were before? Signed Roger the radiographer.
A: Dear Roger. She isn't really your girlfriend is she?

*Reprinted from Nursing Times, ©1996; 92(48):145 with permission from Macmillan Magazines. Edited from the original.

This is one of those made-up relationships normally confined to the royal family. I suggest you forget her and try to get out a bit more.

Q: I am just about to leave school with four GCSEs and a really bad haircut. I would like to work for the health service because I am keen on the idea of working somewhere that has its own canteen. I do not want to do anything too important because I am rubbish at things that are important. Any suggestions? Signed Toby Lightweight.

A: Dear Toby, it definitely has to be a career in hospital management for you. Four GCSEs ought to get you on to an MBA course and, if your haircut is bad enough and you can demonstrate that you are unprincipled and mediocre, the chances are that one of the health authorities will pay for you to do it. Who knows, if you play your cards destructively enough you could be a chief executive before you hit 40.

Q: My boyfriend has become surly and inattentive. He was nice as pie when we first started going out together, but now it is like going out with Darnel Dull, King of the dull people from Dull Mountain. What's more, he is not much cop between the sheets. Signed Lucinda the occupational therapist.

A: Chuck him. You don't spend the day arranging bath aid equipment into alphabetical order and putting the tops back on the felt-tip pens just so you can go home to a man like Darnel.

Mega Hertz*

JOHN M. GARVIN, M.D.

Some days are cursed from the beginning.

As I swing open the ED door, I hear, "I'm dyin' by degrees in here." It's sort of an articulated cackle—a screechy, ominous soprano. Then it comes again: *"I'm dyin' by degrees in here."*

I arch an eyebrow at Sue, one of our nurses.

"She's been screaming that about every 5 minutes for the last 2 hours," she responds with a resigned sigh. "Little old senile lady. Due to be admitted for a foot ulcer, but no bed ready. She'll be down here for about 2 more hours."

God is testing me.

"First patient, Doc," Sue says, handing me a chart. A 7-year-old with a busted lip.

"I'm dyin' by degrees in here."

I wash my hands, walk into the room, introduce myself and reach for the child's face—and the mother slaps my hands down.

Somewhat taken aback, I stare at her in disbelief.

"Did you wash your hands?" she asks me.

"Why? Is it suppertime, Mommy?" the child asks.

"I'm very particular!" the woman explains with a belligerent severity. I don't know about particular, lady, but you've got peculiar locked up tight!

I knew we'd lost the moment, so I had one of my partners see the little girl, with the suggestion that he autoclave his hands in front of the mother. Things were definitely not going my way.

"Second patient, Doc." Sue again.

"I'm dyin' by degrees in here."

"I certainly did well with that little girl and her mother, didn't I?" I ask Sue.

"I'd say," she replies. Sue would lie about anything.

The flow sheet on the chart advises me that one Elmer Hertz has fallen and injured his wrist while visiting in Roanoke.

"Hertz," I tell myself, as I set down the chart and proceed toward him. "Like the car-rental place. Got to remember. Hertz." I have such a hard time with names.

"How are you?" I begin.

"I ain't," he summarizes briefly.

"Warning! Warning!" yells a robotic voice inside my head. "Lethal wit ahead."

*Reprinted from Emergency Medical Services, ©1995; 24(8):70–71 with permission from Summer Communications, Inc. and the author.

"How did you hurt your wrist, Mr. Mertz?"

"Hertz."

"I'm sure it does, sir."

"No . . . my name . . . Hertz."

"Your name hurts?" *Sigh*. This is going to be a difficult case.

"No. That's my name."

I try to make people feel better about themselves; I see it as part of my job. Even when in a bad mood, I try to treat the whole patient.

"No need for self-consciousness, sir. I'm certain that Mertz is a proud name—one with a history of pageantry and high ideals."

"Well, might be. Say, Doc, do you have any trouble with your memory?"

"Not that I remember."

"Kin you check me out for a cold while I'm here? It's in m'bronchials. Been sick about a month. Hate to go to that hospital over home."

"Why?"

"Too little. You can throw a Frisbee over it. No doctor there mos' days."

"You coughing up anything with this cold?"

"Just ol' nuchous."

"Nuchous."

"Yeah. Ol' strangy yella nuchous."

The dreaded ol' strangy yella nuchous! A chill seized me—that and the fear that wells inside each therapist so confronted: Am I man enough to handle a patient laid low by ol' strangy yella nuchous?

"It's cold in this here room, Doc."

"It *is* cold in here." I lean out the door and yell, "Hey! You'all turn on some heat. Me 'n' Mr. Mertz are gettin' pulseless extremities in here!"

"Hertz, Doc."

"I know it does," I soothe. "I'll get you something for the pain in a minute, Mr. Mertz."

"I'm dying by degrees!"

"So, how did you hurt your wrist?" I ask.

It was then that I learned, to my dismay, that Mr. Hertz—or Mertz; I now just thought of him as Nuchous—was one of those patients at his most painstakingly precise when the forthcoming information is least relevant to the purpose of the visit. He began a lumbering, circular narrative that I periodically interrupted to ask: "And that's when you fell on your wrist?"

"Nope, that came later. Y' see, my ex-wife's first husband's present wife's nephew has this dog."

He paused to draw breath and said, "I'm jest tryin' to give you all the information you need, Doc."

"Oh, please continue," I murmured. The diagnosis may pivot on this point.

I was well into making a choice between suicide and putting in for early retirement when he finally finished his story. Probably suffering initial symptoms of respiratory failure from talkin' so much.

"I think we need to x-ray that wrist, Mr . . . ah . . Nuch . . . ah. X-ray . . . x-ray."

"Do you think it's broken or just fractured, Doc?"

"Might be both."

"I'm dyin' by degrees in here!"

Believe me, lady, I know just what you mean!

How to Keep the Operating Room Running on Time

A Surgical Fairytale*
STANLEY A. BROSMAN, M.D.

Once upon a time, in the mythical Kingdom of Surgidom, everything was wonderful at the W.O.S.C. (World's Outstanding Surgical Castle). Well, almost wonderful. True, they had the world's best surgeons, anesthesiologists, residents, nurses, administrators, secretaries, etc., but there was one flaw in the function of this otherwise happy hospital. Surgery never started on time and always ran late. Aside from this, everyone was happy because there was lots of surgery to do, articles were being published by the prestigious journals and, most of all, the surgical housestaff was hardworking, respected, and never asked for vacations.

Unfortunately, this one blemish spoiled the picture since the King, also known as the Chief of Surgery, would develop a scowl on his face and would become grumpy whenever the subject was discussed. Each month the King would call together his trusted advisors for a meeting of the Operating Room Committee. The group comprised the various division Knights, the Princess of the O.R. (head operating room nurse), the Lord of Anesthesia and the senior Knights-in-training (Chief Residents). All of the routine problems were solved with diplomacy and dispatch. But whenever the group was asked why surgery never started on time and why the time between surgeries was so long, each one pointed to the other for being at fault. The Knights claimed that the Lords did not have the patients ready for surgery at the proper time. The Lords said that the Knights were always late. They both blamed the Knights-in-training for not arriving early enough. The Princess would shout that only her subjects were present at the designated starting time for surgery and neither Knights nor Lords could be located between surgeries.

Each month the same complaints and accusations were leveled. The King commissioned studies and investigations to determine the reasons for the problem and who was at fault. Each report came to a different conclusion and only brought more dissension to the group. The Lords would clearly document the tardiness of the Knights while the Knights went to great effort to demonstrate, with statistical significance, that the Lords were agonizingly slow, put in too many unnecessary monitoring lines, and drank too much coffee before and after each surgery.

The King was becoming very annoyed and discouraged. Much of the time there was a scowl on his face. Finally he decided to offer a reward to the individual who could solve the dilemma. He spent hours trying to decide upon an appropriate prize. He had no daughters to offer in marriage. Money would not influence the dedicated surgical staff, although a few suggested he try. Suddenly the answer came to him. The reward was to be the lifetime use of a special restricted parking place built close to the castle entrance with the winner's name prominently displayed.

With a prize like that, everyone hastened to work on the problem. The next operating room committee meeting was held in the large auditorium. The entire hospital staff gathered to hear the solutions that would be offered. In turn, each Knight presented an answer. Each was rejected. The Lord and Princess offered their solutions which were also turned down. Even the Senior Knights-in-training could offer no new suggestions. The King was angry. He ordered his staff to work harder and come up with new answers by the next meeting.

Just before adjourning the meeting, a small voice called from the back of the room. "I think I have an answer to the problem," came the weak, faltering voice. "Just who are you?" roared the King. "I'm a first year urology Knight-in-training," stammered the young man.

The King ordered him to the podium to present his solution. The Knight-in-training announced that he had discovered the cause as well as the solution to the nagging problem. The surgical orderlies were at fault, he declared. They were late in arriving for work, slow in picking the patients up from their rooms, slow to bring them to surgery, could never be found when the patients needed to be moved from the operating room

*Reprinted from Today's OR Nurse, ©1982; 4(1):80, 74 with permission from the author.

THE DIFFERENCE BETWEEN YOU AND ME

table to the recovery room cart, and were rarely available for running errands.

Realizing that they were absolved from blame, the members of the committee stood in unison to cheer and congratulate the lowly Knight-in-training. Everyone, including the King, agreed that this was the answer to the fundamental problem, but what was the solution? There had already been a rapid turnover in surgical orderlies and good, hardworking people never applied for the job.

"The solution is to pay them on a fee-for-service basis," declared our hero. They would receive a set amount of money each time they picked up a patient, for putting patients on and taking them off the operating table, fees for running errands, and tips could be given for special services.

The King was overjoyed. He declared the young man the winner and decreed that the plan should be put into effect immediately. The change was dramatic. Surgery began running right on schedule. The orderlies were even seen escorting the Knights and junior Lords from their homes and offices to be sure they arrived in surgery on time. Everyone was happy, particularly the orderlies. Not only were they working with fervor and excitement, but they were getting rich. They found new ways to provide service. If a patient needed to stop for an x-ray before going to surgery, an extra fee and tip were necessary.

After a number of months, the senior orderly staff decided to organize a guild. The purpose was to set requirements, establish an examination, and control the number of orderlies and their fees. They asked for representation on all of the important surgery committees and became an active voice in setting hospital policy. It wasn't long before the power in surgery was in the hands of the orderlies.

The Knights began to feel uneasy over the turn of events, but as long as the patients were in the right place at the right time, no one complained. It wasn't until the scrub princesses began talking about charging a fee for service for assisting the surgeon, holding retractors, cutting sutures, and handing the correct instruments instead of the ones requested that the Knights really became concerned. So far, the King had been able to keep them in line, but for how long was uncertain.

What happened to our lowly urologist? He quit the program after the second year and became a surgical orderly. After working a few years he was able to retire to a large estate and live happily ever after growing grapes.

The moral to the story: To maintain a successful operating room, remember to follow the rules of Knighthood, or a new guild may arise. Arrive to surgery promptly, help in moving the patients, and always be nice to your scrub princess.

The Relation of the Nurse to the Doctor and the Doctor to the Nurse*

SARAH E. DOCK, R.N.

Some one has said a nurse is born and not made. I would like to amend that by saying a nurse is born and then trained. Woman possesses qualities which naturally make her superior to the average man for this important work, which stands second to the medical profession itself.

The nursing profession is monopolized almost entirely by women. It is about the only thing we are allowed to do without the blame of trying to take away the work from the poor men. In spite of the fact that women are naturally adapted to the art of nursing, superintendents of hospitals often find it difficult to obtain desirable applicants for training. The possible reason for this is the lack of home training and the fact that children are rarely taught the importance of obedience. In my estimation obedience is the first law and the very cornerstone of good nursing. And here is the first stumbling block for the beginner. No matter how gifted she may be, she will never become a reliable nurse until she can obey without question. The first and most helpful criticism I ever received from a doctor was when he told me that I was supposed to be simply an intelligent machine for the purpose of carrying out his orders.

As to the relation of a nurse to the doctor, there can be no relation of the nurse to the doctor other than a strictly professional one. Any other relation will mean disaster to the nurse.

By disaster I mean that any relation not professional will lead to misunderstandings, quarrels or perhaps marriage, and in either case the nurse's usefulness as a professional nurse will be at an end. This is to me a pretty good argument why a nurse should maintain strictly formal relations towards the doctor, never forgetting that her success in the future depends mainly on the doctor's recommendation and influence.

It is true that after several years of doing private duty a good nurse receives many calls through the friends of patients, but suppose she steps beyond the bounds of professional etiquette and commits that unpardonable sin of suggesting to the family that another doctor be called in, perhaps the one she prefers, and in other ways conducts herself unbecomingly as a nurse. Her opportunities will be limited to nursing for that one particular doctor, no matter how qualified and accomplished she may be. Instances have occurred where the physician has been dismissed and the unprofessional nurse retained (but this is very unusual). The professional career of such a nurse is bound to be short. My advice to nurses doing hospital or private duty work would be to maintain a strictly formal attitude toward the doctor.

You may not care for the personality of the doctor who is in attendance but you are bound to respect his profession and obey his orders. If his conduct is such as to offend and make it impossible for you to do conscientious work, make some excuse and give up the case.

After all, no matter how professional or clever a nurse may be, she will never be successful if she lacks common sense, tact and the ability to grasp the fact that her real success depends on the little things in nursing and not on the fact that she may be able to diagnose the case.

A really good, ambitious nurse will prefer the doctor who is particular, even exacting in regard to her work. With a doctor like this an indifferent nurse will be forced to do good work, for she is afraid not to. A careless doctor will make a careless nurse.

Naturally the doctor is or should be the nurse's chief instructor. He should make it his business to know that the curriculum of the training school is what it should be, and that the pupil nurses get the practice required to make for efficiency. By the high standard of the training school both he and his patient will be benefited.

*Reprinted with permission from American Journal of Nursing, ©1917; 17(5):394–396. Edited from the original.

I believe it is the doctor's duty to report a nurse who fails to carry out his orders; but first he should take the role of a kindly critic and tell her of her shortcomings. If this correction fails, then report the pupil nurse; or dismiss her, if she is a graduate and doing private duty. Doctors should never make excuses for nurses who fail in their duty. It is really an injustice to the nurse and can do no possible good.

When he dismisses an unsatisfactory nurse he should tell her why, no matter if it hurts. If she is the right kind of nurse she will do better next time, or be discouraged and give up the profession. When a nurse is doing private duty the doctor should see that she gets the proper amount of rest and recreation. He should also remember that while he is attending several patients, the nurse has only one patient and is wholly dependent on the income from that one patient. If her patient is at all able to pay, I think the nurse should be entitled to the first money, and the doctor should see that she gets it.

If doctors were obliged to spend twenty-two hours out of twenty-four with some of their irritable, nervous patients they would require a few weeks rest at Dawson Springs. Even a machine needs rest and repair. Beyond a certain amount of physical and mental strain the brain refuses to act, and I believe that many cases of neglect on the part of the nurse are due to overwork. Perhaps the over ambitious nurse wishes to carry a difficult case through and refuses to have assistance. Such foolishness the doctor should not allow. Some doctors think nurses require flattery in order to do better work. I do not think so. After all, if she is doing her duty, she is doing just what she should. It is a matter of business with her and to her interest that she do her work loyally and well.

Doctors and Doorknobs*

ANDREW A. ROONEY

Doctors should never talk to ordinary people about anything but medicine. If I were a doctor, I'd never go to another party where there were anything but other doctors present.

When doctors talk politics, economics or sports, they reveal themselves to be ordinary mortals, idiots just like the rest of us. That isn't what any of us wants our doctor to be. We want our doctor to be an intellectual giant who knows all about everything. We don't want him to be someone who has a lot of petty little theories about what's wrong in Washington, or what play the coach should have sent in Sunday when it was third and nine on the twenty-four.

Saturday night, I was talking to a doctor at a party, and he was telling me that the nurses situation is getting desperate.

"Young women just don't want to do that kind of hard work anymore," he said. "A lot of the good ones are quitting," he told me, "because they like nursing but can't take the paperwork." Another thing, he said, was that a lot of nurses resented doctors and often thought they knew as much about a patient as the doctor did.

Well, first thing you know we were arguing about how little a nurse is paid compared to a doctor and how a lot of women ended up as nurses when they should have been doctors and vice versa. I won't tell you which side of the arguments I was on, but neither of us distinguished ourselves. It was the kind of conversation that makes me realize doctors are only mortal men, and it's always a disappointment. I'm looking for a god in my doctor.

Surgeons I meet worry me. When I get talking politics with a surgeon who has done a hundred and fifty open-heart operations, I usually wonder how he ever did it without killing the patients. It turns out he's just as dumb as I am. His opinion of the current Administration is the same as the one I heard from the man who runs the shoeshine stand in the station last week, and

I certainly wouldn't want the shoeshine man fooling around with my heart valves through an incision in my chest.

Years ago, my wife and I were spending the weekend in the house of an old college friend of hers whose husband was an orthopedic surgeon. One morning I started out the front door and the knob came loose. It just twisted around in my hand, so the doctor went down cellar to get a few tools. The doorknob was obviously on the critical list.

All I could think, as I watched him attack the problem, was how happy I was to be a houseguest and not a patient. He fussed with that doorknob for more than half an hour before he got an ill-fitting setscrew in there to hold it. I'd give that doorknob another three days. Here was a distinguished surgeon who had replaced the heads of two hundred femurs with stainless steel balls that enabled patients to walk once again free of pain in their hips, but he couldn't figure out how to fix that one lousy doorknob. What do you make of this?

One problem medical men and women have is one we all share with them. To be really expert in our chosen field takes more than one type of skill, and a person who has one doesn't necessarily have others. The young medical student who masters the details of anatomy and gets the best marks in his class is not necessarily manually dexterous. The dentist who has the ability of a good cabinetmaker to put together perfect, tight-fitting parts that hold together in a person's mouth was not always—or probably even usually—the dental student who finished at the top of his class.

A doctor can't help it if he isn't born with dexterous hands, but if he also has a lot of dumb opinions about the world, the least he can do is keep them to himself so we don't get wondering about his hands.

ACCIDENTS
HAPPEN

Comments Overhead in the E.R.

"I'm uninsured."

"My regular doctor was busy so we came here."

"Wait 'til you see the guy who lost the fight!"

"I take a small pill in the morning and a red one at night."

"Why do I have to wait?"

"I've never seen a doctor before."

"This place looks more like MASH than ER."

"Do I have a pulse?"

"Guess how old I am?"

"I will only talk to a doctor."

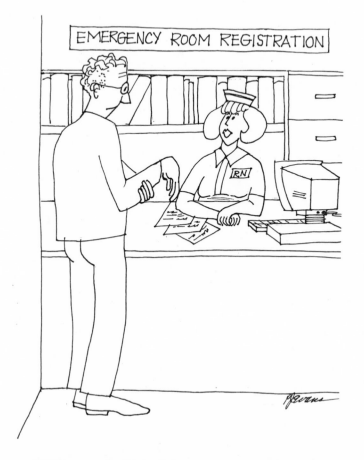

"If it's your check writing hand, it is an emergency."

Official Explanations of Emergency Nursing*

JILL CURRY, R.N., B.A., C.E.N.

Wurtzel's Explanation:

The admission of a patient who arrives in a quilted robe with a packed suitcase supersedes all diagnosis-related group regulations.

Ferrell's Caveat:

Precode patients or those who suffer from bad backs will always arrive in the backseat of a compact, two-door car.

Paul's Axiom on the Conservation of Matter:

The amount of emesis will always exceed the capacity of the container provided for it.

Balluff's Conclusion Regarding Active Labor:

The eminence of delivery is not indicated by the length of time between contractions, but is directly related to the number of times the name of the Supreme Being is invoked by the mother-to-be.

Wysocki's Observation:

Calls placed to physicians on consult will be returned when the emergency physician:

1. Goes to the bathroom
2. Dons the last pair of sterile gloves in his size
3. Is called to an in-house code
4. Receives a call from another physician
5. Sits down to have lunch/dinner

Corollary: The length of time it takes to reach the consulting physician is inversely proportional to that physician's willingness to "hold the line" until the emergency physician can get to the phone to speak to him.

Wysocki's Comment on Language:

Patients are never "brought" or "taken" to the emergency department; they are always "rushed."

V. G. Mills' Scheduling Maxims:

Publication of the ED staffing schedule will result in at least a dozen requests for time off—none previously requested or discussed.

Corollary: Preparing the schedule more than 8 weeks in advance greatly increases the probability that at least one staff member will resign, require major surgery, or be injured on the job.

Wysocki's Admonition Regarding Energy Conservation:

If the lights are turned out in the code room, an unannounced ambulance will appear with a patient in cardiac arrest.

Paul's Law of Extremes:

The degree of dissatisfaction expressed by a given patient is inversely proportional to the severity of illness or injury suffered by that patient.

Corollary: It takes 10 complimentary letters to administration to undo the damage caused by one uncomplimentary letter.

Balluff's Constant of Memory:

The number and importance of the medications a patient routinely takes at home are inversely proportional to the patient's ability or willingness to remember what those medications are.

Corollary No. 1: The patient will always describe the medication he cannot remember as a "little white pill."

Corollary No. 2: If a patient says, "My wife knows what medicines I take," the wife will not have a clue.

Moughan's Observation on Higher Education:

Any college coed who presents for treatment will be accompanied by a friend called "Muffy."

Corollary: Muffy will be more symptomatic.

Carroll's Comment on Mass and Vectors:

The ability of a given patient to move from one place to another without help is inversely related to his or her weight.

*Reproduced from Journal of Emergency Nursing, ©1991; 17(2):120–122 with permission from Mosby-Year Book, Inc. Edited from the original.

Curry's Axiom:

The only good admit is a direct admit.

Corollary: The paramedic whose stretcher patient is a direct admit is worth his weight in gold.

Balluff's Comment on Space and Time:

The chance that a private physician will want to do a complete history and physical, write two pages of orders, and request that at least half those orders be carried out in the emergency department is significantly greater when there is a desperate demand for ED stretchers.

Balluff's Warning:

Don't count your unit beds until they are clean.

Corollary: Don't count your unit beds until they are staffed.

Balluff's Observation on Fluid Management:

You can lead a patient with renal colic to the bathroom, but you can't make him pee.

Corollary: The best cure for diarrhea is a request for a stool sample.

Balluff's Law of Supply and Demand:

Patients in cardiac arrest or with multiple trauma arrive with greater frequency during the lunch/dinner hour.

Corollary: Fewer cardiac arrests and accidents would occur if ED personnel would abstain from eating.

Balluff's "Watched Pot" Theory:

The chances that a high-ranking hospital administrator will stroll through the emergency department unannounced to "observe" are greatly increased during an incredibly uncharacteristic drop in patient census when the staff is in the lounge drinking coffee and shooting the breeze.

Curry's Comment on Opportunity:

The need for a given patient to receive IV fluids is inversely proportional to the number of veins accessible for venipuncture.

ACLS Laws of Time and Distance:

The probability that a patient will suffer a cardiac arrest increases proportionately:

1. With the distance of the crash cart from the patient.

2. With the time elapsed since the ACLS provider last went to the bathroom.

3. As the time before the end of the shift decreases.

ACLS Law of Acid-Base Balance:

The severity of acidosis increases directly with the degree of resistance met when trying to inject an ampule of sodium bicarbonate.

The Ultimate ACLS Algorithm:

If a gross dysrhythmia occurs that is sickening to the ACLS provider, the cardiac monitor should be discontinued at once.

ACLS Law of Medicine:

Drugs used in a medical crisis will be ordered in the least understood unit of measurement—i.e., grains per micrograms per square inch of body surface per millisecond.

ACLS Law of Probability:

The probability of success in using ACLS algorithms is 50%: either it will work or it won't.

ACLS Law of Acceptance:

Under the most rigorously controlled conditions of cardiac index, pulse rate, stroke index, left ventricular stroke volume, right ventricular stroke volume, total peripheral resistance, pulmonary vascular resistance, oxygen consumption, cardiac rhythm, and other variables, the heart will do as it darn well pleases.

Curry's Advice:

In the emergency department, always assume that the question, "How much longer will I have to wait?" is a rhetorical one.

Mills' Theory of Human Resource Management:

Compliments made to reward improvements in a staff member's problem behavior (such as tardiness) result in immediate regression to the former level of performance.

Mills' Observation on Tolerance:

The probability of delays and errors in receiving laboratory and radiologic reports is inversely proportional to the frustration threshold of the particular emergency physician on duty at the time.

Mills' Observation on Truthfulness:

The more effort devoted to the nursing history, the greater the discrepancy between it and the story the patient will tell the physician.

Mills' Discovery Concerning Studied Events:

The decision to conduct a productivity study will result in an immediate and precipitous drop in patient census.

Corollary: At all other times, the number of staff available for work is inversely proportional to the patient census.

Hopkin's Law of Supply and Demand:

The probability that you will need a particular piece of equipment is inversely related to your ability to recall where you last saw that same piece of equipment.

Curry's Admonition:

It is perfectly acceptable to list the patient's insurance carrier as the chief complaint if all attempts to elicit other reasons for the patient's presence at the triage desk have failed.

Wysocki's Law of Inevitability:

If it can't happen, has never happened before, shouldn't happen, and there is no explanation of why it happened, it *will* happen to an emergency nurse.

Official Explanations of Emergency Nursing, II*

KATHLEEN BYRNE AND ELIZABETH L. FEETTERERS

Courtesy Kathleen Byrne, Yonkers, New York:

There is no such thing as a doctor who uses your last available stretcher for "5 minutes only."

If all else fails, read the instructions—they may be in English.

Interchangeable parts are not, unless they have changed the model number—then it may fit.

The probability of cardiac arrest occurring in the waiting room is inversely proportional to the staffing, stretcher availability, and the victim's size and weight.

The sickest patients will forget to register, sit meekly, and quietly wait their turn.

If the patient complains about the noise in the treatment area or the discomfort of the stretcher, he or she is well enough to wait in the waiting room.

If the patient claims that his or her physician knows what medications the patient is currently taking, then (1) the patient will not be able to remember the name of the physician; (2) the physician will not have seen the patient in 2 years; or (3) another physician will be taking the call.

In any emergency department, there is no such thing as too many electrical outlets, too many working portable oxygen tanks, or too many telemetry units.

Never count on your critical care bed until your patient is in it.

The greatest numbers of emergency medical technicians arrive with a patient requiring the least assistance. The sickest patients in history arrive in a basic life support unit.

A patient encountering emergency medical technicians, paramedics, nurses, physicians, registration clerks, x-ray technicians, and laboratory personnel will give the most truthful history of the accident or illness to the environmental staff person cleaning the room.

Always assume that equipment is aware and self-propelled; seek it in the least likely place.

A missing item will always be found at the bottom of the last and dirtiest refuse container or linen bag that is searched.

*Reproduced from Journal of Emergency Nursing, ©1991; 17(6):27A–28A with permission from Mosby-Year Book, Inc. Edited from the original.

If the patient passes the 2-second physical (looks, sounds, and smells okay), assume that the ventricular fibrillation on the monitor is a glitch in the equipment. Besides, an equipment glitch is easier to fix.

Given a choice between a simple and a complex explanation, the patient will opt for the complex one, regardless of its accuracy.

The more a patient's clothing is cut into unusable pieces, the more likely he or she will be treated and released with nothing to wear home.

The more rare a disease profiled on a media health program, the more convinced a patient will be that he or she has this disease.

Expect that a physician will claim "BDZ"—beeper dead zone—when (1) covering for more medical groups than he or she can handle; (2) finishing an exquisite flaming dessert at Le Petit Mal restaurant; or (3) engaged in spouse-unauthorized activity.

Inclement weather of any kind brings in the most and least ill patients—nothing in between.

As you release the stretcher brake for a patient transfer to a critical care bed that you have been waiting for all day, the patient will ask for the bedpan.

Critical care unit beds become available for patients receiving tissue-type plasminogen activator only after they begin reperfusion arrhythmias.

Fertility is inversely proportional to common sense.

Morbidly obese patients always gravitate toward the oldest, heaviest, least maneuverable stretcher and have to be transported to a heavily carpeted unit by a nurse with a documented history of back injury.

If we take literally the working definition of a disaster as "one more patient than can safely be handled," then most emergency departments qualify for disaster assistance.

Courtesy Elizabeth L. Feetterers, technician, Robinson Memorial Hospital, Ravenna, Ohio:

Male psychiatric patients fixated on female genitalia and female patients requiring pelvic examinations will arrive on days when ED staffing is all female and all male, respectively.

The burlap bag containing the live snake that bit the patient will always be handed to the ED staff member with the greatest phobia of snakes.

Off Duty? Hah!*

MARY FERGUSON, R.N.

While others were seeing an old castle moat
I found myself checking the guide's scratchy throat.
As the rest of the bevy fandangoed in Spain
I circled my roommate while strapping her sprain.
When we got to Gibraltar did I visit the Rock?
No, I stayed with a tour-mate who suffered from shock.

I missed all the singing while sailing the Vistula
Because I was hearing of one woman's fistula.
The tour gaily trooped over Rome's seven hills
While I stayed behind giving pills for the chills.
I spent quite a bit of our stay in the Alps
Applying the snow to contusions on scalps.

If I had a rendezvous in Samarkand
It wasn't to hold but to bandage a hand.
Things really got busy when we got to Libya
Where our driver conveniently fractured his tibia.
I really believe if I went to Siberia
The whole Comintern would come down with diphtheria.

So nurses who travel, please hide your vocation
Or be preyed on by people in every location.

*Reprinted with permission from American Journal of Nursing, ©1965;
65(2):198.

Don't Know Nothin'
'bout Birthin' no Babies!*

MARY ALEXANDER, R.N., M.S.N.

Emergency nurses are a special breed . . . not *ever* to be confused with labor and delivery nurses. Labor and delivery nurses have the corner on their share of the market; they will never need to fear me taking over their territory.

At first I thought I was unique; something was lacking with regard to obstetrics in my undergraduate education. I must have been absent the day they explained something pivotal. After several years in emergency departments all over the country, I have decided that my undergraduate education was just fine; it must be a specific obstetric gene that most emergency nurses lack.

How many emergency nurses consider calling a disaster when they get word that a woman is about to deliver in their emergency department? Actually, it would not be a bad idea; there is safety in numbers.

I recall clearly the episode that convinced me that this was not my specialty. My community health experience took place in Appalachia with an extended family consisting of the grandparents, a grown daughter, and her two children. After 2 months of sincere visiting, I suddenly realized that the grown daughter looked a little pregnant. No wonder she had refused all information on birth control! As a good student, I asked my instructor for help in convincing this woman that she should seek early prenatal care. The instructor agreed to accompany me on my next visit. When we arrived, we found that the woman was not pregnant at all—she had delivered a couple of days after my last visit! So much for my assessment skills. I should have known then that I was destined to be an emergency nurse.

Experience has not improved my acumen. On a quiet Saturday morning, radiology requested help in transporting a patient to their department for studies. Because I was not busy, I volunteered to push the patient over.

As the astute emergency nurse, I immediately recognized something unusual about this patient. Did she look a little pregnant? Hmmm. Déjà vu. The chart said her last menstrual period was a month ago. She was a private patient with a kidney stone, waiting for radiographs before her private physician came to see her. Not pregnant. Right. We really should be sure before she gets her abdomen irradiated. (Can't fool me.)

Because emergency nurses always think best in pairs, I asked my coworker to take a look. Grabbing the Doppler equipment and blue goop, we stepped confidently into the room.

The patient strongly protested, even after her mother left the room, that she could not be pregnant. Confidently, in a most professional manner, my coworker attempted fetal heart sounds as I palpated the abdomen. The second I softly put my hand on the patient's abdomen, she exclaimed in a squeal, "Oh! Oh! It's here!"

Lifting the sheet, we were all equally surprised to find a 9-pound baby boy, who responded to stimuli and took his first breath. I am happy to report that mother and baby did fine, the grandmother needed oxygen (emergency nurses can handle that), and the two emergency nurses needed the rest of the day off.

The morals of the story? One, do not *ever* volunteer. Two, *nobody* is just a little pregnant.

*Reproduced from Journal of Emergency Nursing, ©1994; 20(6):596 with permission from Mosby-Year Book, Inc.

Divine Intervention?*

RONALD BRISLEN

The A&E staff thought at first that they'd witnessed a miracle . . . and maybe they had.

Working in the A&E department where death and serious injury are frequent visitors, I have become increasingly aware of religion and the effect that it has on people. We see many people hoping for miracles, but we have yet to witness one—or have we?

Mrs. Aspinall was a fit 80-year-old who had spent almost a lifetime keeping house and looking after her husband, an ex-miner, whose whole existence seemed to be summarised in her comment that 'He needs a new washer for his tap.'

Her story began early one morning while she was standing on a chair cleaning windows. She was reaching for the top panes when she slipped and, unable to save herself, fell to the floor sustaining a fracture of the arm with very marked deformity.

Her husband rushed to her aid, after she had picked herself up and spent ten minutes trying to coax him out of the loo. He immediately assessed the situation and offered comfort and reassurance with the words, 'You silly cow, 'ow the 'ell did you fall?' Looking at the obviously deformed arm he decided that the situation needed his great organising ability which had not seen the light of day since he was acting corporal, Home Guard, in 1944. With a booming voice not unlike that of Churchill, in that it inspired people into immediate action, he pronounced, 'You've broken the bloody thing, better get up to th'ospital,' and doing a quick about turn he retired to his porcelain palace.

So it was that Mrs. Aspinall arrived in the A&E department after first stopping at the WRVS canteen for coffee and biscuits, 'Just in case I was a long time'. Mrs. A, like so many people of her generation, began the explanation of her accident with the words 'I don't want to be any trouble', and in this case she really meant it. But for the convincing argument of her husband, given in the guise of an unquestionable command, she would have stayed at home and just put a bandage on it.

Following an examination and X-ray it was decided that the badly deformed arm would need reduction and the application of a plaster of Paris under a general anaesthetic, but because of the coffee and biscuits it would have to be delayed. Mrs. A was reluctant to while away the time in the department. So after we had applied temporary splints and arranged for a neighbour to take her home in a car, she was allowed to go with instructions not to remove the splints, not to eat or drink anything and to return 20 minutes before the arranged time. So with a cheery smile Mrs. A left the department.

On Mrs. A's return it was obvious that something extraordinary had happened. The arm was no longer deformed but straight. Had Mrs. A's twin sister returned in her place? Was this another test by one of our eccentric consultants? (Both of these have happened before, but they are stories for another time.)

News of the strange event quickly passed through the department and very soon a crowd gathered outside the cubicle in which Mrs. A sat with an all-knowing smile on her face. The consultant barked at the casualty officers, uttering words like incompetent . . . mix-up . . . can't cope. The staff nurse blubbed to sister 'Honestly, I didn't put the splints on too tight.' Student nurses and others smiled at each other, amused at the crumbling levels of management. The radiographer stood at the back of the crowd jumping up, trying to see Mrs. A and waving the X-rays above her head. It was quickly becoming obvious that this situation required the setting up of a committee, a full scale inquiry.

The murmur of voices stopped suddenly as sister pushed her way to the front. If she could sort out 30 steel-helmeted swastika-wearing Hell's Angels, then this present problem was only an irritation which she could sort out in the click of her jackboots. Sister bent down, looked Mrs. A straight in the eye, took a deep breath and asked 'What happened?'

Mrs. A smiled. She had not been the centre of attraction since she was accosted by a sailor, poor man, some 50 years ago and she was obviously enjoying her-

*Reprinted from Nursing Times, ©1981; 77(5):209–210 with permission from Macmillan Magazines, Ltd.

self as much now as she did then. 'Well, dear, when I got home I was sat alone thinking. He was upstairs as usual, y'know one day I'll serve his dinner in there, anyway there I was sat alone when I remembered something that my mother once said and so I thought I would try the bible!"

The effect of the words was amazing. Sister shot bolt upright, her false teeth clicking together nervously; a student nurse stepped back, right onto the consultant's foot but his growl of pain was masked by the staff nurse muttering 'Holy Mary, Mother of God . . . .' Some crossed themselves, others unsure what to do, looked heavenwards. Mrs. A seemed to be bathed in a glowing light. Were we mistaken, or could we hear a host of angels singing? The cubicle seemed to suddenly grow warm. Not a sticky harsh heat, but a warmth that was comforting, relaxing, holy.

The crowd was speechless and yet a thousand thoughts flashed through their minds in the following seconds. Had some heavenly body appeared to straighten the infirm limb? Should we call the hospital priest, or even the cardinal? Would Mrs. A's back kitchen become a shrine to be visited by thousands? Would we be getting a call to Rome where Mrs. A would become a saint? Perhaps even Mr. A would come out of the loo long enough to see his wife appear on the balcony with the Pope. In our minds' eyes we could see St. Peter's Square full to capacity with people in wheelchairs and on crutches all trying to touch her as she walked through the crowd, in the hope of another miracle.

Eagerly we asked if there had been a flash of brilliant light or voices from the heavens. Mrs. A laughed and with that laugh all our dreams, hopes and excitement faded. 'No dear' she said, 'My old mother used to have two family bibles, years old they was, and she told me that her old mum had a fall and her arm ended up all bent, just like mine, so she put her arm on one of the bibles, put the other bible on top and leant on it with all her weight.'

'How did you do it?" asked one. 'Why?' asked another. Yet another asked 'Did it hurt?'

'Well,' she smiled, 'it did hurt a little bit, but all I did was just what grandma did and put it between the bibles. To be honest, lovey, I never did fancy being put to sleep and I had a lovely stew in the oven for dinner. Well, dearie, I pinched a couple of spoonsful of his stew while he was upstairs, but it doesn't matter because he'll never know!'

X-rays showed that the position of the bones was such that all that was needed was the application of a plaster of Paris. Then Mrs. A went home, after we had obtained from her the most firm promise that she would return if she was worried or had any problems.

With the departure of Mrs A a little spark of hope went out of our lives. No trip to Rome. No St. Mrs. A. Mr. A could now stay in his 'stall' uninterrupted. But this spark was to be rekindled into a flame that would be with us for a long time to come.

Two days later a little old man struggled into the department carrying a large and apparently heavy parcel. He dumped it on the reception desk and grunted, 'That's for sister'. Sister was summoned, and meanwhile the old man wandered restlessly around the reception area looking up and down the corridors, obviously very nervous and impatient. When sister arrived all eyes were on her. She began to undo the parcel, speculating on its contents. Was it a bomb, a piece of dismembered corpse or some foul specimen that had been requested?

As the last piece of paper fell away, the little old man straightened, smiled to himself and with a deep sigh of 'Thank God' made a rapid departure in the direction of the gents whose sign he had just spotted.

Inside the parcel were two huge bibles, with a note saying, 'To help in future works—Mrs. A.'

This incident really did happen and today the two bibles occupy a place of honour in the department. They stand alone on a shelf for all to see and beneath them is a little card with the words:

Colles reduction kit
Donated by the lady who last used it.
She disliked the thought of a short GA,
That grand old lady Saint Mrs. A.

The Old Emergency Nurse Reality Scale*

DAWN FENLASON, R.N., BOB KINNEY, R.N.,
SUE MOORE, R.N., M.S., C.C.R.N., C.E.N., DAN MCMULLIN, L.P.N., PAULA
WILSON, R.N., GRACE HAMANN, R.N., AND MIKE MALAY, R.N.†

We were all leaning around the emergency department the other day, waiting for somebody to stand up so we could fight over the chair, and discussing things—educational things, of course—specifically facility design. If we get much older, the conversation went, we are going to have to make some *big* changes around here.

First of all, there will have to be one chair per nurse in the nurses station. At least one chair per nurse older than *40*. We are submitting this as a formal resolution at the next ENA General Assembly.

Patients will need to be on long conveyor belts, rotating slowly around the nurses as we sit in our chairs. . . . If that is not feasible, we will need those little scooters they have in the supermarket. The halls will have to be wider, with rubber bumpers. You know how old people drive. We will have to install seat belts, and helmets will not be optional.

It occurred to us that perhaps other emergency departments are undergoing the same evolution, so we devised the Old Emergency Nurse Reality Scale (see box) to determine whether they too would benefit from facility redesign.

This scale has withstood rigorous testing (we called the emergency department across town). It has been shown to possess fantastic validity and reliability. Feel free to apply it whenever necessary.

OLD EMERGENCY NURSE REALITY SCALE

A "yes" answer to each of the following increases the likelihood that you are an old emergency nurse.
A score of 15 or more, and honey, give us a call. We need to talk.

___The cops you used to date are all retired.

___The current cops call you ma'am.

___You have given meds according to the color of the label because you cannot see the little writing any more.

___You feel like patting new doctors on the head.

___Learning to do it in gloves was harder than learning to do it the first time.

___You remember Quaalude overdoses.

___The Premarin rep is the only drug rep you talk to.

___When you started, nobody heard of ACLS.

___You've noticed that the resuscitation rate in the emergency department is not any different now that we all carry cards.

___You have an uncontrollable urge to lecture 19-year-old women.

___You have given up trying to keep up with new cardiac meds and antibiotics.

___You are taking orders from doctors who used to be your orderlies.

___Your back pain is worse than the patient's.

___To do visual acuities, you have to stand at the 10-foot mark.

___You can start IVs with your eyes closed—which is good, because you cannot see the veins any more.

___The reason you do not want to work on New Year's Eve has to do with the patients, not the desire to party.

___Your first ED uniform included a cap and white nylons.

___You find yourself discussing your children's sex lives instead of your own.

___You have oriented at least one new nurse who asked how you have stayed in the emergency department so long.

___Dr. Scholl's products are a regular part of your shopping list.

___You remember when routine care of head injuries included pneumoencephalograms and searches for the pineal body.

---

*Reproduced from Journal of Emergency Nursing, ©1994; 20(3):250 with permission from Mosby-Year Book, Inc. Edited from the original.
†The authors' combined years in emergency nursing total 128.

Mrs. Moore and the Young Medical Explorers*

PAULA J. WILSHE, B.A.

Let me tell you what happened in *our* emergency department last week. Beginning my shift as unit secretary at 3 PM on a wintry afternoon, I was surprised by the flurry of activity during a normally quiet time of the day. Lights were on in the trauma room, and staff members and ambulance personnel were flying around everywhere. I snagged a nurse in hope of finding out just what was going on. "I was helping out with a code, now I'm going to help intubate the lady in bed 2 . . . talk to you later!" she quipped with a grin as she slipped inside the curtain.

The little lady in bed 2 was an elderly woman, Mrs. Moore,† who had been experiencing some shortness of breath. Her family sat in the waiting room watching *Oprah*, blithely unaware of the activity a few feet away. Despite the best efforts of the ED staff and the pulmonary physician, Mrs. Moore died. The nursing supervisor took the family to the grieving room and relayed the sad news. A short time later she escorted them into the department so they might have some time with their grandmother. The family stayed for a very long time, and it made us all sad to hear the grief-stricken sobbing of Mrs. Moore's granddaughter.

Eventually the family left, the situation in the trauma room was resolved, and several other patients were discharged, slowing the pace of the evening to something more comfortable and steady.

After my dinner break, I received a call from the nursing supervisor, who advised me that there would be more family members coming to say good-bye to Mrs. Moore. Because the body was no longer in the emergency department, she asked that I page her when they arrived.

Shortly before 8 PM, I registered a young woman who was having severe lower abdominal cramping and vaginal bleeding. She was accompanied by her husband and their four small children who, although beautiful, were completely unmanageable and immediately began to run through the waiting room. The father was so upset at his wife's condition that he lost all powers of discipline.

Suddenly I looked up to see a parade of headlights in the driveway. Thinking I was in for an onslaught of patients, I quickly pulled out some bracelets and chart folders. But none of the cars contained individuals in need of medical care. These vehicles belonged to various members of the Moore family, who converged on us simultaneously to pay their last respects to their grandmother. They began quietly milling around the waiting room as I waited for the nursing supervisor to answer my page.

The arrival of the 30 grieving family members only further excited the four children. They continued racing and romping through the waiting room, sometimes even darting through the legs of the Moore family members, who were either so polite or so grief-stricken that they said nothing.

I frantically ran into the department, "I need more tissues! They're crying!" One of the nurses, normally a close and reliable friend, looked at me as if I had lost my mind, while another pointed to the appropriate cabinet and told me to help myself. As an afterthought, she called after me. "Who's crying? The kids or the Moores?" At that point, I could not remember and hurried back to the reception area.

As I tried to finish some paperwork, a movement directly to the left of the window caught my eye. Suddenly there were 40 teenagers in the minor side hallway. They were attending the monthly meeting of the Young Medical Explorers, who were being led through on a tour of the emergency department.

Confusion reigned as the groups began their inevitable mingle . . . the waiting room is not all that big. Some of the Young Medical Explorers may have seen more than their tour had promised, having accidentally followed the wrong group to the morgue to view the body of the late Mrs. Moore. Even those family members who mistakenly joined the teenagers' walk-through and did not have the opportunity to see their late grandmother seemed satisfied with their tour of the emergency department, complimenting us on the neatness and efficiency with which the nurses and an-

*Reproduced from Journal of Emergency Nursing, ©1996; 22(3):261–262 with permission from Mosby-Year Book, Inc. Edited from the original.
†A pseudonym.

cillary staff performed their tasks. The harried husband of the gynecologic patient did not complain when we were unable to find two of his children; they had joined the rest of the Young Medical Explorers (and some hungry Moores) and were headed back to the conference room for juice and cookies.

Eventually all was straightened out to everyone's satisfaction. The teenagers were escorted to the main lobby to meet their parents. The young father was reunited with his missing children. Apparently, their ex-uberance and lack of control were too much even for the stoic Moores, who returned them with curt nods.

As the grieving family members left, they lined up at the door and each one shook hands and exchanged pleasantries with the nursing supervisor. It was a picture not unlike that at the end of a hockey game when competing team members offer one another their mutual respect. I found solace in a cup of coffee and the knowledge that the end of my shift was only an hour away.

You Know You're an Old ED Nurse if You Remember*

TERRY M. FOSTER, R.N., B.S.N., C.E.N., C.C.R.N.
SUSAN E. MILLS, R.N., C.E.N.

You know you're an old ED nurse if you remember . . .

Drawing up 10 amps of bicarb during a code.

Treating SVT by dunking the patient's face in a basin filled with ice water.

When SVT was just PAT.

Defibrillating at 400 watts.

Only one monitor/defibrillator in the entire ED.

Code drugs that were given intracardiac.

When there weren't any drugs in prefilled syringes (and your hands shook while drawing up an ampule of atropine as the heart rate dropped to 30!).

Memorizing the three golden rules of acid base.

When ACLS was for doctors only!

When gloves were for doctors only.

Patients never knew the names of their medicines or what they were for (oh well . . . some things *never* change!).

When blood on your uniform and shoes meant a busy night.

IV bottles.

Keep-open IVs instead of heparin locks.

Rib belts, glass thermometers, and red rubber NG tubes.

Using rotating tourniquets for pulmonary edema.

When casts were made of plaster . . . and only came in white.

Flyswatters in the suture room.

Checking fetal heart tones with a fetoscope.

The only ventilator in the ED was a bag-valve-mask device.

Cold metal bedpans and urinals.

When the ED had only *one* regular drunk and homeless person.

Domestic violence was arguing over whose turn it was to take out the trash.

*Reproduced from Journal of Emergency Nursing, ©1995; 21(4):35A with permission from Mosby-Year Book, Inc. Edited from the original.

When you used to laugh when a patient or visitor said, "I'll get you, nurse!"

Drive-in movies, not drive-by shootings.

How to treat a methaqualone (Quaalude) overdose.

Letting a patient smoke a cigarette (and sometimes the nurse smoking with him!).

Dumping or being dumped on.

QA, CQI, TQM, and TQI were strange letters that we saw after a kid sat at the typewriter.

When no one was certified in anything.

Only needing one page for charting.

Never writing discharge instructions.

Burnout only happened to light bulbs.

When the ED was the ER.

When only the doctors started the IVs.

Freely giving medical advice over the phone *and* over the fence.

Student nurses who worked 8-hour shifts in the ED.

There was only one male nurse in the ED (instead of eight!).

All the physicians were male.

The head nurse *was* a head nurse and always in full uniform (including cap).

Administration's main concern was whether the nurses were wearing their caps.

Nobody ever heard of a director, coordinator, or CEO (or their assistants).

Clinics were the *only* nursing shoe (and never tennis shoes).

Venous cutdowns.

Infusing drips without any controllers.

A central line was a main bus route!

"Main lining" was riding that bus route!

When no one wore a seatbelt—and the speed limit was 70!

"Scoop and run."

When the emergency doctors were moonlighting family physicians.

One RN on night shift.

Introcaths for IV lines.

Glass syringes.

Scrubs were what you did to a wound and not what you wore.

When ENA was EDNA.

Being allowed to write "drunk" as a diagnosis.

Receiving patients from the back of ambulances with fin tails . . . or better yet, hearses that doubled as ambulances and operated from the funeral home!

When an epidural bleed was diagnosed by presentation and not by CT.

When an ectopic pregnancy was diagnosed by a culdocentesis.

No one ever came to the ED for a pregnancy test!

Waiting at least 30 minutes for a serum blood sugar.

Newborn preemies were kept warm inside your uniform next to your chest.

Giving aspirin to kids.

Cold baths or rubbing alcohol sponge baths for fevers.

The *smell* of paraldehyde.

Giving these drugs: horse serum, syrup of ipecac, and IV caffeine.

The fact that a patient was from a nursing home made him or her an automatic "no code."

When there were only two STDs (GC and syphilis).

When STD was just VD.

When AIDS were blue-clad older ladies who helped nurses.

When we let people who were 90 just die peacefully!

The Kidomatics of Trauma*

TOM CARPENTER, NREMT-P

Most of us have attended seminars or read books about sport, occupational or wartime injuries. But somehow, the most common and most underestimated injury group—parents injured by their kids—has been left unstudied and virtually undocumented.

To chart these previously undocumented waters, I have been involved in a nine-year study on the "kidomatics of trauma." So far, the data show definite patterns in the types of injuries parents sustain at the hands of their children. While most parents who are injured by their kids lie about the actual cause of injury, even their fictitious stories show similarities.

Let's start with the basics. As most of us know, "kidogenic energy" does not abide by the standard laws of physics. In kidomatics, the child's mass has little impact on how badly you, the parent, can be injured. For example, a 40-pound child can break your nose with a force equivalent to a car traveling at 50 mph. But does this type of kid-generated injury happen often? To answer that question, I've developed a formula that determines the potential number of injuries sustained in a month:

$$\frac{2(K \times HS\ WWF)}{R} = I$$

The injuries per month (I) is equal to the number of kids (K) multiplied by hours spent (HS) watching the "World Wrestling Federation" (WWF) multiplied by two, divided by the number of relaxation (R) hours. Let's consider the following example:

$$\frac{2(4K \times 40\ HS\ WWF)}{8R} = 40\ \text{injuries}$$

As you can see, this kidomatic problem has the potential to incur billions of dollars in health care expenses. Now let's see if you recognize any of these common parental traumas.

The Good Night Knee

This is also known as the third-degree ligament tear. The parent plants one or both feet on the floor beside the bed and bends at the waist to give the child a goodnight hug. The child grabs the parent around the neck and yanks downward, causing hyperextension of the knee joint. This injury often presents with a parent claiming, "My knee just went out while playing basketball." Be wary of the parent who suddenly dresses in disheveled sportswear during off-seasons.

The Good Morning Traumatic Asphyxia

This injury generally occurs on Saturday mornings (the only day the kids get up before you do) while the parent is sound asleep in bed. The pint-size trespasser strikes suddenly, screaming "Bonsai!" The parent wakes up—just in time—to see a small airborne body heading straight for the abdomen. As the creature pummels the unsuspecting parent, a sudden loss of consciousness and bladder control occur. This type of patient typically presents in a postictal state with exophthalmos, rhinorrhea and a swollen tongue. Of all kidomatic traumas, GMTAs have the highest mortality rate. These types of injuries are usually reported to 9-1-1 as seizures.

Traumatic Testicular Torsion

Have you ever watched a child run, full speed, to give his or her father a hug while the parent is otherwise preoccupied? The parent (unfortunately) doesn't notice the child rapidly closing in at a slightly inferior waistline level—hence, traumatic testicular torsion, commonly accompanied by a gasp and a grimace. This injury is often misdiagnosed as kidney stones due to the way the patient walks post-injury.

Achilles Tendon Interruption

Imagine you are on your hands and knees, busily working on an under-the-sink plumbing project, when a child suddenly jumps on your heel. This injury is easy to diagnose because it is almost always accompanied

*Reprinted with permission from JEMS: Journal of Emergency Medical Services, ©1995; 20(6):82–83.

by a laceration or hematoma on the occipital region of the scalp.

Accidental Tracheal Deviation

No, this is not caused by a tension pneumothorax but by an abrupt karate chop to the anterior neck region. Generally caught by surprise, the patient presents like a choking victim—grasping at the throat, unable to speak and quickly turning blue.

The Good Morning Traumatic Asphyxia

I thought it was a good idea to teach my 4-year-old daughter self-defense. Bad idea. Now when I ask for a hug, I get kicked in the shin and elbowed in the old breadbasket. Symptoms of EA include diaphoresis, shortness of breath and epigastric pain. The patient is likely to state that the pain feels as if someone punched him or her in the chest. (I, too, was hesitant to reveal to anyone just who that someone was.) If the patient lies in the knee/chest position for five to 10 minutes, the pain will usually subside, which is why it is called epigastric angina. A cautionary note: Patients with EA may also be suffering from underlying accidental tracheal deviation.

So there you have it—the injuries most likely to be sustained at the hands (and feet) of those little gremlins. By learning the kidomatics of trauma, you can accurately diagnose those patients who adamantly exclaim, "Honest, I've never felt this pain before."

Incidentally, I am organizing a book, lecture tour and video to further address these enigmatic calls. In the meantime, I can be reached at 900/DAD-HURT. (Calls are $1 a minute, with a minimum charge of 20 minutes.)

Hey, someone has to pay the doctor bills.

Math Quiz for Emergency Nurses*

MYKA CLARK, R.N., C.E.N.

1. You are assisting a primary nurse with administration of charcoal by means of an orogastric tube. The room measures 8 feet × 12 feet. The patient begins to vomit before the tube is removed. Knowing that charcoal can spray in a 5-foot radius (even with a thumb over the opening) and the stretcher is 2 feet wide, how many feet per second do you have to back up to get less charcoal on you than the primary nurse?

2. Doctor A picks up a chart from the rack. He or she finds that the patient is one with abdominal pain who has been seen many times in the emergency department. Doctor A replaces the chart. Doctor B picks up the chart 5 minutes later and also returns it to the rack. Doctor A leaves the nurses' station heading south at 5 mph. Doctor B leaves the nurses' station for the doctors' lounge at 3 mph. How much time will pass before the patient is at an equal distance from Doctor A and Doctor B?

3. You were assigned to cover two large treatment rooms and the gynecologic rooms. By the end of the day you have cared for 10 patients. Four patients were women over the age of 80, all reporting weakness. Two patients were men, ages 72 and 50. The last four patients were women, between the ages of 24 and 40, all reporting abdominal pain. It is 3 PM and time to restock your rooms. How many bedpans will you need?

4. You are the primary nurse for an elderly patient with congestive heart failure. Insertion of the IV needle was exceptionally difficult, but you are able to start an 18-gauge catheter on the second try. You leave the room to check on another patient. A relative thinks that the IV line has stopped dripping and opens the clamp. How much IV fluid will be infused before you return?

5. You are on your morning coffee break. You need to use the restroom but cannot find an unoccupied one and have to walk to the lobby. The coffee pot is dry and you have to make more. When you get to the cafe-

*Reproduced from Journal of Emergency Nursing, ©1995; 21(4):366 with permission from Mosby-Year Book, Inc.

teria, the line extends 10 feet into the hallway. You cannot remember exactly when your break began. How much time do you have left?

6. You are the primary nurse caring for a particularly shy woman in the gynecology room. Her private physician comes to see her, but you can see he is not in a particularly good mood. After much coaxing, the patient agrees to a pelvic examination. How many people will open the door during the examination?

7. You are assigned to the otorhinolaryngology room. A patient needs assessment of a peritonsillar abscess. The otorhinolaryngologist has been paged and expects to arrive in 45 minutes. Three hours later, the doctor arrives and is at the patient's side, asking for a flashlight. Lightly jogging at 22 mph, how many rooms will you be able to search before you find one?

8. You have worked 12 hours on a very busy day. You are ready to leave when you find that your last patient needs to be transferred to the telemetry floor. There is no one else to do this but you. You return the stretcher to the emergency department after the admission. When you look under the cart, how many articles of clothing will you find in the basket?

9. You have been asked to cover a coworker's rooms during her break. One of the patients is an elderly confused man with an enlarged prostate. A catheter has been inserted, and his physician is coming to see him. Somehow the patient manages to get off the stretcher. The drainage bag is firmly hooked to the side rail. Knowing that the catheter is 16 inches long and the drainage tube is 3 feet long, will the patient be able to reach the door?

10. A college student named Muffy is brought to the emergency department with a sore throat. She has no relatives in town. Will you have enough chairs in the room for deeply concerned significant others?

Patients (and Staff) do the Darndest Things*

POLLY GERBER ZIMMERMANN, R.N., M.S., M.B.A., C.E.N.
MARK JONES, R.N.

Interspersed with emergency nursing's excitement and tedium are the unusual episodes that either make us smile or shake our heads. A few examples:

"What's the problem today?"

This basic triage question often yields interesting answers. A woman arrived at 3 AM with an initial report that, "My neck is too thick."

"How long has that been going on?"

"Since I was born."

This is reminiscent of the time a man came at 1 AM to check the cough he had since, "I was in the service in '45."

"Why did you come in *today?*"

"It didn't go away and I thought, 'it's time to get this checked out.'"

The time lapse problem also surfaced when a parent brought in a child for a high fever.

"When did you last give something for fever?"

"I'm not sure. I *think* it was 6 months ago."

Information calls

The barrage of phone calls asking questions frequently reflects current news stories. The outbreak of rat bites on a western U.S. Indian reservation prompted one Chicago mother to call and ask if her children would contract it because they were one-eighth American Indian.

Night shift staff members often receive the more unusual advice calls. One man wanted to know what to do for the burning sensation on his penis after applying Ben-Gay ointment.* He had sought relief from his aching penis after extensive sexual activity.

*Reproduced from Journal of Emergency Nursing, ©1996; 22(3):66A–67A with permission from Mosby-Year Book, Inc. Edited from the original.

*Ben-Gay is a trade name of Pfizer, Inc., New York, New York. No endorsement of this product is implied.

Incoming phone reports are another source of ED oddities. One long-term care facility, reputed to do anything to avoid acknowledging that a patient died in their facility, called in:

"We're sending in a resident for evaluation."

"What are the vital signs?"

"Well, currently he has no pulse, respirations, or blood pressure."

Accurate information

All know the extent of incorrect information provided by patients. One creative individual actually gave the local zoo as his phone number. A newly hired registrar entered the patient's literal response, "I live in the streets," as his address instead of the computer-recognized code of "undomicile." For three mailing cycles, a bill was dutifully sent out, addressed to:

Crazy Bill Johnson
"I live in the streets"
Chicago, Illinois

and returned by the post office each time as "addressee unknown."

Discharge miracle

A discharge stop at the cashier window to finalize billing information tries to deal with such billing problems. One discharged ED patient could barely move or stand and requested an obviously needed wheelchair. As he neared the cashier window by the exit door, however, he looked around and then a "miracle" happened. He leaped from the wheelchair and bolted through the door—hence the term *financial incentive*.

Frequent flyers

It is always a telltale sign when patients walk in and all staff members automatically know their names. Staff joke about seeing them more often than they see their own relatives.

Some of my most memorable people over the years include:

• Eileen,* who wears goggles and appears like clockwork every day to request an eye examination to rule out foreign bodies. She would then sit for hours, patient watching, which came close to a spectator sport for her.

• "Mad Dog" Bade, a street resident, who thought-

fully brought flowers for the nurses, which he carefully selected and picked from the professionally manicured gardens in local city parks.

• Enit, an elderly man who ate daily in the cafeteria and took the time to stop at the ED nurses station to sing an impromptu little tune.

• Claude, who would offer a token of his gratitude by giving the nurse a choice of the "treasures" he found in the trash that day (an empty pretty jar, a dry pen).

• Bertha, who always called 911 for an asthma attack after a fight with her daughter ("See what she does to me!"), but not until she carefully applied her makeup. She thoughtfully tried to minimize the "bother" by walking to the street corner to meet the paramedics.

• Lollie, a stylishly groomed woman, who nonchalantly changed her birth date every year. She literally remained 65 in our computer for 3 years running.

Believe it or not

"The husband" came to the emergency department in full cardiac arrest. "The wife," notified at work only that her husband was in the emergency department, walks in unprepared for the gravity of his condition. Finding her husband in the middle of the code, she immediately collapses to the floor in full cardiac arrest herself. There is a twist. He survives; she does not.

Then there was the time one woman became aware of her husband's long-kept secret when she came home to find him dead from an apparent heart attack . . . dressed in her underwear.

Do you understand?

Instructions given but not correctly understood or carried out frequently serve as an interesting reminder to never assume anything.

A teenager who recently started to use oral contraceptives came to the emergency department with lower abdominal pain. When the pelvic examination was performed, a large "glob" of white matter was found. You guessed it: she had been faithfully inserting the pill vaginally. In the same vein, a young man with a urinary tract infection called to say he was having trouble inserting the prescribed sulfamethoxazole (Bactrim) into his urethra.

A young teenager was pregnant despite swearing her boyfriend always used condoms. After more in-depth discussion, it became apparent that the couple was ap-

*All names are pseudonyms.

plying the condoms not to his penis but his thumb, just as demonstrated in their sex education class.

And concerning sexual behaviors . . .

Perhaps the unusual is most evident in other "adventuresome" sexual activities. Universal stories about objects inserted in bodily orifices abound. Some involve everyday household objects: shampoo bottle, wine glass, cherry tomatoes, and olive jar with the olives still in it. The normalcy of the objects is exceeded only by the patient's casual attempts to explain the mechanism of injury as a normal accident. "I must have slipped and fallen on it."

The "nothing unusual here" approach was also taken by the man who called 911 at 3 PM to report that his "friend" had just had a seizure. The paramedics found them in a hotel parking lot. The miniskirted, heavily madeup woman was unconscious in a kneeling position on the front seat floorboards; the flushed man's disheveled clothing featured an open pants zipper. He could not remember his "close friend's" name or age. Our conclusion about the circumstances seemed confirmed when he fled the scene as the police arrived.

Another incident involved the stuck vibrator that kept turning itself on and off with every position change of the patient. All the staff could hear coming down the hall was an intermittent buzzing that became louder and louder. The buzzing "peaked" as it was removed and placed on a metal stand. "Turn that thing off!" the male doctor barked. The female nurses all stood back; no one wanted to appear that they knew how to operate it.

Stories also become funnier afterward because of staff comments. An unpeeled potato removed from a patient's rectum became great "raw material":

"What happened to the potato?"

"It's in pathology; they're mashing it."

And who but an emergency nurse could create this party game? One emergency nurse made a copy of an x-ray film showing an inserted unopened beer bottle and had staff guess the brand for a prize at the Christmas party.

Not quite with the program

One known schizophrenic patient would be found wandering around our department. Wearing a purchased white lab coat, he would stand at the ambulance entrance. He would authoritatively direct all incoming traffic, from patients with sprained ankles to empty stretchers, "Go straight to the OR, they're waiting for you!"

But he made the eternal hall of fame in our minds when he walked up to a patient sitting in the waiting room, calmly looking him in the eye and asked in a most therapeutic tone, "Can I help you? I'm God."

In 1 month three different grandiose delusional patients each believed he was "God." This was the capstone of religious "visitations" for our department. The brand-new registrar mistakenly entered one patient's name just as he claimed, "Jesus Christ." The staff eagerly notified public relations that we had a VIP patient. One nurse suggested we call pastoral care to inform them that their boss was doing a site visit. Another nurse asked the agnostic emergency physician how it felt to meet someone whose existence he had denied for so long.

One of our "Jesus Christ" patients became agitated when a name band bearing "John Doe" was placed on his arm. "That's not my name!" he screamed as he started pacing. After one nurse quietly whispered something to him, however, he winked and immediately became quiet. The nurse who whispered to the patient revealed his strategy: "I told him that I knew he was 'Jesus Christ,' but that we had to give him this name because we had some unbelievers here." All the funnier because the physician was a yarmulke-wearing Orthodox Jew.

It's a strange world

These incidents are passed down and kept alive through an emergency department's oral tradition, proving once again that truth is stranger and funnier than fiction. Patients not only say the darndest things, they *do* them.

Patients (and Staff)
Still do the Darndest Things*

POLLY GERBER ZIMMERMANN, R.N., M.S., M.B.A., C.E.N.
MARK JONES, R.N., C.E.N.

Emergency departments are the arenas for health care's unexpected and quirky occurrences. While remaining empathetic to a patient's need, the ED health care worker also detaches enough to appreciate the humor, irony, or bizarre nature of the situation.

Triage

"What brought you in today?" is always a key question to discern the acuity and condition of the patient. One wife shared the subtle clue she discerned about her husband's behavior. "I knew something was wrong when he started to bring in, rather than take out, the garbage." Another related she knew there was a problem when her husband with chronic obstructive pulmonary disease insisted on wearing his nasal cannula prongs in his ear.

Sometimes the familiar questions evoke a surprise response.

"Date of birth?" the psychiatric patient was asked.

"I don't have a birthdate. I'm from the planet Zenon and we're hatched."

Another routinely asked question is, "Do you have an attending doctor?" One frequent ED patient replied, "Of course! I come here every time I need one."

Patients with respiratory conditions are frequently asked the follow-up question, "Do you smoke?"

"I used to," replied the wheezing patient, "but I quit."

"Good for you!" exclaimed the nurse. "When did you quit?"

"Today."

Registration

One wealthy VIP frequent patient had a widespread reputation for his arrogant attitude. When asked his name and birthdate on coming to the emergency department, the man rudely snarled, "You ought to know who I am. They named the whole darned building af-

ter me!", referring to the major hospital wing called the _____ Pavilion. He did, that is, until one registrar responded, "Oh, OK, Mr. Pavilion. I just need to verify your current address."

The patient was pronounced dead by the emergency physician, but the funeral director left before the paperwork was complete. Needing to finish the forms, the registrar chose the options of "refuses to answer" for religion and "unable to sign due to condition" for consent.

But that is nothing compared with the bureaucratic confusion concerning one patient who left without a proper discharge. He was brought by the funeral director to the emergency department for a death pronouncement, but subsequently was taken to another hospital by the funeral director because of the supposed wait at the first institution. So now the quality improvement records show that there was a dead patient who registered but left without being seen (LWBS).

Our drug "reps"

Drug seeking is a well-established pattern among some of our clientele. These people typically have "incapacitating" pain that can only be assessed subjectively with, "regrettably," so many allergies to everything but narcotics. And, by the way, the doctor who usually prescribes their narcotics just happens to be out of town. The extent that this is presented as normal and believable is bemusing to the experienced nurse, who easily pierces the facade.

Some drug-seeking patients become more aggressive in their quest. One patient screamed at the physician who refused his request, "This is malpractice! I want your name and DEA number!" Another took to literary skills, changing his prescription for "Tylenol #3 (three), dispense 4 (four)" to "Tylenol #5 (five), dispense 40 (four)ty." The prize for the best forgery at-

*Reproduced from Journal of Emergency Nursing, ©1996; 22(6):39A–40A with permission from Mosby-Year Book, Inc. Edited from the original.

tempt, however, goes to the pharmacist-flagged prescription that literally read "Morfin (morphine), 1 pound."

What we have here, I think, is a failure to communicate

ED health care workers develop a jargon and sometimes forget the patient may perceive a different meaning. For instance, one nurse announces a new patient with a febrile seizure as a "shake and bake." Then, there's the common experience of informing the patient he or she has a fracture, only to be asked, "But, is it broken?"

The German psychotic patient needed medical clearance before placement. "Does anything hurt?" the nurse asked in a rote manner. "Yah," the patient replied. "I have to go to the bathroom and I was told I hauft to wait a minute. *That* (placing his hand on his heart and hanging his head) *hurts* me."

One couple kind of appeared out of nowhere and began asking the nurse detailed personal questions about the Yugoslavian patient's condition. Finally, the nurse stopped to inquire, "How did you say you are related to Mr. Kutlesig?"

"Oh, we're not relatives. We're here visiting someone else. But we're from Yugoslavia, too!"

The elderly patient was not able to hear the physician speaking or read his written communication. "This isn't working!" he states. "Get a sign language interpreter." Activating the on-call system, one finally arrived 90 minutes later. As she began the gestures of sign language, however, the patient looked at the nurse and exclaimed, "What in the world is that lady doing?" No one had clarified that she did not know sign language.

There was the psychiatric patient who was escorted to the single-room department bathroom. The nurse waited outside the locked door, but then realized it had been very quiet for a long time.

"Are you OK?" she asked while knocking.

Dead silence.

Her voice rose with concern. "Is something wrong?" Silence.

When her continued pounding and calling brought no response, she feared the worst. A key could not be located, and engineering was paged stat. Finally, after 10 minutes of noisy work, the bathroom door was removed. There was the patient, sitting serenely on the toilet, looking at the door.

"Why didn't you open the door?!" the nurse demanded, feeling both relief and anger.

"You never asked me to *open* the door," the patient replied matter of factly.

But the most frustrated individual in miscommunication was probably the psychiatric patient who walked up to the nurse, holding the phone he had literally ripped out of the wall. "This phone needs to be fixed," he announced with exasperation. "I cannot reach the commander of the CIA on Internet!"

Prisoners

Then, there are the just-arrested criminals who decide to postpone seeking treatment for their "chest pain" until after they commit a robbery and are arrested. (They wanted to be able to pay cash?) The desire to avoid the inevitable jail is especially evident when the symptoms keep growing. One prisoner was able to come up with eight medical complaints by the time his triage session was over, including chest pain, low back pain, headache, urinary burning, penile drainage, constipation, ear pain, and an ulcer "acting up." And the police had just brought him in to have his laceration sutured.

CHAOS AND COMPLIANCE

Who are the patients and why are they here?

Patients are everyone, regardless of race, color, sex, religion, age, disability, marital status, sexual orientation, or national origin. The sick person is seeking solutions to the universal problems and experiences of illness. Dual challenges for all patients seeking quality, holistic nursing care are to wish to recover and to cooperate with treatment.

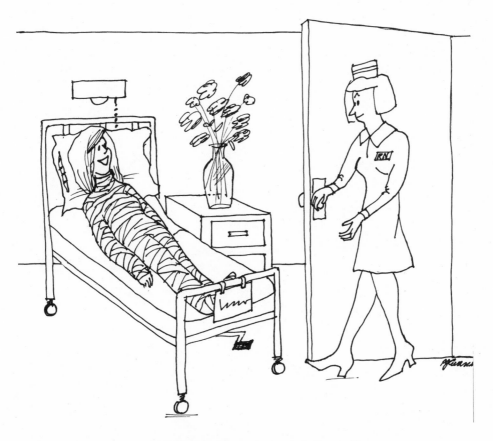

"Can you give me a sponge bath now?"

A Grammatical Overview of Medical Records: The Write Stuff*

COREY D. FOX, PH.D.

The following quotes were lifted verbatim from the medical records of a general hospital in a large metropolitan area.

"Patient suffers from headaches while menstruating on the top of her head."

"There is a pressure bandage on the hip which is markedly swollen and tender."

"Patient is a newborn infant delivered over an intact perineum which cried spontaneously."

"Patient experiences difficulty swallowing tires easily."

"Patient had bronchoscopy today. Exam showed normal bowel to 25 cm."

"History: Patient was shot in head with .32 caliber rifle. Chief Complaint: Headache."

"Patient has difficulty walking on Digitalis."

"Patient had a D&C a year ago and all of her eyebrows came off."

"Patient referred to hospital for repair of hernia by a social service worker."

"Patient sent to hospital for erosion of the cervix by a local medical doctor."

Dictated: "Patient had a Pap smear today." Transcribed: "Patient had a Pabst Beer today."

"This was a nonsterile delivery by the nurse in the bed of a five pound male infant."

"Patient was struck by an auto while she was walking across the street at approximately 45 miles per hour."

"Patient complains of worsening acne and itching rash as well as nasal congestion of his trunk."

"Patient referred to hospital by private physician with green stools."

"This 54-year-old female is complaining of abdominal cramps with BM's on the one hand and constipation on the other."

"This mother of a 2-year-old desires a circumcision."

"Patient has been married twice, but denies any other serious illnesses."

"Patient's wife hit him over the head with an ironing board which now has six stitches on it."

"Patient is separated from his wife, and he also is allergic to Penicillin."

"This 8-year-old came to the GU clinic with his mother who has an absent right testicle since birth."

"Patient has no children and she doesn't smoke or drink either."

"She moves her bowels roughly, three times a day."

"This GU patient states he urinates around the clock every two hours."

[Male patient] "Pelvic exam: Deferred."

"Rx: Mycostatin vaginal suppositories, #24, Sig: Insert daily until exhausted."

Who Needs Money?*

STEVEN PACK, R.M.N.

If I could get back all the money I have lent to psychiatric patients over the five years I have been working in nursing I would probably have enough to retire on. Well, at least enough to spend a constructive afternoon care planning in the staff association club.

I do not know if other psychiatric nurses have had the same experience, but most of my patients seem permanently broke, out of cigarettes or both.

Being 6ft 3ins tall and weighing 16 stone, I cut quite an imposing figure but as I have always been receptive to my patients' needs I am regarded as a soft touch.

Now, don't get me wrong. I don't just go handing my hard-earned money over to patients on request, but I find it difficult to ignore a plea for some loose change for the payphone or a quid or two for some fags, especially if I know the person is broke. Why do I do it? Picture the scenario: a patient, having tried unsuccessfully to obtain money from fellow patients, comes to me for a loan. He thinks (I hope) that I am a great guy for helping him out. I feel happy because I have shown compassion for his needs, and I've been promised faithfully that as soon as his giro cheque comes through I'll be paid back.

Failing this, the coming weekend is the one and only in the year on which the patient's relatives visit, and they always bring loads of money.

So the deal is clinched, hands are shaken and everyone is happy. The difficulty comes in recovering my assets.

When reminded of the loan, most patients appear to experience short-term memory loss or they are up to their eyeballs in debt with the charge nurse and he takes preference over me.

When I was two months into my nurse training I escorted four patients into town on a Saturday afternoon.

Very soon they were all complaining of severe hunger so I took them to a big department store restaurant. Having dutifully queued up and purchased my sausages, chips and beans and fought my way through the shoppers to a table, I heard my name being called by one of the patients, who had just reached the cash desk. Surprise, surprise, having piled on a huge mountain of food, he had no money. With a frustrated queue behind him and all eyes on me awaiting my reaction, I approached the cashier. Needless to say, four-and-a-half years later I am still owed the money.

Later in my training I worked in a long-stay ward and struck up a good rapport with a loveable rogue of a patient. While helping him do his washing I discovered that he possessed only one pair of underpants. I explained his predicament to my wife, who promptly sorted out several pairs of my underpants for him.

Having discreetly presented them to him and been thanked profusely for my kindness, I discovered a few days later that he had sold them to other patients in the ward and spent the money on cigarettes.

Still, it hasn't been all doom and gloom. There have been numerous occasions on which a patient's generosity to me has surpassed my expectations. I once struck up a relationship with a patient in a medium secure unit. As he had 'parole' to walk the hospital grounds, we used to wander over to the general hospital canteen for a pot of tea and biscuits.

Initially I always paid as I felt this was expected, but very soon, on his suggestion, we took it in turns on alternate weeks.

I was flat broke (and still am) but my patient was even poorer than me, so there we would sit, surveying the kingdom of the hospital 'Ritz', drinking tea and munching biscuits, and very nice it was too.

*Reprinted from Nursing Times, ©1996; 92(41):201 with permission from Macmillan Magazines, Ltd.

Battle Hymn at Bathtime*

MARY FERGUSON, R.N.

Mine eyes have seen the contents of the linen closet go.
All my patients are left sheetless for I moved a bit too slow.
And since their beds are dampish this will really be a blow.
So I'll go searching on.

I have scrounged around the dresser drawers of every empty room.
I have stretched to scan the closet shelves so full of dust and gloom.
I have peeked into the cupboard where we always store the broom.
The blasted stuff's all gone.

So it looks as if to make their beds I'll have to improvise.
At least until the laundry cart appears with fresh supplies.
But that's why nurses pray each night that God will make them wise
To grab the sheets at dawn.

*Reprinted with permission from American Journal of Nursing, ©1965; 65(6):198.

A Little Medical Madness (According to U.S. Newspapers)*

WILLIAM BURMESTER

I am not in the medical profession; however, my great-grandfather was a general practitioner and I have a cousin who was a corpsman in World War II. So you see, I do have strong ties to the health field.

I am an avid newspaper reader and because of my special interest in health care, I have been clipping articles concerning unusual medical happenings. Some of the stories I have collected left me curious as to how individual cases may have been handled. For instance, just how was the patient of this accident treated? I've never heard, but according to the article, here is what happened:

"... *Mrs. Frances Blanc, 45, of Maple Street, escaped injury when her* can *went out of control and hit a parked station wagon at 12:01 a.m. today at the corner of Fifth and Main."*

Then some years ago the New Castle (Pa.) News reported another puzzling automotive mishap:

"Firemen from Central Department were called to Jefferson and Grant Street where a parked couple *was found smouldering about the floor boards."*

An Ohio woman was reported to have suffered some ill effects from an unusual accident which happened out in a rural area:

"... she was looking back to see if there was any traf-

*Reprinted from Emergency: The Paramedic's Magazine, ©1985; 17(2):18, 20, 22 with permission from Bobit Publishing, Torrance, CA.

CHAOS AND COMPLIANCE

fic coming, in order to cross the road and started to walk when the car of Leo Blank of Lame County knocked her up *on the bridge.*"

In my collection of dubious diagnoses, I have the story of an accident which may have required the services of either a doctor, plumber or mechanic; you decide:

". . . Mrs. Malone is in fair condition at Butler County Hospital with a fractured hose *and ribs which she suffered in the collision."*

Although the diagnosis is dubious in many such stories, the prognosis is puzzling in many others. In Scranton, Pa. nonmedical persons undoubtedly questioned the wisdom of the local physician when they read:

"Prompt action of a physician probably saved the life of Warren Tretheway, 2-year-old son of Mrs. and Mrs. Tretheway of Scranton yesterday, when the child swallowed a quantity of lye, which his mother was using in cleaning household articles. The boy's mouth was badly burned up and sold as junk."

I must admit I have some serious reservations about the staff of another hospital for this bit of hanky-panky:

"Cleora Smith suffered a broken leg in the collision. She was taken to Riverside Hospital where her arm *was treated and put in a cast after which she was sent home."*

Of course many baseball fans will recall the day when Yogi Berra was struck in the head with a fast ball. According to one newspaper account of the event:

". . . Berra was rushed to Ford Hospital. X-ray pictures of the popular baseball figure's head showed nothing."

We are not really sure about this one either:

"Mr. and Mrs. Jerome Smith and children left Sunday for Wichita, where they will take treatments for his ears, and the family will enjoy the show."

And there are probably those who may have considered this treatment a bit harsh:

"Both men were examined by veterinaries and immediately shot by Humane Society officers."

Occasionally we run across advice offered by specialists which we find something less than profound.

Like the advice that some "do-gooder" gave mothers in a popular medical column:

"When the baby is done drinking, it should be unscrewed and laid in a cool place under a tap. If the baby does not thrive on fresh milk, it should be boiled." . . . Really!

And just picture this bit of fiendish advice, if you can:

"To remove coffee stains, place stained part over a bowel and pour boiling water into it from a height."

For this bit of information, all the baldies of the world can probably feel eternally grateful. I found it under a garden column, but I presume it was written by a scalp specialist:

"Baldness may be caused for many reasons: a local attack of disease, shallow soil (a rock present underneath the sod) cinch bugs or the doings of a dog."

And you can imagine the consequences of an action such as this:

"Possibly the worst thing that could happen to a voodoo believer is for the leader to put a nurse *on* him."

A "Dear Abby" column as published in one newspaper offered advice which Abby was forwarding from a prominent psychiatrist:

"Police records show that almost every sex offender has had an early record of "peeping." While "peeing" itself may not be a serious crime, it is only fair to society to let the police know who these offenders are. Wives and families cannot always be depended upon to get the sick person to the psychiatrist in time."

In my efforts to better understand the health profession, I have happened upon some startling and unusual happenings. For example, consider the reaction this prominent actress got after a visit to her plastic surgeon:

". . . She returned to Hollywood last week, called her friends to a party and unveiled the new nose. Her guests toasted it."

And look what happened when an English teacher tried to practice medicine:

"She upended the child and shook him in a vain effort to dislodge the participle."

And a vote of shame to the doctor who took part in this orgy as depicted in a newspaper headline:

"Blind Woman Donates Eyes To Blood Bank."

In 1981, Pennsylvania readers were startled to read:

"Nation's First Test-Bube *Baby Due In January."*

I would also like to ask how the medical profession responded when confronted with this tally of suicide methods used in one year in one area of the country:

"Poison, 50; poison gas, 29; hanging, 185; drowning, 30; firearms, 124; cutting or piercing instruments, 18; jumping from high prices, 7."

I also found that some hospitals go to unnatural extremes to avoid labor trouble:

"An execution session of the hospital board was called last night when news of the union's contract rejection was revealed."

Finally, my reading has led me to the words of many people who are grateful for favors received from health care people in their time of need. I would like to share some of the little homilies which are made public as "Cards of Thanks" in local newspapers throughout the country; for example:

". . . and in addition to all those very fine people who looked after me in St. Joseph's Hospital, I also wish to thank the many kind ladies of the church who took care of my husband while I was sick."

And another:

"We wish to express our appreciation and thanks to all those who helped in the illness and death of our husband, father and brother, George W. Jones. We especially want to thank the doctors and nurses at general hospital."

A dear lady in Iowa probably said it best, as she echoed the sentiments of patients the world over, summing it all up in but a few words:

"I would like to take this opportunity to thank all the many kind friends for their thoughts of me during my illness. Tomorrow I am scheduled for major surgery. Dr. Blank and Dr. Jones are my physicians, so you see I do need your prayers."

Keep up the good work doctors . . . we'll be reading about you!

My Glove Is Quick*

EVETTE GRINS, R.N.

The clamor of the phone drilled through my skull and dragged me awake. My mouth felt like it was filled with the gauze packing I'd pulled out of the lanced abscess on my last patient's butt.

I squinted at the clock. Eleven AM. The phone was still ringing, my head was pounding and I figured I might as well get up. I picked up the receiver. A cool, businesslike voice asked if I was Tess Tosterone, if I was a private RN for hire, and if I'd be interested in picking up a few bucks on an easy case.

"Yeah, yeah, yeah," I said. I didn't really want to take on a new case right then, but I needed the money—the bills on my table were piling up faster than the dust on the dishes in my sink. I scribbled the information on the back of an old patient ed sheet and mumbled something about being over there in an hour.

I showered and put on my last clean uniform. The jar of instant coffee was as empty as my bank account, so I just chewed up some coffee beans and swished the gritty stuff down with boiling water. Nursing isn't for sissies.

I headed out, feeling almost human. But questions about the case were starting to bother me—especially when I got to the address I'd been given. It was a stone mansion that screamed of big money. I walked up the driveway and all I could think was, "WHY?" Why

*Reprinted with permission from Journal of Nursing Jocularity, ©1994; 5(4):6–8.

would someone this rich, who could afford a whole staff of flunkies-in-white, want to hire a hard-bitten loner like me? There was only one possible answer—the job would be dirty. I didn't know just how dirty, but it didn't matter. In this racket, you learn to take the cases as they come.

I rang the bell and a for-real butler showed me in and left me in a hallway where each marble tile must have cost more than I earned in a year. A few minutes later, six feet of trimly built, blow-dried manhood came down the curved stairway, and suddenly my body told me how long it had been since I'd had something hard inside me that wasn't a speculum. "Hi, gorgeous," I said, trying not to leer too much.

He said, "Miss Tosterone?" His voice sent little ripples of excitement up and down my spine.

"Call me Tess, sweetheart," I cooed in my huskiest tone. "And what do people call you when they want you real bad?"

"Bert Hansom."

"You sure are, honey," I murmured appreciatively. "Are you the one who phoned?"

"No, that was Ernie, my partner."

"And are you the patient?"

"Oh, no!" he laughed.

"Too bad," I said. "I could really take care of you."

"The patient is upstairs," he coughed. "Come with me, please."

"I just might, Bert," I said meaningfully. "But let's take care of business first, okay?" I followed him upstairs and finally got a look at my patient—suddenly I knew just how big the stakes were in this case. There on the bed was Donald F. Rump himself, America's premier corporate raider, supposed to be worth better than a million bucks for each of his 400-plus pounds. He lay there like a whale out of water, gasping and in pain.

Sitting by the bedside was a slightly healthier-looking version of the patient. Maybe 300 pounds, sweaty and unshaven, but breathing normally. He stood up and greeted me.

"Miss Tosterone, I presume? I'm Ernest Rump. I called you in to take care of my brother, Donald."

Something about the way Bert went over and took Ernie's hand and held it against his cheek told me that I wouldn't be dancing the silk-sheet samba with Bert after all.

"What's the diagnosis, Rump?" I snapped.

Ernie looked at me carefully before answering. "I don't suppose I need to inform you that this matter is highly confidential."

I managed to stop myself from slamming him up against the wall. Instead, I just said, "You already know

the answer to that one, Rump. You called me in because you heard I'm a pro. So I have to figure it's something big, something so big your regular staff couldn't handle it. Now suppose we quit wasting time. Just lay it out for me."

"Tell her, Ernie," Bert urged. "I think we can trust her."

"All right. As you see, my brother is in considerable pain. The doctors say he's badly—uh—impacted, and they want to operate to relieve what they have called an intestinal obstruction. But we'd prefer to take care of this little problem without hospitalization. Can you help?"

I gave the patient a quick but skillful abdominal exam. He had increased bowel sounds but no rebound tenderness. I looked back at Ernie. "How long has he been in this way?" I gritted.

"His last—uh—number two was over a week ago."

"And what have you done about it so far?"

"Well, we gave him some Ex-Lax, but . . ."

Something inside me finally snapped. I grabbed his shirtfront and shoved my nose in an inch from his face.

"Listen, Rump," I hissed. "You ever so much as look at a box of Ex-Lax again and I'll tie your arms into a knot around your neck, you hear me?"

"Ooh!" exclaimed Bert. "Could you show me that?"

Ernie struggled to get loose, then yelped, "I hear you. Please, let me go!"

I released him. He fell into a chair, then tried to regain his composure as I grilled him about his brother's diet. I wasn't surprised to hear that Donald Rump lived on rich foods—high-fat meats and refined sugar, but almost no fresh fruits and vegetables. I also wasn't surprised to hear that the doctors who had seen the patient hadn't asked any questions about his diet. Typical.

"Can you help?" Ernie asked anxiously.

"Yeah, Ernie, I can handle this." I told him how much I charge.

He looked surprised. "That's all?"

"That's all. You see, unlike your brother here, some people just want to make a fair living for their work. But I guess you wouldn't understand that." Donald Rump groaned loudly, and I wondered if what I'd said had gotten to him.

"What are you going to do?" Bert Hansom asked me.

I opened my case and took out a bunch of Chux, a basin, fresh gloves, an enema set, and my institutional-size tube of K-Y jelly. "You don't want to know," I grunted.

"Oooooohh!" swooned Bert. "Could you show me that?"

I chased Bert and Ernie out of the room and got to work. From his moans and groans, I guessed Donald Rump wasn't enjoying it any more than I was. But I did what had to be done. That's what they pay me for. Then I helped the patient walk to the bathroom to finish the job. He took a while—he had a week's worth of it inside him. Meanwhile, I stuffed my gloves and the soiled Chux into a plastic bag.

Rump looked pale but relieved when he staggered out. I helped him back in bed. Then I washed up, but I knew it would take more than soap to make me feel clean again after this job. Finally, I let Bert and Ernie back in.

Ernie rushed to his brother's side. "Are you all right, Donald?" The patient nodded. Ernie turned to me. "I don't know how to thank you, Miss Tosterone."

"You want to thank me?" I growled. "Then get him on a proper diet. That goes for you, too, Bozo. Low-fat vegetarian, lots of fiber. Maybe the two of you can still

head off coronary artery disease, diabetes, cancer and a rerun of this situation. That's how you can thank me. That, and pay me."

I wrote out a report for the doctors, collected a check from Ernie and handed him a patient ed sheet on diet and nutrition. Then I got out of there. Back out onto the streets, into what passes for fresh air in the city. The rain was coming down hard, but I didn't mind. I figured it might wash away the stench of the Rump brothers by the time I got home.

The dirty dishes were still marinating in my sink, but they'd have to wait. I took a long shower and tried to clear my mind for the next case. Maybe, for once, it would be something clean and easy. But somehow I doubted it.

Would You Mind Repeating That?*

JEANNETTE M. HILL, R.N., M.S., C.E.N.

Everyone needs humor. If you are a good listener, the people around you will provide some humorous moments. Be prepared to listen and enjoy.

Nurse: "Who is your doctor?"
Patient: "The one who is taking care of me."
Nurse: "How do you know that?"
Patient: "His name is on my name bracelet."

Patient: "I have a red bead in my ear."
Nurse: "How do you know there is a red bead in your ear?"
Patient: "I put it there."

Nurse: "What medications do you take?"
Patients:
- "I take latex every morning." (Lasix).
- "My doctor knows."
- "My wife knows." (Wife has no idea).
- "My husband has the list." (Husband left the list at home.)

- "I take three white pills every morning."
- "Nurse, that's a very good question. I take the medicines my doctor has prescribed."

Patient: "How long will this take? I have an appointment in 10 minutes."

Doctor: "You will need to be in a cast for 4 to 6 weeks."
Patient: "Forty-six weeks????"

Nurse: "Why did you come to the emergency department?"
Patients:
- "My doctor sent me."
- "I was in the area and thought I'd stop by."
- "I've been vomiking (vomiting)."
- "I've been to three other emergency rooms and they can't find anything wrong with me."
- "The other hospital wouldn't admit me."
- "You are here to help me."

*Reproduced from Journal of Emergency Nursing, ©1995; 21(5):45A with permission from Mosby-Year Book, Inc.

Nurse: "How long have your legs been swollen?"
Patients:

- "A long time."
- "Always."
- "Are they swollen?"

Nurse: "How do you feel?"
Patients:

- "Not 100%."
- "I feel fine."
- "I'm so sick, I could just die."
- "My wife knows."
- "I don't know."

Nurse: "How long have you been sick?"
Patients:

- "Forever."
- "Quite a while."
- "For days on end."
- "This episode started exactly 13 minutes ago."

Doctor: "What did your mother die from?"
Patient: "She died in her 90s."

Doctor: "What did your sister die from?"
Patient: "She died in her sleep."

Nurse: "Do you have pain?"
Patients:

- "I just feel thick in the head."
- "No pain, someone is standing on my chest."
- "No pain, I can't catch my breath."
- "No pain, my wrist is just dangling."
- "No pain, there's just this arrow sticking in my chest."
- "No pain, but you should see the other fellow."

Doctor: "You will either get better or you'll get worse."
Patient: "Then I'm not coming here anymore."

Visitor: "Could I borrow a wheelchair to take my friend to the fireworks? He's not supposed to walk."

Nurse: "Why did it take you so long (8 hours) to come to the emergency department after you fell and lacerated your head?"
Patient: "I had to wait for a ride. My friend was busy so I drank beer while I was waiting."

Statements by Patients:

- "I'm glad it's not broken, only fractured."
- "You never know what you might catch in a heavily wooded area."
- "I don't need help. I was just testing my Lifeline button (Lifeline Systems, Inc., Watertown, Massachusetts)."
- "My psychiatrist tells me I'm crazy."
- "My nose started to bleed after I was aggravated."
- "The blood was coming out like from a garden hose."
- "Could you feed me? I haven't eaten for 3 days."

At 10:30 PM, the person on the phone says, "Would you make an appointment with my physician for tomorrow morning?"

At 6 PM on a Saturday night, the person on the phone says, "I need my vasectomy reversed now."

After a nurse has spent 2½ hours caring for an elderly woman with acute congestive heart failure, her friend, who has been at the bedside, asks, "Will you be taking care of my friend until she gets a hospital room?"

A patient wishing to avoid a speeding ticket runs into the emergency department and asks, "Could the doctor write me a note stating I had to hurry here because I had a nosebleed?"

Another Troublesome Patient*

KATHLEEN HUDSON, R.N., B.S.N., M.I.C.N., C.E.N.

Really! The people we have to put up with! The shift began with a bang. As soon as I walked in the door, we got a call from Medic One stating that they were rolling to a motor vehicle crash, with an estimated time of arrival at 10 minutes. I waited . . . and waited . . . I did not want to get involved in anything lengthy. I knew that as soon as I did they would give us call.

An *hour* after the first call, they finally contacted us. They said they were at the scene of what appeared to be a major crash, but could not locate the vehicle or any victims. Some trees were down, scraps of lumber and debris were scattered around, and a dead animal lay on the road. It was too confusing for me. If they could not find victims, they were not bringing me any. I turned off the lights in the trauma room and went back to work.

While pondering that call, I answered the triage light. There stood this guy—a man covered with blood and mud, with twigs stuck in his hair. He was a real beauty. He told me that he had hurt his arm and had to see a doctor right away because he had to be in Santa Rosa in an hour. (Right. They all say that.)

I brought him immediately back into the department because he was obviously injured. For a mechanism of injury, he told me that he was flying low and hit a tree. (I've heard this before, too. Haven't we all?)

I brought him a gown and asked him to get un-dressed. You would have thought I was asking for his firstborn child. He initially refused, and I did my nursely best to convince him that it was necessary. In the midst of my pleas, he winked at me and then asked if I had been a good little girl. (Oh great, another one of *those*!)

I instantly became a cool professional and informed him that I would cut his clothes off if it was too painful to remove them otherwise. He then insisted on removing them himself, saying that they were the only set he had.

When he was finally undressed, my assessment found an obese elderly man with an open airway, rapid, shallow respirations, and tachycardia. He had oozing lacerations to his head, right lower leg, and right forearm. Bleeding was controlled with direct pressure.

He was oriented to person and time, but unclear about place. His pupils were constricted, his face was flushed, and his nose was bulbous. He was restless and agitated, mumbling about comets and dashing somewhere. His attention span was short. He kept putting his finger alongside his nose and saying that he needed to be on his way. Was it a head injury? Was it just drug or alcohol intoxication? Maybe hypoxia? Hypoglycemia?

I put his chart up to be seen and recorded his name on the tracking board—Claus, S.

My Stiff Leg Matches My Cane!*

PAULA BUE, SHARON SIVERSTON, ANGIE MCBRIDE, BECKY IHLE, AND JEFF LUCEY

Stiff as a board, ugly as heck
I don't bend there anymore, oh well.
Turn my head! Lift my feet!
I'm too darn stiff to get on my feet.
Help! Help! There's three men in my bed!
Arthur-itis, Ben-Gay, and Charley Horse!

Snap, crackle, pop.
You don't know what I'm going through!
If only my heart would stop.
When it's cold and it's raining
I feel it the most; the burning,
the pain, I'm just an old post.
The toilet's too low! The paper too high.
I can't hit the pot no matter how hard I try!
So all you nurses, handle with care because
my bones will break and my skin will tear!

*Reprinted from Journal of Nursing Education, ©1993; 32(4):191 with permission from Slack, Inc.

A Rapid Screening Test for Neuropsychological Function*

ROBERT S. HOFFMAN, M.D.

Purpose: Rapid screening of medical and psychiatric patients for evidence of organic mental disorder. Requires 2 minutes and pencil.

Standardization: Norms generated by administration to 50 consecutive patrons of Doggie Diner, West Geary Branch, San Francisco.

Instructions: If patient is lying down, have him/her sit up, and vice versa. Remove all distractions from the room. Ask the following questions:

1. What was the closing bid for ITT common stock at 4 P.M. on February 12th?
2. What is the world indoor speed record for the 100 yard dash performed with dog sled and 10 huskies?
3. How many times did Hughlings Jackson divorce and remarry?
4. What starring role brought Wallace Beery to national prominence?
5. What makes this test different from all other tests?
6. Who was the inventor of the Unna Boot?
7. What is the pressure per square inch of Mount St. Helens in full eruption?
8. What was Freud's comment to Fliess regarding the unconscious symbolism of pistachio nuts?
9. Which color has the lowest frequency in the light spectrum, infrared or ultraviolet? And why is this?
10. How often does a Venezuelan armadillo change his/her protective coat?
11. What is the difference between a duck?
12. Why is it hotter in the summer than in the city?
13. Name all of Rula Lenska's professional acting credits excluding television commercials.

Scoring

Number Correct	Interpretation
11–13	Mensa membership recommended
7–10	Qualified to dine with William F. Buckley
3–6	Tune T.V. set to "Bowling For Dollars"
2	Dementia
1	Anencephaly, or 100% false transmitters in cortical neurons
0	Aberrant tonsils with neoplastic change have replaced entire brainstem

Patience, Patients*

ROBERTA GRAHAM POWALSKI, R.N.

Patient in the waiting room: "Have you forgotten me?"
(*Thought: "No, but I'm working on it."*)
Reply: "Now Mr. Whitehead, you know I can't forget you, you're one of my special friends."

Patient in the waiting room: "You called me. Is the doctor in?"
(*Thought: "No, he's not in. I'm going to treat you myself and give you a cut rate."*)
Reply: "Yes, he is. Sorry, we're running a little late."

Female patient: "Do you want me on the table?"
(*Thought: "Actually, I don't even want you, but the doctor made me call you."*)
Reply: "Yes ma'am. I'll have to drape you before the exam."

Male patient: "Do you want me to give you a specimen?"
(*Thought: "No, if I wanted one, I'd take the time to collect my own."*)
Reply: "Yes, sir. Start in one bottle and finish in the second one."

Patient: "Is the doctor delayed due to surgery?"
(*Thought: "No, he's playing golf, but he won't let me tell you that."*)
Reply: "I'm afraid so. You know emergencies don't make appointments."

Female patient: "Do I have to take off my panties?"
(*Thought: "No, let's just work around them and surprise the doctor."*)
Reply: "Yes ma'am. Just put your things over behind the screen and I'll put this sheet over you."

Patient: "Does the doctor want to see me in his office?"
(*Thought: "No, he wants to see you across the street at the donut shop because he's hungry."*)
Reply: "Oh, yes, but he's with another patient right now. I'll let you know when to go in."

Patient: "Do you want to see me again?"
(*Thought: "Not me—I didn't ask to see you in the first place."*)
Reply: "Yes, just stop at the front desk and the clerk will make another appointment for you."

*Reprinted from Today's OR Nurse, ©1984; 6(1):48 with permission from Slack, Inc.

LEARNING
TO LEARN

Learning to be an effective nurse is never a smooth road. By accepting that learning is real work, one can then begin to develop healthy habits for lifelong understanding. The purpose of learning is not only to acquire knowledge for immediate use, but also to serve as an incentive for continued growth.

Ability and resourcefulness in practice will depend upon an ever-expanding skill base. There can be no compromises along this pathway to becoming an accomplished practitioner.

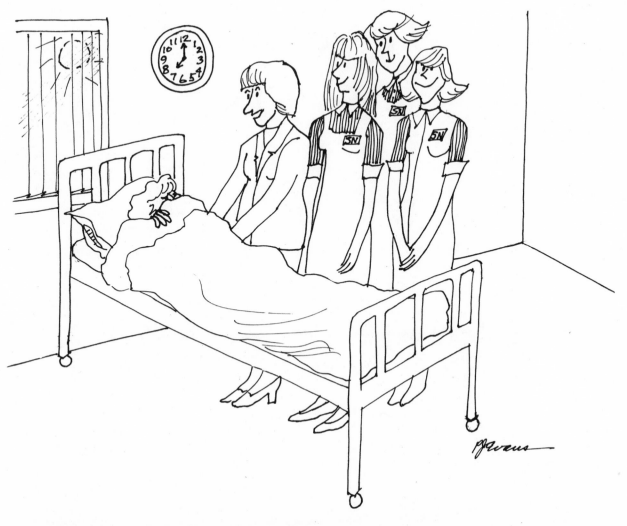

Mrs. Hyde, you're in ICU; no matter what, we'll see you.

Funny Things Happen
on the Way to Becoming a Nurse*

NORMA PETERS THOMAS, R.N., M.S.

For all her fumblings, the student nurse is truly the most unselfish of God's creatures. In an age when a young lady can choose from a variety of attractive careers, she chooses a career so demanding and so exhausting that I am constantly amazed that schools of nursing still recruit so well.

These are beautiful people, special people. I record a few of the many humorous things that happened during my years as a teacher not to laugh at students but with them—and to take you back to those frightening but fond years that we all remember. Perhaps my recollections may also help you show a bit more tolerance the next time you're with a student who puts her foot in her mouth.

I taught on a male unit. A person who has never been there cannot imagine the effect a 19-year-old girl has on a sick man. He perks up, he's fine, he's not sick, he protects the student right or wrong, he laughs heartily, he makes passes. The unit becomes a social affair with me the villain, constantly reminding the students that they are there to care for the sick, to learn procedures, to transfer classroom principles into hospital reality.

Picture a man turned on his side, buttock exposed, awaiting an injection from a student. Shakingly she grasps the syringe, looks to me for support, pauses for long minutes—then, before I can intervene, takes her index finger and tactually divides the buttock into quarters.

The man jumps, swears, and says, "What the hell's going on back there!" Or, more smoothly, "Having a good time, girls?" Add embarrassment to trauma.

Or, after all the above has taken place, the student says in a stage whisper: "I can't do it." My line: "Yes, you can." Hers: "No, I can't." With a dangerous gleam, I state: "Do it."

Speedier than sound, quicker than the eye, she jabs the needle into the skin, sighs with relief, and pulls it out. The patient didn't even feel it.

Rightly so, since in her quest for speed and skill she had forgotten something. "Would you mind injecting the medication this time around?" I stage-whisper through gritted teeth.

Two other notable injection boo-boos remain vividly in memory. A girl who has since become an excellent nurse was the most nervous student I ever had. I walked into a unit one day just in time to see her taking the patient's blood pressure—without a stethoscope. She was so nervous that when I'd watch her doing a dressing she'd have great difficulty holding the instruments in her shaking hands. I swear you could sing a song in time with the clanging of the instruments against each other.

Her first injection was something else. She couldn't seem to grasp the patient's skin in her shaking hand to give the needle. Good soul that I am, I removed her hand and held the patient's skin to make it easier. There followed a fantastically beautiful injection, right through the skin of my hand and into the patient!

Then there was the slow, hesitant student who tried everyone's patience. During her junior year, she was caring for an elderly stroke patient on a rubber air mattress, and she asked me to go with her to give an injection because she wasn't sure of the proper site. I was anything but happy, and it was a hot summer day, but in we went. She pointed to the area, and I nodded. Slowly she gave the injection. I couldn't believe how slowly she gave it, as though wishing to prolong the pain.

Angrily I snatched the syringe from her and said: "An I.M. should be given just as though throwing a dart. You need much more speed, much more wrist movement, like this."

Down darted the needle—and hissing air blew up in my face, as though to cool me off. Neither of us said a word. I quickly taped the hole in the mattress and called the supervisor. That day at noon a loud hissing sound permeated the cafeteria as I passed the students' tables.

Strange things also happen when student and doctor get in the act together.

We had a neurologist from Italy—Italian temper, accent, the whole thing. Instead of saying "Smile" to the patient so he could check facial symmetry, this doctor always said, "Show to me your teeth."

One day a lady did just that—took out her false teeth and showed them to him. He was so angry at the uncooperative patient that he began to bark out orders. Wanting to check the patient's writing ability, he told the student: "Give to me a piece of paper!" The quaking student dutifully tore the corner off a sheet of paper and handed it to the good doctor. Wow!

Scene: Doctor about to incise and drain a localized foot abscess. He works quickly, injecting 2% Novocain to anesthetize the area, and then picking up the scalpel.

Doctor: "Notice the inflamed area with its localized purulent center. I will incise the center, and by using antibiotics and soaks the affected area will begin to heal very nicely."

Student: "Does Novocain work so quickly?"

Doctor: "Huh?"

Student: "When I have a tooth filled, the dentist waits several minutes for the Novocain to take effect before he drills."

Doctor: "Oh." And proceeds.

Student: "That's O.K., Mr. Jones. Try not to think about it. Here, let me hold your hand. Maybe it won't take long. Try to hold still even when it hurts."

Doctor: "Good God! Let me have more Novocain and we'll do this right!"

So it goes, year after year. Wherever there are nursing students there are stories, some funny, some sad. But how caring, how sincerely concerned these young students are—yes, even today.

Practical Potpourri*

LINDSEY HALPERIN

Last summer I became a fool,
I decided to go to nursing school.
I thought that it would be so fun,
I counted the days one by one.
I went to the doctor and checked out just fine,
He gave me the shots seven, eight and nine.
The first day of class I felt kind of queasy,
Making friends here might not be so easy.
They gave me my schedule, told me what to wear,
What would happen if I was absent, even how to do my hair.
I thought, "I can do this, it will be a breeze."
Then they said "79 on a test will bring you all E's."
The panic set in, but determined as ever
I began all my classes, "I'll never fail. Never!"
The teachers, they lectured, and hard as I tried,
I couldn't keep up, I felt sick inside.
All these papers, these tests, how can I get through it
The instructors kept saying, "I know you can do it."
A good kick in the pants is just what I needed,
And a shoulder to cry on, then I proceeded.
Take one day at a time, hour by hour if I must
Maybe minute by minute, I just missed my bus.
I forgot the kids piano lessons, how to get them to the game,
The dinner with the Smith's, now, what was my name?
I know that I'm in here but can't see through the fog.
All these books and the readings, I'll just kick the dog.
The patients are grumpy, but once in a while
They'll look right up at me and give me a smile.
Now wait a minute here, this isn't so bad.
I just can't remember what made me so sad.
This nursing, that I thought was for the birds,
Is turning out to be too wonderful for words.
Another few months and school will be done
And the grandest prize I will have won.
I will have run hard and finished the race
And conquered my goal with poise and grace.
The friends I've made have been so true,
Are all by my side, they've made it too.
And on the day that I leave school
I'll realize that I'm no fool.

*Reprinted with permission from Journal of Practical Nursing, ©1991;
41(1):59.

I'm one of many with a desire to care,
To help, to heal, to take a dare.
The uniform I'll wear with pride
And know that God is on my side.
And so to nurses, your lives in route
With much respect, to you, I salute.

You can all become good students, a few may become great students, and now and again one of you will be found who does easily and well what others cannot do at all, or very badly.
— William Osler, *Aequanimitas,* 1904

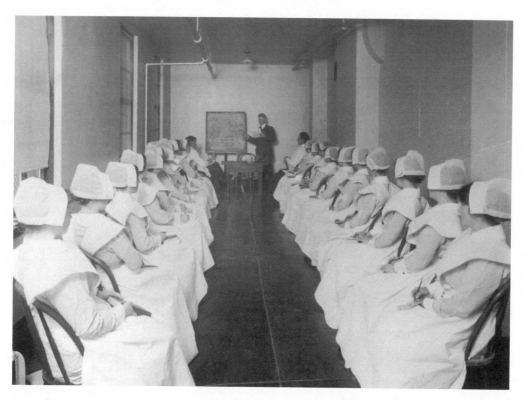

Lines of student nurses seated in nurses' lecture room; State Insane Hospital, Nebraska, 1914. Reprinted with permission from Nebraska State Historical Society.

My Most Humorous Moment in Nursing, Second Place Essay*

MERILYN D. FRANCIS

Nursing is a second profession for me, and there was no hesitation in my exchanging designer corporate suits for a simple yellow and white bibbed student nurse uniform. My feet were definitely happier being placed in cushioned sensible shoes rather than the high-heeled torture chambers they were accustomed to.

Autumn in my area of the country can feel like spring late into October. This particular day was clear and balmy, so I decided to take the Metro to my clinical rotation instead of fighting the city traffic. I would have a hearty walk to and from the train, and a chance to review some notes while someone else did the driving. My uniform was starched and pressed to a grandmother's standards and my shoes were whiter than sterile gauze. I looked professional and I felt professional.

During my fifteen-minute walk to the train station, I thought about how well school was going, how much I enjoyed the pediatric rotation, and how in another year I would be a nurse. My posture became more erect and my steps began to acquire a lilt as images of nurses I had worked with and read about crossed my mind. The idea that one day with hard work and dedication I too could become a part of this group of excellent women and men, put my imagination into overdrive. Thoughts of being part of a trauma team, or being a nurse on a transplant team, gently holding the hand of a dying patient or seeing the faces of parents holding their newborn for the first time, put a smile on my face. I thought of a nurse from England I had recently met and her mentioning the Queen Alexandra's Royal Nursing Corp. What a marvelous name! It evoked a flight of fancy which took me to the deck of a ship, with me dressed in white with a royal blue cape, sailing the seas looking for people to be nursed back to health. Even though I had descended to the dark station of the Metro, my outrageous daydreams were still shining. I was still sailing to exotic ports, my cape flapping in the wind.

"Excuse me. Excuse me, miss?" A scruffy man in his twenties interrupted my cerebral journey. I turned to him ready to blurt out proudly, "Yes, I am a nursing student," but waited for him, with a knowing smile, to ask the expected question.

"Miss, nice uniform. What hotel are you a housekeeper at?"

From then on, I drove.

*Reprinted with permission of the National Student Nurses' Association, Inc., Imprint Magazine, ©1993; 40(5):62.

Acing that Interview*

DAVID PAGE

For the past month, you have been receiving interview advice from your mother, your friends, and every teacher and mentor you have. List your strengths, they say. List your weaknesses. Be yourself. But the truth is, when it comes time for the interview, nothing helps.

By their very nature, job interviews make your heart tachy and your self-confidence drop to shock levels. To do well in an interview you need to do something different. Something irreverent, fun, feisty and foolish, like the advice I'm offering here. I can't guarantee any of this will get you a job, but it may make you laugh and relax—the thing you need most to ace that interview.

Piece of Advice 1 Interviewing is a lot like taking the National Registry exam; it is more about learning how to fulfill expectations than actually demonstrating your skills. So, long before your interview day, start practicing. Grab a friend, a classmate, the person next to you on the bus—anyone who will ask questions and look at you blankly—and put yourself in the hot seat.

Job interviewers always ask three basic questions: "Why do you want to work here?" "What do you have to offer?" and "Who are you?" With these questions, they are looking for more than just discovering whether you are a Ricky Rescue or a reformed ax murderer. They are looking to uncover your true potential as an employee. Practice constructing answers the interviewer would like to hear. Think of something flashy like, "Since I was 4 years old, I have had a deep interest in resuscitating my fellow man and have found your organization to embody the excellence and quality suitable for utilizing my superb medical skills." Really, it works.

Most interviews also include a scenario that asks you to respond as you would in a real emergency situation. These scenarios usually have no right or wrong answers. Instead, they evaluate your ability to walk through a tough situation, using good judgment. The answers are not as important as the process you use to reach them. The interviewer wants to be sure you are capable of making a decision based on good observation skills and that you can keep a cool head. To prepare, have your practice partner make up all kinds of bizarre emergency scenes, and then talk your way out of them.

Piece of Advice 2 Before the big day, drag out your favorite suit or dress—the one that makes you feel smart and confident. Get it cleaned, and take the Star of Life off the lapel. Dress up. That way, the interviewer cannot possibly imagine how awful you will look on a night shift with your hair sticking up and your shirt untucked. Be sure to wear loose, comfortable underwear. How you feel underneath makes all the difference.

Piece of Advice 3 The night before the interview, eat a sensible dinner and leave yourself plenty of time to run out to Kinko's to make extra copies of your résumé and certification cards. Stop by the video store, and rent one of those action movies in which the burly hero stands off a whole army of thugs. As you drift off to sleep watching the movie, imagine yourself as the hero and the interviewers as the thugs.

Piece of Advice 4 On the day of the interview, give yourself plenty of time to prepare. Consider sewing your zipper or buttons shut before you leave home. This eliminates the danger of walking around with your fly open or your dress undone. Do not drink any fluids before leaving home. This way, you will not need to remove clothing to use the toilet, saving any ripping prior to the big moment. You may suffer some slight dehydration as a side effect, which might make you feel a little off-balance, but your forehead and armpits will perspire less. Place a paper towel in your pocket or purse to take care of those sweaty palms.

*Reprinted with permission from JEMS: Journal of Emergency Medical Services, ©1995; 20(8):81–82, 84. Edited from the original.

Piece of Advice 5

Stop at your local 7-Eleven convenience store en route to the interview, and assemble an Interview First-Aid Kit. This includes breath mints, strong anti-perspirant (applied to forehead, palms and arm pits), Clearasil, Pepto Bismol, Alka-Seltzer, ChapStick and Beano (which the vegetarian underground considers the cure-all for bad flatus).

Piece of Advice 6

Your interview really begins when you arrive in the building lobby. Check out the scene carefully. Sagging furniture in the lobby is not a positive sign of organizational health, and you probably should begin searching beneath the cushions for lost change or scissors. These may be the only things you get to take away from this particular interview.

Check in with the receptionist, smiling at least twice. If she offers you doughnuts, don't be tempted. Eating at this time is fatal due to interview stomach-churn. Look interested; your interview isn't just occurring in front of the interview panel, there are secret cameras watching your every move.

Piece of Advice 7

The actual interview usually is conducted by a panel that includes a director, a supervisor, a field provider and, sometimes, a medical director. Sitting across the table from you, this panel can produce a heightened state of panic, but don't let yourself be intimidated. Imagine that everyone in the room has misplaced oral airways hanging from the corner of their mouths and traction splints on their arms.

As they begin to question you, do not be surprised if you feel as though you know more than the interviewer. But do not trust this feeling. Keep your answers simple, and even if the interviewer makes a stupid statement, do not say, "No . . . Bonehead, you are dead wrong," or

"Duh! Hello! Is anybody home?" And do not point out the jiggling piece of doughnut frosting on the medical director's mustache. A typical ego will not appreciate such helpfulness.

Piece of Advice 8

When you reach the end of the interview, turn the tables and ask a few questions of your own. This really impresses potential employers. Sit up straight, and act as if they are hoping you will consider working for them. Ask the interviewers about their patient care philosophies, their work schedules, and, just to throw them off, ask how their CQI program has developed during the past year.

Piece of Advice 9

Once the interview is over, shake everyone's hand—but not before using the paper towel you stowed in your pocket. Resist the urge to ask what you really want to know: "How many more candidates are you grilling today?" "When can I start?" or "Please, would you hire me—*right now*?"

Home Free

Head for the restroom. Your interview is not really over until you are safely in the nearest bathroom either throwing up or relieving yourself of copious amounts of diarrhea. Now is the time to give yourself a break. You have been through a traumatic experience, and you need CISD (crazy interview stress debriefing). Find a good friend and go bowling. Imagine the interviewers' faces on the pins. Then forget all about it, and do not sit at home by the phone.

The key to interviewing success lies within you. You are definitely a lot better at it than you think. Lighten up, and let yourself relax. Because the truth is, there really is no such thing as a perfect interview.

Memorizing the Cranial Nerves with a Funny Story*

JIM COMPTON, R.N., C.E.N.

The message from my old flame Lola was short and to the point. "I think it's my nerves, Johnny. The emergency nurse said something about 'cranial nerves' and you know how bad my nerves can get. She tried to explain but I got all confused. It was too hard to remember! I need you to help me, Johnny."

She wanted to meet me at our old hangout and give her the lowdown. My last A&P class seemed a long time ago. I only hoped that I could remember them myself. It wasn't going to be easy—remembering those cranial nerves, I mean. Or seeing Lola again, for that matter.

The *first* thing I sensed once inside *"The Ol' Factory* Tavern" was Lola's perfume. It was a unique scent, a *smell* quite easy to identify.

A *second* later I found her, two rooms over, in the *"Up-Tech* Lounge." Well, instantly I could see the writing on the wall, as clear as a hand held in front of my face. Simply put, I could see the light. "A confrontation is coming," I thought, as I glimpsed Lola's approach out of the corner of my eye. She came close, gradually looking deep into my eyes, looking through them as if to see what lay behind.

"Nice to see you too, Lola," I said evenly. "Where ya been stayin' while you're in town?" "The *Oculo-Motor* Inn," she purred. "*Third* floor. . . . Room #3." "Nice accommodations," I replied. Lola moved in close again, and my eyes narrowed reflexively. My *pupils constricted* in the light of her steady gaze.

"The place is packed tonight, Johnny. Look around." Lola motioned with a slender finger. I followed her lead, *looking around* in every direction, seeing little of interest, with two exceptions. Glancing *down* and to my *side*, on Table #4, I saw a cold bottle of mineral water waiting for me—*True Clear*, my favorite. And *looking straight sideways*, at Table #6, I spotted Lola's flashy boyfriend, a guy known to most as *Abe Ducens*. Now I'd seen it all.

"Nobody else in here can help me, Johnny," Lola said softly. "Only you." I put a fiver on the bar and thought about ordering up a *fifth* of rotgut. "Maybe Abe's boys can help you," I said. "*Try Jim an' Al,*" I hissed through *clenched teeth* and a *tightened jaw*. Lola *touched* my *face* lightly—on my *forehead*, my *cheek*, and my *jaw*—trying to calm me. Her touch *felt* soft and wispy, then *sharp* like a pinprick, as Abe got up and started to walk toward us.

I felt like giving him a facial—no *seven facials!* But I'm a nonviolent sorta guy so all of the action was in my face. I *forced* a smile that quickly became a *frown*. I *closed* my eyes tightly, puffed out my cheeks, and *blew* out a breath, all in an attempt to compose myself. The bartender gave me a sip of rotgut. The *taste* of it on the front of my tongue made my mouth water. My eyebrows *rose* in surprise and my *eyes* teared up. It was awful stuff.

As Abe came closer, I had a clear sense of being behind the *eight* ball, so I looked to protect myself. Behind the eight ball? Ah, *a cue stick.* "Put that down, Johnny, and be nice," Lola whispered to me, *first* in one *ear* and then in the other. "Abe and I are history," I heard her say. I couldn't believe what I was *hearing* and reeled at the news, *dizzy* and off balance.

"Sorry, Johnny, I thought you knew," Lola continued. "He left me for a showgirl. They're getting married on the *ninth* of next month. To my '*glossy-fair-angel,*' he says. Or, wait, maybe it's on the tenth. On the *tenth*, in *Vegas*, I think. I'm really not sure. Ninth or tenth—not much difference, I guess."

I felt like a fool. I took a sip of mineral water to buy some time. It *tasted bitter* on the back of my tongue, making my mouth water again. I swallowed hard and almost *gagged*. I managed to say a few simple words of apology to Lola as my heart rate and my blood pressure went down. "*Vegas,* huh?" I thought. "That's wandering unusually far away." I sensed something visceral going down through my chest to the pit of my stomach.

Maybe things were turning out all right, after all. A band came onstage (an *eleven*-piece punk outfit called "The *Spinal Accessories*") as Abe said goodbye and left with the showgirl. I *turned* my head toward their de-

*Reproduced from Journal of Emergency Nursing, ©1996; 22(3): 248–249 with permission from Mosby-Year Book, Inc.

parture and then *back* the other way toward Lola. "Are you all right?" she asked. I *shrugged* my shoulders and *pushed* my head forward to watch the band, trying to look unaffected, the way us guys do.

Lola laughed. "You're so silly, Johnny," she said. "Well, at least now we can talk about those horrible 'cranial nerves' . . . though I must say, they seem oddly more familiar now than when I first got here." Lola paused for a moment. "Except," she said slyly, "for the last one, the *'big hippo'* nerve."

"The what?" I said incredulously.

"You know, the last one, *#12*, the one they call the *'hippo-colossal'* nerve," she giggled, *sticking* her *tongue* out at me. I'd been set up!

"You know, Johnny," Lola said, laughing again, "While I was away, I became an RN like you. I only made up that story about my nerves to make sure you'd come and see me. Am I forgiven?"

I used my own "hippo-colossal" nerve to return her gesture in kind and we both laughed now. And we drank a gentle toast to old friends and those damnable cranial nerves.

My Most Humorous Moment in Nursing, Third Place Winner*

GAIL G. CLOWER

Each week on pre-clinical day, we receive our patient assignment and have the opportunity to prepare for clinical rotation by reading the patient file, checking the Kardex, reviewing laboratory reports, medication cards, the surgical schedule, and meeting our assigned patients.

My assigned patient was scheduled for surgery the following morning at 8:00 AM. I went to my patient's room to introduce myself and speak with him about his surgery. I did ask about his family and he mentioned his brother would be at the hospital in the morning to await the outcome of his surgery.

The following morning, I reported to clinical at 6:30 AM. As usual, I peeked in my patient's room and he was sleeping. After attending morning report and speaking with my co-assigned nurse, I went to check on my patient. It was 7:30 AM and I wanted to take vital signs before he left for surgery.

Upon entering my patient's room, I found him sitting up in a lounge chair, dressed in tan slacks and a short-sleeved shirt, and ready to eat from a breakfast tray on his lap. I immediately removed the breakfast tray, explaining that he could eat later but no food at all at this time. He looked at me with a confused expression. I asked if he had taken his morning shower. He replied that he had already bathed. I asked if he had taken his medication. He answered that he had already taken it. I assumed that the mild tranquilizer had confused him.

I explained that he needed to take off his clothes and put on a hospital gown. I offered my assistance with this task, since he still seemed confused by my request. Apparently the sedative was taking effect.

Reluctantly, he removed his shirt and T-shirt and put his arms through the gown. Following my tying the back of the gown, he removed his shoes, socks and trousers. I helped him to bed and asked that he remove his boxer shorts so I could wash his abdomen with a special pre-surgical cleaner. At this moment, he started to laugh. I asked him what was so funny. He replied that I had him mixed up with his brother—his twin brother that had been taken to surgery at 7:25 AM!

*Reprinted with permission of the National Student Nurses' Association, Inc., Imprint Magazine, ©1994; 41(1):95.

Verses Rap MRSA*

SUZANNE ROGERS, R.N., C.R.R.N.

We wrote a "rap" song to teach the importance of hand-washing to unit nursing personnel. We then went to each nursing unit, dressed in baseball caps with buttons about handwashing, handed out copies of the rap song, recited it in spirited alternating verses, and required the audience to join in the chorus. Initially seen as outrageous and funny, the rap song caught their attention and produced long-lasting effects. A year later we surveyed staff who had attended and found most could still recite the chorus and often did so without prompting.

Here we are, the Clean Hands Crew—
We got a little rap to show you
　　what to do.
You join in when we reach the chorus;
Gotta learn the words and sing
　　them for us.
You gotta . . .

(Chorus)
STOP—PROTECT YOURSELF—WASH YOUR HANDS

Well, we're the crew and we're here
　　to say:
You gotta get with it the clean-hands
　　way.
Wash your hands a lot each day.
How much? When? What's a lot?
　　you say?
Listen up. Learn the way.
Infection control is the issue.
It's not enough just to use a tissue.
The germs you leave are not going to
　　miss you,
They'll spread around and then you'll
　　wish you
Took the time to:

STOP—PROTECT YOURSELF—WASH YOUR HANDS

Fifteen seconds of water and soap,
You scrub and you rub—don't be a dope.
Wash 'em off, rinse 'em off, learn to cope,
Gotta drown a germ. It's not a
　　vain hope.
Gotta break the chain,
It's no pain.
Scrub away and look at the gain.
You gotta . . .

*Reprinted with permission from American Journal of Nursing, ©1992; 92(7):41.

STOP—PROTECT YOURSELF—WASH YOUR HANDS

Help wash out MRSA.
MRSA is strange, MRSA is a cursa.
It gets in a patient and makes
   him worsa.
It's a little word for a great big phrase,
And it's bad news for us these days.
It's Meth Resistant *Staph Aureus.*
It is real and so the story is . . .
Cross infection is the spread of
   its direction—
Gotta wash it out with your inspection.
And a simple action that's a correction.
You gotta . . .

STOP—PROTECT YOURSELF—WASH YOUR HANDS

Don't need music and you don't
   need bands,
Just a simple message—Wash your
   hands!
Before you start and when you're
   through,
In between and on the run,
Every time you leave a patient—
Before you go you must have patience.
You look, you think, you don't go yet.
Stop at the sink and get your hands wet.

STOP—PROTECT YOURSELF—WASH YOUR HANDS

The Muddy Waters
of Clinical Teaching*

CAROL ROE, R.N., M.S.N.

With more and more patients being discharged early rather than later, we often are teaching about medicine and self-care as the patient goes out the door. It's tempting to assume that our instructions are clear—and we don't always have the luxury of evaluating whether we're assuming correctly. Unfortunately, nearly every nurse can recall an occasion when what seemed as clear as water to her was as clear as mud to her patient.

A young mother whose baby had a diaper rash called a pediatric clinic. According to the clinic records, mycostatin ointment and a suspension for oral candida had recently been prescribed, and the nurse told her to begin treatment with mycostatin. At a routine checkup two days later, not only did the child still have a rash, but it had worsened. When the office nurse asked about treatment, the mother promptly pulled out a bottle of mycostatin oral suspension. The cap had an eyedropper attached. The nurse explained that the preparation was for oral use. Somewhat indignantly, the mother said, "It says right here, put one milliliter in each cheek daily!"

Another child, brought in with fever and cough, was diagnosed with otitis media. The pediatrician prescribed a liquid antibiotic; the directions said, "Give 1 teaspoon twice a day until gone." Late in the day, the mother called the office, saying that something was wrong: The child screamed every time she put the medicine in his ear.

Then there's the case of the elderly woman who had sought relief for persistent nausea and vomiting. Baffled, she called the office, wondering what to do with the "silver bullets" that were to be inserted "one every four hours as needed for nausea."

The nurse explained that when the suppositories were inserted into the rectum they would dissolve and enter the bloodstream. "How can something made of foil dissolve?" the puzzled woman asked. The nurse had neglected to tell her to remove the foil.

Similar misunderstandings arise in the hospital. For example, a patient newly diagnosed with insulin-dependent diabetes had been taught self-injection using normal saline and an orange. A week later he was hospitalized with a blood sugar of 680 mg/mL. After he was stabilized, a nurse brought him an insulin vial and asked him to demonstrate his injection technique to assess his readiness for this discharge.

The client drew up to the correct dosage without difficulty and then looked around with a confused expression. "I can't give this," he said. "I don't have an orange." After a short conversation, the nurse discovered that he had been injecting an orange with the prescribed dose and then eating it.

We can all relate examples of errors and anxieties that could have been avoided by telling the patient comprehensively and intelligibly what he needed to know. Sometimes, though, we can thoroughly cover every base we can think of and *still* miss one. Consider Mr. B, for example, who had been hospitalized for chest pain. After an acute MI was ruled out, a cardiac catheterization was scheduled. The nurse gave Mr. B a booklet and questioned him closely about his understanding of the procedure and its diagnostic purpose.

After the catheterization, she found him looking somewhat depressed. Asked why, he blurted out, "Well, I know what's wrong with me. I have heartworms. I saw one on the TV screen!"

*Reprinted with permission from American Journal of Nursing, ©1992; 92(7):20.

Do They Really Understand Us?*

DOROTHY A. COCHRANE, R.N., M.N., KATHLEEN OBERLE, R.N., M.N., SUZAN NIELSEN, R.N., B.S., JODY SLOAN-ROSENECK, R.N., BScN, KATHY ANDERSON, R.N., AND CINDY FINLAY, R.N., M.N.

A nurse was stopped by a patient on a stretcher in the hallway.

"Nurse, do you know where I'm going?"

"No, Mr. C. What did your nurse tell you?"

"Well, she said I was going to the O.R."

Indeed, the patient *was* on his way to surgery. But further discussion revealed that he didn't know what "O.R." meant. He had signed his consent, and apparently knew he was to have "an operation," but didn't realize that he was going to have it *now*.

This incident started us thinking about whether patients understand what we say. That is, how does jargon interfere with our communication? We—a clinical nurse specialist, a research coordinator, and three staff nurses—decided to do a study to find out.

For two weeks, the project nurses, who were all working at the bedside, listened to themselves and to their colleagues in conversation with patients. Each time a word or phrase that might be considered jargon was used, it was recorded. From that list, we selected 34 of the most common, and constructed sentences using each. The sentences were acontextual—that is, without clues to the meaning of the key word or phrase; for example, "I am going to take your *vitals*" and "You are going to be *NPO* after midnight."

We surveyed 101 adult patients, 50 on the first day of admission and 51 on the fourth day in the hospital. In scoring the responses, we were not looking for technical explanations but, rather, the general sense of the term. If a patient defined "taking vitals" as "taking my blood pressure, pulse, and what not," we marked the response correct. The response "taking my vital organs" was marked incorrect.

What *does* 'ambulate' mean?

Although none of the words tested were correctly defined by all patients, most were defined correctly by more than half of the respondents. Correct responses ranged from 16%, for "flatus," to 98%, for "O.R.,"

OFF THE MARK

Here's a sampling of how our participating patients defined frequently misunderstood terms:

What we said	What they heard
Vitals	Organs
	Personality
	Name, age
BM	Basic metabolism
Analgesic	Salve
	Enema
	Sedative
	Laxative
Stool	Like a chair
Meds	Medical records/chart
	History
Sutures	Dentures
	IV
Ambulate	Move me to another floor/hospital by ambulance
Nauseated	Sleepy
	Dizzy
Void	Throw up
Flatus	Infection
	Fluid or phlegm
	Stuff in your urine
Hypertension	Nervous
	High strung
	Stressed out
	Overactive

"stethoscope," and "bloodwork." "Analgesic," "meds," and "hypertension" were other puzzlers.

Not surprisingly, words that have more than one

*Reprinted with permission from American Journal of Nursing, ©1992; 92(7):19–20. Edited from the original.

LEARNING TO LEARN

149

meaning—that is, those used commonly in different ways by health care personnel and by laypeople, such as "stool," which is "like a chair" outside our particular world—were often misinterpreted, sometimes quite creatively: "Vital" was defined as "personality," "organs" ("I'm going to take your vitals" takes on a terrible significance!), and "name and age" (from "vital statistics," probably). "Ambulate" became "move me to another floor/hospital by ambulance" and "to void" was "to throw up"—not really so far-fetched an answer.

Using jargon every day as we do, it's easy to forget that not everyone speaks our language. (And, after all, neither are *we* "native speakers.") But for the patient confronted with "foreign" words, an already unsettling experience may become downright frightening. For 14% of the newly admitted patients we queried, "radiology" meant "cancer treatment"; to them, the statement "We're taking you to radiology this afternoon" could conjure up alarming thoughts of "Oh no, I've got cancer and they haven't told me!"

ACADEMIC
APTITUDE

Flourishing in an ivory tower is very different from a mere visit while a student. Success here means learning universal academic politics in addition to the unique cultural norms that operate on every campus. Academia is a microcosm of the working world, but with its own unique set of complex rules.

Among the many demands of this reflective life are research and publication, curriculum development, committees, fund raising, and knowledge of technologic advances. However, it is effective teaching that enriches both student progress and clinical practice.

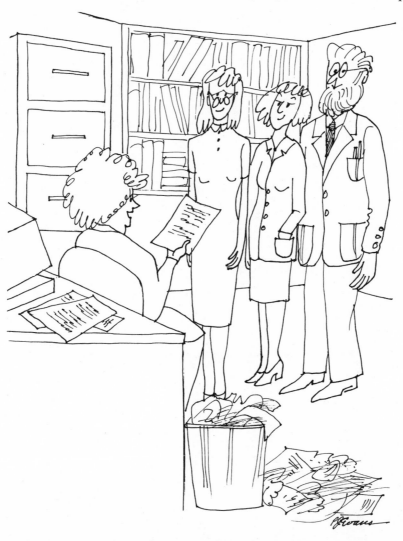

After months of agonizing research, the committee has concluded nothing.

The Three "R's" in Nursing Education*

CAROLE A. SHEA, R.N., PHD

From an educator's point of view, the world seems to be obsessed these days with the three "R's." However, these three "R's" are not the traditional ones—reading, 'riting, and 'rithmetic—but instead are three new ones—redesigning, restructuring, and retooling.

A New Student Body

Despite the uncertainty of health care reform, people are flocking into nursing education programs. Those new to nursing come from diverse backgrounds. Some enter nursing school upon graduating from high school. More are choosing nursing as a second career. The diversity of the nursing student body bodes well for the profession, but sometimes makes it difficult for students and faculty. Undergraduate programs are changing not only the content, but also their traditional teaching methods to stimulate and facilitate learning for different student populations. Therefore, nursing faculty are undergoing the retooling process, too.

Experienced nurses are turning to education to find new ways of dealing with the changes in the workplace. Because they are often in mid-career, with family responsibilities and established ties to a community, these prospective students find themselves with fewer options when choosing an educational program. A commonly used strategy is to "go local" because it is friendly, familiar, and relatively inexpensive. However, this strategy ignores the potential for a good fit between the needs of the student and the programs of the educational institution. It also may lead to a poor investment in the long run.

It is well known that adult learners tend to be self-directed, oriented to practical considerations, and highly differentiated. Baccalaureate and master's programs for RNs should be designed and structured accordingly; unfortunately, many are not. Nurses who return to school should avoid the following types of institutions.

Types of Institutions

The Hoop School of Relearning. Students achieve success by jumping through hoops to relearn what they already know. Hoops may take the form of complicated admission processes, nonstandardized tests, many challenging exams, and two or more courses in chemistry.

The Great Mountain Academy. Students have the privilege of learning to make a mountain out of a molehill by studying nursing through the conceptual framework of a lesser-known nursing theorist. Renaming common terms, writing 250-page care plans, and designing research studies that require multiple regression analysis are featured.

The Quick-and-Dirty Certificate Institute. Students learn to speed read the Procedure Manual and to hone their skills in an afternoon. Tips are provided on the art and science of framing the certificate.

Seeking a College of Dreams

All joking aside, returning to school can be a nightmare or the stuff of which dreams are made. Nurses should seek the way to their own "college of dreams." As applicants, they would find that the college personnel treated them as valued customers, easing their transition to the student role. As students, they would be able to build on their previous experience and develop their creativity in meeting their educational goals and objectives. Curriculum would be visionary, and teaching methods would allow for individual differences. Faculty would understand that because students have a personal life outside class, they need options for part-time study, flexible curriculum plans, leaves of absence, and deadline extensions. Psychiatric nurses would study advanced psychiatric nursing at the cutting edge of research and practice. They would also take courses in "the big picture," "how to be system savvy," "starring roles in advanced practice," and "Total Quality Management" (or the latest version) to prepare them for a fulfilling future.

*Reprinted from Journal of Psychosocial Nursing, ©1994; 32(5):7–8 with permission from Slack, Inc. Edited from the original.

This "college of dreams" is not a fantasy. Some nursing programs already feature many of the elements that are necessary for success and satisfaction for adult learners. By means of satellite programs, summer programs, long-distance learning, and self-paced programs, nursing colleges are striving to increase access to quality education that is affordable and convenient.

Education is a life-changing process—some say it is a life-long project. It may seem like a momentous decision, but investing in yourself is always a wise decision. Call your state nurses' association for information about the nursing programs in your area of interest. Become one of the retooled psychiatric nurses who are making an outstanding contribution to the mental health of our nation. Just do it!

That'll Learn'em *

ROSEMARY COOK, R.G.N.

If you have ever thought that those who can, do and those who can't, teach, here's your chance to see if you could make it in the groves of academe. Answer all questions—your time starts now.

1. **What is a 'module'?**
   (a) part of an academic course
   (b) the example set by teachers
   (c) a harmless lump under the skin
   (d) one element of a space rocket

2. **What characterises the first semester of a course?**
   (a) core modules
   (b) expenses
   (c) morning sickness
   (d) sleeping sickness

3. **What is a 'first degree'?**
   (a) an academic award following undergraduate studies
   (b) the body temperature at 6 am
   (c) a superficial burn
   (d) a member of a female pop group

4. **What is the ENB Higher Award equivalent to?**
   (a) a degree
   (b) half a degree
   (c) climbing Everest
   (d) an OBE

5. **For what would you use Medline?**
   (a) conducting a literature search
   (b) telephone advice on health problems
   (c) catching fish in southern European waters
   (d) checking late availability holidays

6. **A summative assessment is one which . . .**
   (a) counts towards a final award
   (b) tests arithmetic
   (c) is only taken by some students
   (d) is taken between May and September

7. **'Student centred learning' means . . .**
   (a) students take responsibility for learning
   (b) students spend more time in the library
   (c) lecturers have an extra day off
   (d) there aren't enough lecturers

8. **Pedagogy is . . .**
   (a) the practice of teaching
   (b) the practice of teaching standing up
   (c) a qualification for chiropodists
   (d) child pornography

9. **What is APL?**
   (a) accreditation of prior learning
   (b) phonetic spelling for Granny Smiths
   (c) a new record label
   (d) a Far Eastern guerilla movement

*Reprinted with permission from Nursing Standard, ©1996; 11(13–15):18.

10. What is CD-Rom?
    (a) a computerised information system
    (b) a musical information system
    (c) the twin of CD Remus
    (d) a lesbian pop icon

11. What is preceptorship?
    (a) a period of support for newly qualified nurses
    (b) advice for women planning a pregnancy
    (c) the command of a Roman legion
    (d) a score of 46 in Scrabble

12. **What is the difference between preceptorship and mentorship?**
    (a) preceptorship is for newly qualified nurses
    (b) mentorship is for women after the birth
    (c) a pointless conceptual exercise
    (d) about four nautical miles

13. What is the purpose of NVQs?
    (a) to recognise levels of competency
    (b) to re-introduce second level nursing
    (c) to create jobs for assessors
    (d) to qualify people to empty bedpans

Your score:

Mostly As: You are probably already in nurse education and reading the library copy of this journal. Shouldn't you be reading something more academic? Or taking out a personal subscription?

Mostly Bs: You have a tenuous grasp of the basics and you could probably make up the rest. Do you fancy a career in education? Someone has to prepare the next generation of nurses and you are ideally underqualified for the task.

Mostly Cs: It is rather worrying that you are loose in the NHS with this sort of theoretical background. Are you sure you attended your own training? If not, consider a rapid move into management.

Mostly Ds: You have no idea, have you? Your conception of nurse education is the annual fire lecture. On no account should you be allowed to take on the mentorship of students; you might not survive the experience.

Dear Journal Editor, It's Me Again*

ROY F. BAUMEISTER

Dear Sir, Madame, or Other:

Enclosed is our latest version of Ms # 85-02-22-RRRRR, that is, the re-re-re-revised revision of our paper. Choke on it. We have again rewritten the entire manuscript from start to finish. We even changed the goddam running head! Hopefully we have suffered enough by now to satisfy even you and your bloodthirsty reviewers.

I shall skip the usual point-by-point description of every single change we made in response to the critiques. After all, it is fairly clear that your reviewers are less interested in details of scientific procedure than in working out their personality problems and sexual frustrations by seeking some kind of demented glee in the sadistic and arbitrary exercise of tyrannical power over hapless authors like ourselves who happen to fall into their clutches. We do understand that, in view of the misanthropic psychopaths you have on your editorial board, you need to keep sending them papers, for if they weren't reviewing manuscripts they'd probably be out mugging old ladies or clubbing baby seals to death. Still, from this batch of reviewers, C was clearly the most hostile, and we request that you not ask him or her to review this revision. Indeed, we have mailed letter bombs to four or five people we suspected of being reviewer C, so if you send the manuscript back to them the review process could be unduly delayed.

Some of the reviewers' comments we couldn't do anything about. For example, if (as reviewer C suggested) several of my recent ancestors were indeed drawn from other species, it is too late to change that. Other suggestions were implemented, however, and the paper has improved and benefited. Thus, you suggested that we shorten the manuscript by 5 pages, and we were able to accomplish this very effectively by altering the margins and printing the paper in a different font with a smaller typeface. We agree with you that the paper is much better this way.

One perplexing problem was dealing with sugges-tions #13-28 by Reviewer B. As you may recall (that is, if you even bother reading the reviews before doing your decision letter), that reviewer listed 16 works that he/she felt we should cite in this paper. These were on a variety of different topics, none of which had any relevance to our work that we could see. Indeed, one was an essay on the Spanish-American War from a high school literary magazine. The only common thread was that all 16 were by the same author, presumably someone whom Reviewer B greatly admires and feels should be more widely cited. To handle this, we have modified the Introduction and added, after the review of relevant literature, a subsection entitled "Review of Irrelevant Literature" that discusses these articles and also duly addresses some of the more asinine suggestions in the other reviews.

We hope that you will be pleased with this revision and will finally recognize how urgently deserving of publication this work is. If not, then you are an unscrupulous, depraved monster with no shred of human decency. You ought to be in a cage. May whatever heritage you come from be the butt of the next round of ethnic jokes. If you do accept it, however, we wish to thank you for your patience and wisdom throughout this process and to express our appreciation of your scholarly insights. To repay you, we would be happy to review some manuscripts for you; please send us the next manuscript that any of these reviewers submits to your journal.

Assuming you accept this paper, we would also like to add a footnote acknowledging your help with this manuscript and to point out that we liked the paper much better the way we originally wrote it but you held the editorial shotgun to our heads and forced us to chop, reshuffle, restate, hedge, expand, shorten, and in general convert a meaty paper into stirfried vegetables. We couldn't, or wouldn't, have done it without your input.

Sincerely,

*Reprinted with permission from Dialogue, Newsletter of the Society for Personality and Social Psychology, ©Fall 1990.

Epidemic: Overheaditis*

GLORIA JEAN GROSS, PHD, R.N.

Aargh! I thought I was safe, but I think I've caught it! I've just returned from a conference where it was impossible to avoid.

The conference drew participants from a wide geographic region, including several Midwestern states, and included speakers from across the United States. The speakers were all recognized experts in their respective fields and spoke knowledgeably and even eloquently on their topics. I recognized that they were also, unfortunately, all afflicted with a condition that seems to be pandemic within the American community of speakers, teachers, and trainers.

Although I've thoroughly perused the various sources that label illnesses, injuries, and medical conditions, I've been unable to find an official name for this condition and have therefore taken the discoverer's prerogative to label and christen the disorder as "Overheaditis," an inflammation of the overhead. This dreadful affliction has the unusual characteristic of not affecting its primary victims (speakers) much, but uses them as vectors to spread the symptoms of confusion, irritation, and anxiety to all those within a sphere of influence, the ultimate victims (participants).

Overheaditis may manifest in one or a combination of several distinctive presentations. Each evokes certain signs in the vector. One of the most common indicators is an abundance of overhead transparencies carried in an open-ended folder. The vector will be seen trying vainly to keep all pieces within the confines of the folder while continuously muttering, "Oh, I hope I have these in order." The victims display an early symptom—apnea (holding their collective breaths) from the moment they see the overflowing folder. Just as the speaker is announced and stands to begin the lecture, at least one half of the contents falls on the floor. The victims moan in concert with the vector. A minion hurries forth to collect the varied pieces and tries, in whispered conference with the speaker, to reorder them while the anxiety levels of the victims go up and up as they anticipate being subjected to out-of-order, upside down, and/or backward pictures.

A second sign is often displayed at this point. The participants begin to exhibit disordered thought following a sequence of events. Vector is at the lectern, which is placed several feet from the projector and from an assistant who will display the transparencies at the appropriate times during the lecture. The assistant has neither been consulted ahead of time nor been provided with a copy of the speech, so must rely upon appropriate cues from the presenter. "Uh, Joan, could you show number 6 now, please . . . oh, make that 5, yes . . . no, perhaps it's right before that one. That's it . . . now, could you place 33 over that? What . . . no, not that one . . . just three down and put it on top of . . ." By this time, at least one third of the victims are thinking about their next break or yesterday's meals. The assistant often suffers from auditory hallucinations—"Destroy! Destroy! Destroy!"

A different presentation almost always appears only in the vector who is either an expert in some very complicated field or who *isn't* an expert, but wants everyone to think she or he is. The overhead transparency used by this speaker has the entire formula for the composition of the universe on a 10-inch square, usually drawn by hand with 75 arrows using six different colors. The vector "discusses" the contents of a *single* transparency for 60 minutes saying at least three times, "You probably can't follow this too well there in the back, but . . ." In the worst cases, the screen is the only light in the room for the entire time, leaving the victims in the dark, literally and figuratively. They exhibit squinting, strange positioning of the head, and constant muttering, "What is that in the corner? Can you tell what AZ leads to?" More than three fourths of the victims will develop drowsiness and fall asleep.

Much more common are the vectors who are compelled by their particular form of overheaditis to put everything ever printed in the English (or other) language on transparencies in the original form. When the victims are members of this vector's class, they get the original text of the *Encyclopedia Britannica* on the overhead transparencies in itty-bitty print (itty-bitty syndrome).

*Reprinted from Journal of Continuing Education in Nursing, ©1994; 25(1):46–47 with permission from Slack, Inc. Edited from the original.

This speaker has a delusion that no one will read a given assignment unless it's presented on an overhead. The victims are not amused and become paranoid, believing that the vector is lazy, thoughtless, and "out to get 'em." The vector often demonstrates a tell-tale verbal symptom of repeating "I know you can't read this, but I wanted to expose you to it." *Expose* us to it? No!

The vectors afflicted with itty-bitty syndrome are very often paralyzed and unable to function (if one calls this functioning) when the bulb on the projector burns out. It does so with monotonous regularity because the life span of the bulb is considerably shortened when the projector runs all day long. Even though the speaker should know how often burnout occurs, this particular vector appears surprised each time and never learns how to replace the bulb. Therefore, the participants always get a well-deserved break while "someone" locates and replaces the bulb.

The converse of the vector who has itty-bitty syndrome (IBS) is the vector who appears quite healthy. Every overhead transparency has been made professionally using high-resolution graphics, delineating only important points, and is clearly marked. Symptoms in the victims have an insidious onset. The vector begins the lecture slowly, while turning over each transparency in concert with the appropriate parts of the talk. As the speech progresses, transparencies are flipped in split-second succession to become a blur in the speaker's efforts to "get done on time or give you all this material." Not surprisingly, the symptoms in the victims mimic those seen in itty-bitty syndrome, with the exception that plaintive cries of "Slow down!" replace the yawns of itty-bitty syndrome.

Some vectors escape with milder forms of the disorder. Their symptoms include:

- using colored "transparencies" that aren't (transparent, that is) so only a pleasant blur is shown;
- leaving one transparency on for 15 to 30 minutes that has absolutely nothing to do with the subject at hand;
- standing in front of the projector to point at some item, thereby effectively blocking the view of at least one half the participants;
- putting transparencies on upside down or backward; and
- placing the transparency so that only one half is visible—only the half not being discussed.

To date, no fatalities have been reported from overheaditis, but given its rate of spread and increasing virulence, it is probably only a matter of time. Therefore, it is important to institute public health measures that will prevent such a tragedy.

Of course, all sufferers of overheaditis have one characteristic in common—the disorder will only manifest in the presence of that ubiquitous environmental hazard, the overhead projector. Therefore, an obvious solution to this pandemic is to ban the sale and purchase of overhead projectors. However, given the distinct unlikelihood of that happening, other measures will have to be taken to control the spread of overheaditis.

If the Plan is put into effect immediately, perhaps there is hope for complete eradication or at least a remission before the year 2000. In the meantime, I've just had a report that there is an outbreak of another incipient epidemic—Whiteboardemia . . .

Jargon Jaundice*

JANE WARNER, R.G.N.

Jane Warner explains the style of writing required for an exciting new nursing title, the Journal of Advanced Jargon.

Over the past few years, a spirit of commercial rivalry has entered the NHS. All over the country competition between health trusts appears to be the norm. Therefore I bring you good news and bad news.

The good news is that at long last greater competition will soon exist between health care publications, so leading to increased consumer choice. The bad news? As executive director of this exciting venture, I am as yet uncertain of its proposed title. But the *Journal of Advanced Jargon* strikes a pleasing note.

Already, potential contributors are busy leaving their ivory towers in order to make a conceptual approach to my front door. All seem to be anxious to be featured in the first edition, which, due to the intrinsic nature of the publication process, should be available during late summer, as befits such an august body of work.

Although I strive to welcome new writers, I prefer the more tried, trusted and esoteric types. Alas, I have had to reject a number of submissions for the simple reason that the aspiring writer has used plain, comprehensible English, which is totally at odds with the intended house style of the journal.

I strongly believe that constructive criticism is helpful to inexperienced contributors. My blue pencil, however, is almost down to the stub from writing 'What does this mean?' in the margin where words like 'bed-making' have been used.

Naturally, I would be the first to admit that I am 100 per cent committed to the practice of nursing, provided, of course that it has first been adequately defined. I mean, can you imagine the chaos that would be caused if one of our potential readers were to clear a patient's obstructed airway without recourse to a lengthy period of reflection on the prioritisation of care and the ensuing literature beforehand?

Golden rules for writers

Although it may be too late for nurse experts to contribute to the first edition of the *Journal of Advanced Jargon,* in my editorial capacity, I consider it a duty and a privilege to offer a few golden rules to those intending to grace its pages.

The first rule concerns the choice of title. This does not necessarily have to be connected to what follows. Ideally, I recommend that it should be at least as long as the main body of the submission. There are two simple ways of achieving this. The first is by the utilisation of that oft-neglected punctuation mark known as the colon. By its judicious use, you are at once free to link a series of completely unrelated concepts into your work. A hypothetical example might be: 'Trans-dimensional quality assurance: a critical framework for reflection on semi-professional attitudes towards the care of elderly clients.' The second, which relies on the question mark, is less popular as it dramatically reduces the optimum length of the title in direct proportion to any chance of having your work accepted for publication. For example: 'The implementation of care. Why?' It is important to note that both titles included the word 'care'; categorical proof that you are clinically credible.

The second golden rule can be summarised thus: think of your submission in terms of a gourmet restaurant meal. Your reader will be hungry for knowledge, and so your introduction should tantalise the brain cells in the same way as the taste buds. Of course, the entrée should be solid and indigestible, but the dessert should be so featherlight that after the bill has been paid the diner immediately wonders what he or she ate.

Imaginary reference

The third rule concerns the all-important rule of referencing. *The Journal of Advanced Jargon* will use a modification of the Harvard system in which one reference per published article is totally fabricated. A truly influential piece of work will lead to the imaginary reference being widely cited by students of nursing desperate to give an impression of erudition while meeting imminent assignment deadlines.

Finally, I must express my sincerest thanks to *Nursing Standard*'s editorial team, who have permitted me to launch a serious rival publication. I wish them well, and hope their circulation figures do not suffer as a result.

*Reprinted with permission from Nursing Standard, ©1994; 8(37):38.

Computer Randomized Academic Promotion System (CRAPS)*

DENIS R. BENJAMIN AND KENT OPHEIM

The conferring of titles cannot be taken too seriously. One's appellation not only determines how the world perceives one's work but must also be designed to preserve one's identity and uniqueness in an institution or organization. Standard old fashioned titles no longer fit the bill. There is always the dangerous possibility that someone will be able to pigeonhole you if you are merely called Professor or Director. Not even the Teutonic Herr-Professor-Doctor is any good any more. Our institution, like most others with an academic bent, has evolved a long way from the traditional, simple and straightforward approach to the naming of positions, but there is as yet no scientific way to establish satisfactory titles. The technique outlined in this paper fills a desperate need in academia and is readily adaptable for government and industry. It will ensure that no one, either inside or outside the organization will have the faintest clue as to what the people really do.

Words are arranged in three columns and each column should be used (see Table 1). Under exceptional circumstances only two columns can be used, but this greatly decreases the value and the level of obfuscation. Never ever use a single column alone. Merely select one word from each column of Table 1 by using the random number generator on your personal computer. The words can be arranged in at least six ways; A + B + C, B + A + C, A + B, B + A, A + C and B + C, thereby considerably increasing the number of possibilities. Because of the number of words available and the ways of arranging them the possibilities for titles approach the hundreds if not thousands. This number should be ample for all organizations up to and including the Federal Government apart from the Drug Administration.

Table 1

Column A	Column B	Column C
1. Research	Associate	Professor
2. Deputy	Assistant	Director
3. Acting	Advisory	Head
4. Co-	Coordinating	Supervisor
5. Clinical	Facilitating	Instructor
6. Visiting	Training	Administrator
7. Chief	Project	Facilitator
8. Post doctoral	Consulting	Coordinator
9. Interim	Program	Lecturer
10. Senior	Executive	Adviser
11. Junior	Under	Chairperson (-man, -woman)
12. Principal	Technical	Specialist
13. Graduate	Administrative	Consultant
14. Academic	Managing	Counselor
15. Distinguished	Financial	Analyst

The use of the suffix "emeritus" deserves special attention, since its addition will allow the individual to carry his title in perpetuity, while treeing the original moniker for recycling.

CRAPS has received the whole-hearted support of university administrators, since the conferring of prestigious titles can often substitute for salary increases during times of tight budgets. Automating the title selection process using just a personal computer offers significant savings to department chairpersons and Appointment and Promotion Committees. Additionally, making the computer coin-operated could also add significant revenue to the department.

*Reprinted with permission from Journal of Irreproducible Results, ©1996; 41(3):28.

A Standardized Method for Determination of Who Should be Listed as Authors on Scholarly Papers*

RICHARD B. RAFAL, M.D.

A handy method is described of selecting among the inevitable onslaught of 100 to 200 potential coauthors that mysteriously appear whenever a journal article is submitted for publication. The "relative authorship weighting scale" helps to decide who actually qualifies as an author and serves as an objective means of determining the appropriate order in which these various goldbrickers should be listed on the manuscript.

In order to eliminate the guesswork and subjectivity that are so often a part of the coauthor selection process, the relative authorship weighting scale (RAWS) has been devised. Utilization of this new method is easy (Table 1).

For each potential coauthor, check all items that apply, and then total the corresponding RAWS values in the right-hand column. Using this number (the RAWS raw score), final analysis is made with Table 2, which is self-explanatory.

It is the author's firm belief that strict adherence to this new system will simplify the selection of potential coauthors. Standardized criteria should eliminate political conflicts, reward only those who merit selection, and weed out those sneaky, sniveling parasites who pad their resumes with the work of others.

Should a person be miraculously selected as a coauthor utilizing this technique, another pesky problem is the order in which authors are listed on the paper. This is sometimes a source of friction. Such unpleasantness is avoided by judicious use of Table 1; simply list the authors according to numerical order of their point totals (after your own name, naturally).

It is recommended that for every article, each person's RAWS score should be recalculated. This will enable various lackeys, underlings, and inferiors to improve their chances before your next journal submission. More important, this maneuver buys additional time for a larger gift or higher "bid" to roll in.

Keywords: Bum; lazy; freeloading; obsequious; boot licker; leech

Reprint can be obtained by putting dimes into the nearest photocopying machine.

*Reprinted with permission from Chest, ©1991; 99(3):786. Edited from the original.

Table 1—RAWS

Potential Coauthor's Qualifications/ Duties Performed	RAWS Value
Resident that conceived the idea, researched, xeroxed, and wrote the paper	+2
Simple car wash	+5
Simonizing	+10
Vacuums car interior (including mats)	+15
Generalized posterior kissing (must be of >2 year duration)	+8
Blatant brown-nosing	−4
Benign neglect	+25
Prior listing on his or her paper as an author	+150
Bribe (generic)	+30
Cash bribe	+75
Whole lotta money	+200
Shoe shine	+3
Dry cleaning (must include pickup AND dropoff)	+10
Relative	+14
Blood relative	+21
In-law	−25
Peels grapes	+6
Sexual favors*	+25 to +500
Arm twisting by Department Chairman	+31
Takes "on call" for you	+35 per night
Actually contributed to the paper	+2
Female	+10
Young female	+25
Young, attractive female	+65
Has pictures of you in compromising positions	+185
Holding hostages[†]	+29 to +45

*Depends on specifics.
[†]Depends on number and who is being held.

Table 2—Final Status

RAWS Raw Score	Status
Over 10,000,000	Qualifies as a coauthor
≤10,000,000	Sorry Charlie

God, the Cosmos and Support Letters*

KRISTINE M. GILL, R.N., PHD

*This is a story about trying to get letters of support for a grant application. It's also about keeping life's aggravations in perspective. **Please listen.***

Thursday

It's been 2 weeks since I first called consultant A for a support letter. She forgot to dictate the letter to her secretary before she went on Christmas vacation. That's OK; I have 2 weeks before the grant is due. All three consultants and the three participating agencies have agreed to send their letters next week. Two letters finally arrive. The grant is written. It looks good; this is some of my best work. All I need are the letters. I planned this well.

Friday

I turn in the grant for the dean's signature and other university approvals.

Monday–Friday

What a great vacation!

Monday

It's Martin Luther King, Jr.'s Birthday: No class, no mail.

Tuesday

I'm still missing four letters (3 consultants, 1 agency). Consultant A says: "Oh, did I forget your letter? Tell me again what to write and you can pick it up after 4:00 p.m." Consultant B says her letter was in the mail last Friday. I leave a message for consultant C.

The agency manager says: "Oh yes, we're very busy today, but it has been dictated. You can pick it up in the morning." I leave a message for consultant B that the letter has not yet arrived. I pick up the letter from consultant A. The grant was ready at 8:30 a.m., but was not taken to the university's research office. I need the letters first. I'm tired and frustrated!

Wednesday

I call the agency from home to be sure the letter is ready. There is no letter. The manager will be in soon. I drive to the office hoping to have time for a letter to be completed while I wait. She's not there; she's sick. Tears are near. My throat is so tight I can hardly explain my dilemma. I go out to the car and cry. I may not be able to submit this grant because I don't have a letter!

I drive to consultant C's hospital office to get her letter. I page her several times and wait an hour. She doesn't show or call. I leave an urgent message. This seems so futile.

Later in the day, I receive a message from the agency. The manager had called and dictated a letter. But there's still no letter from consultant B and no message from consultant C. I pick up the letter from the agency.

It's lunch time. I'll get a hamburger, and call consultant C. I finally locate a phone in the shopping mall and I'm told that the letter will be ready when I get there. I'm overjoyed! But when I get there and read the letter I find that it needs to be revised. She used a wrong title. She can't find the letter in the computer. She'll bring it to my office this afternoon.

The letter from consultant B had been in the university's mail system. It's found! The letter from the agency is wonderful! A note from consultant B says she will fax her letter. I'm tired, but the grant went in today.

I laugh and tell two of my colleagues about my comedy/tragedy! We think everything that could happen has happened. We laugh! It's a great relief.

I wait until 5:15 p.m. No letter. I go home and tell my husband that I have learned a lot. Tomorrow will be

*Reprinted with permission from Image: Journal of Nursing Scholarship, ©1994; 26(4):332.

better. I won't let it get me down. Everything happens for a reason. Everything happens in its proper time.

Thursday

I walk into consultant C's hospital through the Emergency Room and see a dear friend. Her 3-month-old granddaughter just died. The baby's brothers skip by with pictures they colored. My friend and I hug and we talk. She says they have a faith that sustains their family.

We hug again. I watch the sobbing mother leave with her family holding her. Five minutes earlier or later and I would have missed them. This is no coincidence. It was meant to be.

I share with consultant C that this sort of thing has happened a lot in my life, especially the last couple of years. God is telling me something. I'm listening, but I don't always know what it is. I will keep listening, and hope I hear. The letter seems so insignificant now, yet I finally have it! The grant is done. I was there for a friend. I pray for the baby. I am thankful that I was there to learn whatever was intended for me.

I'm putting things into perspective. I worked a limited number of hours and days on the grant. I didn't let a need for perfection get to me. I took a vacation.

Perhaps this is a reminder to keep a healthy perspective on life and work and the fact that I'm a part of the cosmos and its human family.

I notice a typo on consultant B's letter: wrong year. I get her permission to change the date. Then I laugh.

Friday

The university's research office calls while I'm in class. I reassure them that the human subjects' approval is pending just like it said in the grant application.

Postscript

In March, I was told I was not awarded the grant. But in July I won a $275,000 house in a raffle sponsored by a local hospital. Later I found out that an administrator in the university's research office saw a television news report about my good fortune while sitting with her sick father at the hospital. She was thankful for the diversion and told the nurses (who also know me) about my winning. Even though it was midnight, they celebrated.

God . . . the universe . . . the cosmos . . . is indeed wonderful and mysterious! Listen.

Understanding Your Advisor: A Survivor's Guide for Beginning Graduate Students*

ALAN FEINGOLD, ED.M.

New graduate students can be easily distinguished from the more seasoned ones—the new arrivals are the ones flashing broad smiles and exuding unwarranted optimism. Beginning students like yourselves often harbor erroneous beliefs about graduate school. For example, you may associate politics with Washington—not with academic departments. Or, you may assume that the function of your advisor is to offer "advice." In graduate school, as in the business world, what you don't know can hurt you.

Success in graduate school largely depends on your ability to develop effective communication with your advisor. Unfortunately, advisors employ an argot that is confusing to most first-year students. Misunderstandings often occur between student and advisor, sometimes resulting in an abrupt and untimely end to the student's promising career. The author presents here a translation of "advisor-speak" into ordinary English, hopefully providing fledgling graduate students everywhere with the tools necessary for at least a fair chance of surviving the first year of graduate school.

What Your Advisor Says	What Your Advisor Means
The students in our program are competitive.	The students in our program stab one another in the back.
The students are friendly but competitive.	The students smile at one another—and then stab each other in the back.
You're expected to live on your student stipend.	You're expected to take out thousands of dollars in loans—and still be forced to do years of teaching for us at wages that would embarrass the manager at the local McDonald's.
There are rules and regulations that must be obeyed.	There are rules and regulations that must be obeyed *by you*. The faculty can do whatever the hell we want.
You're surprisingly honest.	Boy, are you naive!
It's important that you have a powerful advisor like me to "protect you."	This department is run like a jail. Weak newcomers must quickly find a tough "protector." And you know what the price is for that protection.
Don't ever forget, I'm your advisor.	Don't ever forget, I'm your boss.
You're expected to pass a comprehensive oral examination.	This is the only exam you'll ever have to take in your life where the examiners have decided whether to pass or flunk you *before* the test has begun.

What Your Advisor Says	What Your Advisor Means
An important part of graduate education is learning to interact productively with faculty.	Graduate students must learn how to curry favor, grovel, and mindlessly concur with every prevailing belief.
If you don't follow my advice, you will have trouble getting your degree.	If you don't follow my advice, you will have trouble getting your degree.
This is only a suggestion.	Of course, I can also suggest that you find another advisor.
I like the students in my class to participate in group discussion.	I "get off" on watching my students cut one another to pieces, especially now that cockfighting has been outlawed.
That's a very interesting question. Maybe we should discuss it some more—at my place.	I don't take seriously the university policy on sexual harassment.
I have tenure.	I can be tyrannical, duplicitous, and irresponsible—and nobody can do a damn thing about it.
Your paper is interesting and worthy of publication, after correction of a few crucial omissions.	My name isn't on it!
Your paper is interesting and worthy of publication, but it first needs some professional polishing.	I want to make some trivial changes—so I can justify putting my name on it.
Remember, your financial aid is provided by my grant.	Remember, if you give me any problems, you'd better be prepared to cough up 20 grand a year to continue in the program.
Your assistance on my project will afford you important research experience.	Your assistance on my project will add another publication to my vita.
You seem to be having some problems with statistics.	Nineteen out of 20 students who displease me never get their degrees.
The department expects you to write a thesis that will make a contribution to the literature.	The department expects you to write a thesis that will take up space in the university library.
You're required to defend your thesis in an oral examination.	That's the last chance the faculty gets to take pot shots at you before granting your degree.

Understanding Your Doctoral Dissertation Committee: A Survivor's Guide for Advanced Graduate Students*

D. L. PIERCE, M.A.

If acumen is required to correctly interpret the verbalizations and signals of the graduate advisor in the early portion of the doctoral program, then advanced techniques of translating "advisor-speak" are absolutely vital in dealing effectively with a whole committee during the most sensitive and crucial stage of the doctoral track—the oral defense of the dissertation. As a public service for graduate students everywhere, the author presents here an in-depth guide for interpreting the often enigmatic comments of the doctoral dissertation committee.

What Your Committee Says	What Your Committee Means
Look on this as a learning experience.	You're going to suffer.
Let me explain the format of the defense.	Let me waste time so you become more nervous.
We're here to support you.	We're here to destroy you so that you don't compete with us for grants and publications.
I found the overall concept interesting.	This is a token compliment before I rip you to shreds.
I would have liked to have had more time to study this.	I didn't read it.
There are particular aspects of the study that I would like to hear more about.	I read it, I just don't remember it.
I have some concerns about this whole area of research.	I hate your advisor, but he/she is too powerful to insult personally so I'll use you as a proxy.
Your hypotheses were not tied to the existing literature.	You came up with a creative, new idea and we want to make sure you never do it again.
Your research is an interesting extension of my early work.	Why didn't I think of this?
You fail to take into account some relevant research.	You failed to cite my article(s).
The biological information you present does not add to an understanding of the concept.	I learned psychology in the 1950s so I don't know what you're talking about.

What Your Committee Says	What Your Committee Means
I'd like to point out a couple of minor inconsistencies.	I'd like to tell you in detail about every mistake you made—as well as about your shortcomings as a person.
Explain . . .	I have tenure. I don't have to think for myself.
Your statistics do not support the hypotheses.	I don't understand anything other than a one-way ANOVA.
Your statistics are simplistic.	I'm the only one here who knows statistics and I want to rub it in.
How did you randomize your sample?	I had to come up with at least one question.
I don't think the time is right to try and publish work in this area.	At least not until I get something published in it.
Let's wrap this up.	I'm getting hungry.
Could you step out of the room so we can discuss this?	We decided beforehand to give you your Ph.D., but we want to make you sweat a bit more.

A PATIENT'S TALE

How often do nurses really get to hear what their patients are saying about them? After they leave the room, patients will express their point of view on all aspects of their care, real or imagined.

Due to their own vulnerability, the patients' perception of problems in health care delivery is magnified. In many instances, these complaints are valid and accurate. All of the stories strike a common cord, because each and every one of us will probably be a patient at some time. View these personal accounts from the other side of the sheets and judge for yourself.

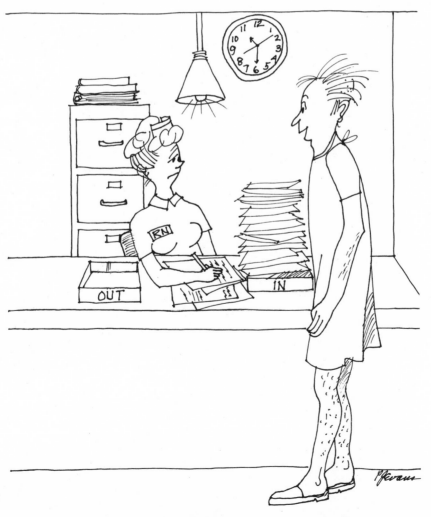

Why am I a GI patient when I'm not even a veteran?

Grave New World*

JAMIE MALCOLM, R.M.N., R.G.N.

This was serious. The only way I could get out from under the duvet was to be rotated round, full length, on my bottom. The hip joints were gone, the balls and sockets crunchy and corroded. All that blasted marathon running in the early 80s had done for me.

I could not afford private surgery from the health-care conglomerates. Monopoly markets had made routine surgery the preserve of the BMW classes. Pre-used Ford owners like me could only finger the glossy brochures with their colour plates of very clean, crisp nurses and dedicated 'your life in their hands' surgeons and dream of the plush, carpeted, private hospitals. You know them, the ones that people mistake for pizza houses? The receptionists don't half get cheesed off being asked for a deep-pan green chilli and pepperoni with a side order of Hawaiian salad every few minutes. Plays havoc with the corporate image, having representatives of the underclasses hanging around the smoked glass doors.

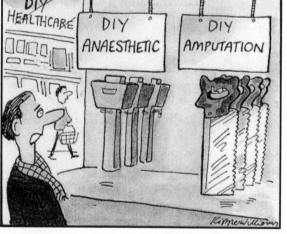

The NHS couldn't help me. With a waiting list of 26 years for wart removal there was little hope of my hip joints being replaced, unless they dug me up and did a retro-fit after I had shuffled painfully off this mortal coil. Not surprisingly, really, with that once great national institution now consisting of a small outpatient department on a level field just off the M6 at Southwaite Services. Former NHS employees like me could only dream of the smoke-filled duty rooms of our youth and curse the market forces, whatever they were.

No, there was only one thing for it. I would have to dip my toe, or rather my atrophied joints, into the DIY health-care market.

I had not been down to the superstore for a while; my home-decorating days were long past. At first sight the big red hangar-like building seemed the same but then I noticed that the four parking spaces near the

door were marked 'for able-bodied only'. The other 600 places all had those neat little person-in-a-wheelchair logos stencilled on them in yellow paint. I hauled myself on to a wheelchair from the trolley bay and rolled myself through the entrance. A crisp young man in a white coat, looking uncannily like Dr. Kildare, asked me what I was looking for. 'Hips are shot,' I hissed through teeth clenched with pain. 'Ah, yes sir, third aisle on the left, orthopaedics. Hip joints are on the third shelf down,' he smoothly intoned in a therapeutic voice. I set off down the broad aisles passing the Spear & Jackson home vasectomy kits and the Hozelok catheterisation packs.

The pain was getting worse. All this stress was doing me no good at all. An unfamiliar feeling was edging its way down my left arm.

There they were. Serried ranks of 'Walktall' steel and Teflon replacement hip joints. Another Dr. Kildare clone appeared, his lips moving in sales-speak: 'Hip replacement? Could I recommend that you consider buying a Black & Decker Op-Mate, only £199.99 a must for the home surgeon? It comes, for this month only, with a free copy *Orthopaedic Maintenance for the Newly Old*.

I pushed myself round the store filling the trolley, gazing at the displays: butane, propane and anaesthetic gasses, Rawl-plug skin closure and stitch sets, a remarkable self-assembly flat-pack commode. I lingered in the lighting department marvelling at the Duracell home endoscopy set (not recommended for use on domestic pets).

That radiating arm pain was intruding into my thoughts but the trolley was full with everything you could need for a DIY home hip replacement (except the Hitachi compact disc player with integral ECG monitor that you can only get at Comet). I had ticked every item on the checklist given to me by a slick as-

*Reprinted from Nursing Times, ©1993; 89(5):37 with permission from Macmillan Magazines, Ltd.

sistant at the customer services desk. The sign above his head boasted quality and a money-back guarantee. Money back? I couldn't see myself hopping across the car park clutching a defective replacement hip joint in one hand, and an assertiveness training pack from the mental health department at WH Smith in the other, ready to tackle Kevin ('your friendly in-store manager') with a demand for my money back.

A group of jobbing surgeons and out-of-work the-atre nurses were hanging around the exit, touting for work as I approached the checkout.

Maybe it was the effort of lifting up the Op-Mate. Maybe it was the market forces finally grinding me down. Anyway, as the crushing chest pain pushed me to the floor, I could hear Tracy at the till speaking into the microphone in that bland monotone of the consumer age: 'An assistant from the cardiac department to checkout 15 please.'

An Aural Assault*

BARBARA L. FINCH

It's funny how childhood memories can lie dormant for decades and then suddenly surface to shed light on something seemingly unrelated. This happened to me recently, when I spent five days in a hospital recovering from surgery.

As my morphine-induced euphoria began to fade, I suddenly had a vision of a large yellow sign, about the size of a stop sign. It was imprinted with bold black letters reading:

QUIET
HOSPITAL ZONE

I knew this sign. It used to be on Washington Street near the Charleston General Hospital in the southern West Virginia town where I grew up. And when I was growing up, I never understood the sign. Did it mean that kids from the nearby high school should be quiet when they got close to the hospital? Could people lying in bed inside that enormous red brick building really hear us talking outside? Or did the sign refer to noisy cars and trucks? Or maybe it was supposed to signal a moment of silence in tribute to all the poor sick souls trapped inside?

Today, I think I know the answer. Whoever erected the sign made a mistake. It should have been *inside* the building.

My recent postsurgical stay (which, incidentally, was not in that West Virginia hospital) was an experience in aural assault. Although I received superb care from competent and caring doctors and nurses, I was astounded by the level of noise that surrounded me. And I was in a private room!

What did I hear? As soon as I could sit up, I made a list:

Visitors talk, laugh, and argue in the hallway outside my door. Monitors beep. Physicians are paged. Food and laundry carts rattle. Phones ring. TVs blare. Toilets flush. Nurses and aides give and take orders in the hall. Patients moan. The ice machine clucks and lays its cubes. The nursing station searches for staff members by paging them in each room. Visitors drag wooden chairs across uncarpeted floors. Volunteers hawk newspapers. The clock on the wall ticks so loudly I ask to have it removed (not an unusual request, according to my nurse).

No wonder I remembered that sign from my childhood as I lay considering whether I needed pain pills or ear plugs.

In an age where so much attention is focused on patient satisfaction, I was surprised at how little effort had been made to simply create a quiet environment where I could rest and recover. Most of the most aggravating noise could have been easily and economically controlled:

*Reprinted with permission from Health Progress, ©1993; 74(4):72, 71 and the author. Edited from the original.

- Families do not have to stand in the hall and talk; every floor has lounges away from patient rooms, and hospital staff members should direct them there.
- Physicians do not have to be paged every few minutes; most of them wear beepers and can be easily summoned that way. Similarly, nurses could be outfitted with beepers, so they would not have to be paged in every patient room.
- Television sets can be turned down, squeaky wheels greased, and chair legs tipped with felt or rubber to make them less noisy.
- Volunteers can be instructed to tap gently on the door and quietly inquire if patients would like to purchase a newspaper.
- And, yes, it would be nice if patients could be kept comfortable, so they wouldn't have to moan.

A Consumer Speaks Out About Hospital Care*

ANONYMOUS

An outraged patient describes the omissions and commissions that made two weeks of hospital care anything but holistic, personalized, and humane.

Hospital employees talk too much and they talk too little. They ask patients questions that are none of their business; they fail to ask patients questions that they should. On occasion they give more of themselves than we might expect; on occasion they fail to act even remotely humane. They decline to communicate information about the patient's condition to the patient; they volunteer information to the patient which is no patient's business.

To protect the guilty, I choose to remain anonymous, but my identity is known to the editor. I'm past middle age, a professional person but not a physician or a nurse, have extraordinarily acute hearing but must wear trifocals, and have almost total recall, a photographic memory for faces and for illustrations in the PDR, and a working knowledge of biochemistry and physiology. My sex is irrelevant to this article.

When the surgeon, properly certified, recommended elective surgery for late spring, 1975, I marked off two weeks on my calendar.

An admitting clerk telephoned for preliminary information, observing that I would be called "on Monday before eleven" with definite word about a bed being ready. At one Monday afternoon, I called admitting, where a clerk insisted I had already been admitted.

"Funny thing . . . I haven't signed any papers and no one has taken any blood from me and I'm still sitting here at home."

"Well, I don't know . . . I must have you confused with someone else. C'mon down right now and I'll find you a room somewhere."

By four o'clock I was in a semi-private room, at $130 per day. At six, a tray was brought, with apologies: "This is the dinner the patient before you ordered before the heart collapse. They took the body out just before you came, you know. If you don't want this, I'll find something else." Assuming that the previous occupant of my bed had not died of botulism, I ate the meal.

At ten o'clock an unidentified nurse appeared: "Your medication." I said none had been prescribed. She was adamant. I asked her to read the orders again.

"Aren't you X?"

"No—I'm Y."

"Wow!" she blurted, "Wrong room again!" and disappeared.

My operation was scheduled for nine o'clock on the third morning, and the expected NPO sign went up on the doorway at bedtime. At midnight an orderly awakened me to announce that he was removing my water carafe because of the pending surgery. Luckily, I sleep easily and am not nervous.

*Reprinted with permission from American Journal of Nursing, ©1976; 76(9):1443–1444. Edited from the original.

At six I was rolled onto a cart and wheeled to a "holding ward." Without glasses, paper or pencil, and expecting a long wait, I began focusing on the conversations going on around me, and on the staff's actions. Some of the aged patients were so frightened they were shaking. Some of the blacks were screaming about discrimination, saying that they had been kept waiting too long.

An aide asked the RN at the desk for instructions about one of the shouters. "Do as you think best," said the RN.

"But *you're* in charge. I don't have any authority."

"Listen, G," said the RN. "You *know* this is only my second day on this job and you've been here a month. *I* just don't know. Why the hell can't you handle the situation?" Shrugging her shoulders, the aide did what she thought best—nothing.

Shortly afterward, an anesthesiologist in a green scrub suit sauntered over to the RN, now injecting something into the hip of a pre-op patient. Putting one hand over her eyes and wrapping an arm around her waist, the doctor said, "Guess who, honey." The statistical probabilities of the nurse bending or breaking the needle would make an interesting study. Fortunately for the patient, she did not.

"My God, my God, please take me *now* instead of after the operation" was the next cry I heard. Fear spread quickly to the woman on the adjacent cart, who began sobbing that "they" wouldn't let her keep her rosary.

"Anyone for coffee?" came a cheerful query from an off-duty aide passing through.

And so it went, on and on. If TV sitcom writers climbed into hospital gowns and, tape recorders at the ready, spent a morning in a holding ward, they could collect enough material for a full season.

Nine o'clock and unconsciousness really came too soon for this observer. About an hour later I woke up, not in a recovery room but in a "post-anesthesia room" that looked like an auto-repair shop: 40 carts with 40 patients, each with I.V. apparatus on high, parked parallel. At each cart station were four jets: air, water, oxygen, and God-knows-what. At each station, emergency tools lay atop spanking-white towels; above each station, a cabinet held tape, hemostats, scalpels, bandages, and all the miscellaneous "just in case" paraphernalia. When I was billed $25 for "use of PAR," I knew the auto-repair shop analogy had been correct.

Three nights later, well after eleven, an orderly woke me, insisted I was being operated on in the morning and that he was, therefore, removing my water carafe.

While I had a uneventful recovery, not a day went by without someone trying to give me medication meant for someone else. One midnight, however, a nurse appeared with medication I knew was intended for me. She asked my name and then, with a flashlight—thus showing compassion for my roommate by not flooding us with overhead illumination—checked my name and patient number on the wrist identification band. "We seem to make *so* many mistakes," she explained. "I like to be sure, because I'm not always on this floor."

A young lady with a badge identifying her as a "prenursing student volunteer" came in one afternoon, unaccompanied, called me by name, and said she had to take my blood pressure. While I knew this was a teaching hospital, I had not been aware that it was a self-teaching institution. Stating that she was still in high school, the girl fumbled with the cuff. When, after five unsuccessful attempts, she confessed, "I just can't seem to find the artery," I adjusted the position of the stethoscope and gave her a standard reading. She went happily on to another victim.

Daily, some staff member offered to give me a bath; others proffered back rubs. On one of the 14 days of my stay, the "Bookmobile" was trundled through the hall on its much-advertised "daily" rounds. An underdeprived and overfed matron from suburbia suggested I might enjoy a magazine or book "and there's no charge," but she didn't have a list of what was available, didn't know "for sure" what she had, and didn't wheel the cart to my bedside. At the moment, I was absorbed in the current issue of *Science,* so my reply probably spoiled her day, as she had spoiled my concentration.

After visiting hours, nightly, nurses would come in to inspect the shelf of books I had brought with me and would casually relate the peccadilloes of the nursing staff, the idiosyncrasies of the medical staff, the brash advances allegedly made by some resident physicians, and the disdain with which most nurses regarded medical students. I learned of the practical jokes played on the more pompous surgeons, of the substitution of specimens for new members of the tissue committee, and of general adolescent behavior by all but a few prune-faced ancients.

Would the staff have told me what they did if they had known that my surgeon was my cousin and that many of the RN's had been to nursing school with my daughters and nieces? Or were they so open *because* they knew of my relationships and hoped I would repeat their tales? Whatever the answer, nothing can change the facts that for 14 consecutive days I was offered the wrong medication and that only one nurse positively identified me before giving me a drug.

Would the horseplay outside the operating room have continued if the staff had been aware that a keen ear was listening, albeit coupled with spectacle-less, unfocusing eyes? Would the RN in the holding ward have told the aide to do as she thought best if the nurse knew she was being overheard by, say, a newspaper reporter or a plaintiff's lawyer in a malpractice suit? Would an aide have asked me a few days later, in hushed tones of confidentiality, whether urology had anything to do with urine, if she had had an understanding supervisor?

And what can one say of the staff member who, confusing two people with similar surnames, administered mineral oil to my roommate—sedated and in traction—and then vanished for four hours? During that time, the oil proved it was fresh, viscous, and efficacious, but the poor patient's signaling to the nursing station brought no response whatsoever.

To See Ourselves*

LEAH L. CURTIN, R.N.

The message received is not always the message intended, and the message intended is not always the message sent.

While I can think of many organizational miscommunications, I can think of none as hilarious or as humiliating as this allegedly true story. Last week I had occasion to speak to one of my sisters, who also happens to be a nurse. In the course of our conversation she told me about one of her co-workers whose 75-year-old mother was preparing to have her very first Pap smear. A dignified and modest matron, it had taken the combined efforts of her doctor, her daughter and her husband to convince her to make an appointment with a gynecologist. She was so nervous that her daughter offered to drive her to the gynecologist's office. And so it happened that this modest and somewhat elderly matron spent the night before her morning appointment at her daughter's house. She had packed a little suitcase in which she put clean underwear, make-up, stockings and the like. She was sure that she had remembered everything. However, as she was preparing herself to dress after her bath, she discovered that she had forgotten the feminine deodorant spray that she had bought especially for this occasion. When she couldn't find it, she hunted around her daughter's bathroom desperately searching to see (she did not have her glasses on) if her daughter happened to have some on hand. In short order, she

found a spray can that looked just like the one she'd forgotten and sprayed the area in question.

Carefully attired and coifed, she entered the gynecologist's office for her scheduled visit. In due course, the physician left the room and she undressed and a female assistant put her up in stirrups. The physician entered the room and sat down on the stool at the end of the examination table. Looking slightly nonplussed, he said, "My, aren't we dressed up today!" and proceeded with the exam. Our modest matron was perplexed by his comment, and the more she thought about it the less she liked it.

By the time she reached her daughter's home, she had worked herself into an indignant rage. As she recounted the tale to her, the daughter said, "Mom, I've known this physician for years, and I don't think he would deliberately embarrass or insult anyone. Did you do or wear anything different?"

"The only thing I did differently than I usually do was to use some of your feminine deodorant spray."

"But, Mom, I don't have any feminine deodorant spray."

With that, they both headed to the bathroom to look for the spray can in question. It turned out that what her mother (quite inadvertently) had used was her 13-year-old granddaughter's sparkle hair spray!

Oh! to see ourselves as others see us!

*Adapted with permission from Nursing Management, ©1995; 26(9): 7–8. Edited from the original.

View from the Pillow*

ROBERT B. RUSSELL

Eight hospitalizations led this patient, who thinks nurses are superb, to this heartfelt "But . . ."

During many hospitalizations, I have observed that patients have three principal topics of conversation. The first is themselves—what is wrong with me, what is wrong with you, what has been done about it,what is going to be done about it. The second is the doctors—who they are, what their specialty seems to be, when they're going to visit, and what we plan to ask them. But it is the third subject which really dominates patient talk. That topic is the nurses—who and what they are, what they're doing, and how they do it.

Make no mistake about it; nurses are constantly being appraised by the patients. The patient's world is a small one, cut off from the familiar "outside," and so he tends to magnify the significance of little things that occur within his world—that small part of the hospital he is able to observe. Since it is the nurse who does most of these little things, it is important that the nurse know on what basis the patient makes his judgment of her.

Let's grant, at the very beginning, that the patient's estimate may be as erroneous as the 1948 poll on Truman's chances against Dewey. And let's establish for certain that, if any patient were asked to generalize his observation about nurses, he would be unlikely to qualify a statement about how wonderful he thinks nurses are and what a superb job they do for their patients.

For the generalization is true. Nurses *are* wonderful. And nurses do in fact perform superbly. What I'm concerned with here, however, is not the generalization, but the evidence upon which the generalization is made, and more particularly the areas in which, in the patient's judgment, individual nurses have fallen short of perfection.

Housekeeping Fever

The nurse's personality, real or professional, has a lot to do with this judgment. I remember Miss Simmons very vividly, even though it has been eight years since I was under her care. Each morning, seemingly before the cock could crow, she virtually burst into our ward with "GOOD morning, everybody! Rise and shine! Let's all be awake and get this room shipshape!" She meant to be cheery, no doubt, but we did not appreciate it. It was much too early in the morning for so much energy to be bursting out. Nor could we understand why, the day being as long as it is, there was any necessity for rising (impossible for many of us) and particularly for shining.

We suspected the truth to be that Miss Simmons was a demon housekeeper. She had many an argument with us: we contended that we were the important matter, not the general neatness of the room; she countered that the neatness of the room was important to our morale. We argued that our morale would be just fine if she'd let us sleep a bit longer and leave the housekeeping until later. However, Miss Simmons was not to be denied. During her tour of duty we had the most meticulously neat room in the hospital, but I am glad to say that I've met only one Miss Simmons in all my experience as a patient.

A Question of Age

Miss McInnis is another case in point. When she came to take a patient's temperature, she might say, "Get that thing out of your mouth!" Now there are other ways of asking a man to stop smoking his pipe. And perhaps even those words may be used, if said with a twinkle in the eye and the proper shading of voice tone. But Miss McInnis achieved neither the twinkle nor the shading—merely the reaction, "Who does she think she is? Isn't she aware that I'm old enough to be her father?"

"Under your tongue, now, that's a good boy" is all right for brother Willie or for a senile uncle, but not for the general run of adult patients.

And that "we" so many nurses use ("We must lie still now." "It's time for our medicine."). That word might

*Reprinted with permission from American Journal of Nursing, ©1961; 61(12):88–91. Edited from the original.

well be dropped from nursing vocabulary. The patient knows the nurse means "you," and the "we" smacks of the kindergarten. One nurse had the difference taught to her rather embarrassingly. When a patient laughed uproariously at a question she asked, she was momentarily nonplussed. "Do you realize what you said?" he asked. She hadn't realized before, but her blushing indicated she did now: using the first person plural, she had asked Mr. Jackson to get back into bed!

The Human Touch

But back to personality. Miss Zelon had it, in the sense that I mean it. It wasn't glamour or anything of that sort, but a certain sense of relaxed fun. One morning she piqued our curiosity by looking out the window each time she came into the room. "Five patients here now," she said. We were in a four-bed room; who was the fifth? We spent the morning on the subject, but got only a smile from her. In the afternoon she pointed out the fifth—a brand-new Valiant she had just purchased. Thereafter, the car became a conversation piece, and we had many days' fun out of it.

She even made fun out of her name. What was the nationality? She let us guess. We inquired her first name of other nurses, hoping for a clue. We found it out: Jeannette. The game went on; it took a whole morning. The proper answer was Lithuanian, and nobody had guessed it. And so it went: we had to guess where she came from "north of Boston"; we discussed the operation of the Valiant; we found her capable in sports talk. We all liked to see her come in; efficient to begin with, she added sunshine to her job.

Yet what in the world is to be feared? Perhaps there's an answer to that, too. Perhaps Miss Wells expressed it one day as she was wrapping a patient's abdominal binder tighter than he wished it. Continuing to wrap as he protested, she at length concluded the job and winked at him, "Never let the patient get the upper hand." Even the protesting patient laughed in appreciation of her devotion to orders. Maybe that's the answer. And there may be other answers, too, that I don't appreciate.

Technique and Timing

The nurse's technique in doing her job is, of course, the most important element in the patient's appraisal of her. There are nurses who can give a hypodermic injection absolutely painlessly; there are others whose very approach causes the patient to stiffen in terror. A backrub administered by Miss Quinn was a gentle coating with massage cream and a dusting with powder;

she might as well have coated and powdered her desk top. Miss Arbett put her fingers into it, rippling up and down the muscles, relaxation emanating from her every finger.

Miss Kress heard a patient's complaint about bowel gas with a so-much-pain-is-inevitable attitude and advised a grin-and-bear-it-philosophy—a stoic superiority to pain perhaps possible to a captured Iroquois. Miss Lasker, despite steaming summer weather, brought a hot-water bag. But Miss Ring provided relief with a rectal tube.

Nurse after nurse treated the ulcers on a patient's feet, but only Miss Zelon thought to cut his half-inch toenails. A bed bath given by Miss McInnis was perfunctory; Miss Ring's technique was at once thorough and loving. Most nurses, in leaving a dose of pills, did just that; only Miss Kilburn and Miss Arbett remained to see that the pills were actually taken. And yet all nurses must certify to the taking, not the leaving with the patient. (Some doses are so evil-tasting that few patients fail to have the momentary temptation to flush them down the toilet.)

But however perfect the technique, it won't be appreciated if ill timed. Miss Jones used to stride in, vigorously shaking a thermometer, just as breakfast was arriving. I've had blood samples taken during my evening meal. I've been approached with an enema set during visiting hours. After being up for the prescribed limit of one hour, I've climbed into bed for a nap, only to have Miss Ginn tell me it's time to make my bed. I've been awakened to take a sleeping pill. And, three hours after I've taken the pill, I've been awakened to have my temperature taken.

Less Mystery, Please

During my last hospitalization I developed a staphylococcus infection, and separation from other patients was indicated. When the matter was explained to me, I made no objection to isolation and was transferred to a two-bed room in which another patient with a staphylococcus problem was lodged. Never had it been thoroughly explained to Mr. Lynn that he was to live in relative isolation. Ambulant and a great visitor, he roamed rather too freely in the wards. When I attempted to explain to him the necessity of our isolation, he attributed his isolation in part to me and in part to "Hitler," his name for the head nurse, and made a point of leaving the room when she was not about. Matters came to a head, as they had to. His own doctor, mincing no words, explained the danger of spreading infection and told him to "stay put." The whole situation might have been avoided had somebody explained to Mr. Lynn at the very start of his isolation.

There are many other instances of needless mystery in hospital procedures. A patient's dosage is changed, and a new pill is left for him—no explanation. Why the mystery? The patient takes his pill, and does not question. But he always wonders what he's taking and what it's supposed to do for him. Can he not be told?

Too Great Expectations

A doctor once told me that he had often wondered why patients read the "junk" they do read—detective stories, pulp magazines, and the rest—when they had so much time that might be put to better use. He discovered why when he, himself, had to undergo the removal of his gall bladder. He had entered the hospital armed with "serious reading," foreseeing a wonderful opportunity to catch up on professional reading and even tuck in a literary classic or two. He found, to his considerable surprise, that he had absolutely no interest in the books he had brought and spent his hospital period with magazines! Now, it would have been a mistake to judge Dr. Jack by the way he spent his hospital leisure. Hospital sluggishness had smothered what I can assure you is an undeniably brilliant intellect. It is a mistake to judge any patient on the lassitude he displays in the hospital or on his abnormal self-concern or petulancy.

Experience and Empathy

Nurses know what pain is, in the abstract; but can they *feel* the patient's pain unless they have themselves experienced pain? I certainly should not recommend that each student nurse undergo an operation as part of her training; but I do feel that, if the nurse has herself had an operation, she is much better equipped to feel the patient's pain and to understand the patient.

Something like this lack of feeling for pain caused Miss Kilburn to misinterpret my situation entirely. I had had a subtotal gastrectomy and was coming out of it nicely, clear-eyed and lively, when an abscess developed within my abdominal wall. Two days after the operation I was hanging onto the siderails, feeling that something had gone wrong, but not knowing what. For all I knew, this was normal postoperative pain. Three days and three nights my situation persisted (I discovered later that the doctor suspected the cause, but was hoping the thing would break of itself) before the abscess was punctured for drainage.

But Miss Kilburn, in response to my wife's "What's

wrong with him? His eyes are popping from his head, he's very warm, and he looks drawn" confided in her that I was a very tense man and insisted that I must be secretly worried about something. She had, apparently, but one reason to assign for the tension—some romantic hidden life, I suppose, some subtle schizophrenia, some Jekyll-Hyde business. I don't blame her too much, for that could have been so; but might not physical pain be a symptom of something wrong physically? I'm sure that to this day—if she remembers me at all—Miss Kilburn is convinced that I was something in which Alfred Hitchcock might have been interested.

When a nurse asks a patient, "How do you feel?" what answer can be given her? The question has, outside the hospital, almost no significance. "How are you today, Joe?" asks his friend at the shop. Joe's answer is invariably "Fine," even though he has spent half the night walking the floor with the baby or worrying about a pain in his back. For "fine" is the only answer expected or desired. To the nurse's question, "How do you feel?" the patient's answer ought, of course, to be the very answer he avoids giving in other circumstances; yet he'll say "fine" just the same unless the nurse is specific in her questions.

Then, too, the answer may be a relative one: "Fine" said to a nurse may be "not so good" to a wife. Compared with how he felt yesterday, the patient may be "fine"; compared with the standard of normal good health he may be less than that. "Fine" said postoperatively may mean merely that the patient expected to feel much worse. Yet I have heard many a nurse respond to a patient's "fine" solely with "I'm awfully glad to hear it." What should her comment have been? "And what about that pain in your side? Do you still have that? You said yesterday that you were having difficulty moving your bowels; any luck yet?"

Superwomen

I fancy many of you nurses have been asking, "What does the man think we are—superwomen?" My answer is that I do indeed. I think the nurse *is* a superwoman. She proved it by becoming a nurse in the first place, for only women on a plane above the average can hope to qualify. I admire nurses tremendously, even those who may have rubbed me the wrong way, for I appreciate both their motivation and the delicate difficulty of their jobs. If I have seemed to accentuate the negative, it is only because the negative, being the unusual, calls attention to itself. The nurse as a human being may err on occasion—and who does not? The nurse as nurse is incomparable.

Cover Your Rear

DENNIS KNEALE

And other words of advice for those who have to suffer the indignities of a hospital stay.

When it comes to bedside manner, my neurologist at New York University Hospital favors the blunt approach. Checking out fierce shooting pains down the back of my thighs, he squints at a telling MRI scan: It shows a chunk of vertebral-disk shrapnel that had "extruded" (read: burst) into my spinal canal.

"*Jesus!* You got one big *jamboni* in there," he says. Avoiding surgery was no option. "That thing ought to be out of there and in a scrap bucket by the end of next week," another doctor advises.

So it was—and oh, the agony: the loss of autonomy, the pain and ineffectual painkillers, the tyranny of those damnable, butt-baring hospital gowns. Not to mention the whininess that makes those who love you hope for higher hospital mortality rates.

Let's try not to be a baby about this. But it *huuur- rrt*. This was, after all, my third major surgery and hospital stay since 1989—and my second in four months. All before hitting age 39.

December 1989: kidney surgery at Mount Sinai Medical Center in New York to fix a blocked drainpipe, leaving behind a gaping scar that bisects the spare tire on my left side. February 1996: knee surgery at St. Luke's-Roosevelt Hospital to replace a blown-out ligament and repair cartilage (the only surgery that makes me sound a little cool, like I'm a middle linebacker or something). And June 28: back surgery at NYU, the most delicate operation leaving the most embarrassing scar. It starts just below my waistline and rises northerly a few inches along my spine. Makes me look like one of those beefy-boy refrigerator repairmen who wear their jeans way too low, displaying the wrong kind of cleavage.

Soon, maybe, it will be your turn. So in the interest of helping those who come next, as well as offering me yet another venue in which to complain, here are a few pointers.

Brace for a loss of control.

Minutes before being wheeled into the Mount Sinai operating room, I lodge a simple request to use the bathroom. Doctors actually debate this: "What do you think?" says one. "Nah, he's gonna have a catheter anyway," the second one answers, letting slip a truly unpleasant disclosure. Ultimately my mom intervenes: "*Please!* Let the guy go to the bathroom." They relent; doctors have mothers, too.

The obvious lesson: Having your mom, or your tough-talking spouse, as your second at these duels is crucial. Someone has to fight for you.

Take back control in meaningless ways.

Hospitals often fail to treat us like the paying customers we are. We must take back the night, and the little things count. Order takeout deli heroes in protest of cafeteria gruel. Refuse to go to sleep. Bring your own new pair of jaunty pajamas to fight the humiliation of those hospital gowns. And use your own toiletries: Tony shampoo and moisturizer, a gift from my wife, were much nicer than the junk that hospitals buy in bulk.

But this one was particularly fun: For doctors who visit you, introduce yourself and ask their names and specialties; it lets them know when they have ignored the social graces.

What do you think this is? "E.R."?
(Or: Don't be an extra in their drama.)

Chances are your hospital will have legions of medical students practicing on patients. (They are called "residents" because they pretty much live there.) Which is fine if you feel like being used for education. Not me, in light of a morning-after humiliation at Mount Sinai. My one goal 24 hours post-op was to deny the existence of that catheter—the long, thin tube that extended under the blanket and entered, upstream, into a very uncomfortable area.

Then this clipboard-toting stud in a white coat enters my room on "rounds," leading a few other residents. I had never seen him before, and he doesn't bother to introduce himself. He recites my particulars (name, age, procedure), then the kicker—"He's got a catheter"—and suddenly yanks back my blanket so everyone can see. I look down and gasp; a female resident winces and looks away.

It turns out you don't have to subject yourself to this. If you don't feel up to it, just say no.

Be nice to doctors, but be even nicer to nurses.

You probably think that when you go into a hospital, you're under your doctor's care. Wrong. That's the nurses' job.

My surgeons were great; worked wonders, all. But after they are done, they move on to other customers; nurses get you well.

Suck up to them unashamedly. They are beleaguered by paperwork, dissed by doctors and tormented by kvetching patients. Ask them their names, how long they have been at the hospital, where they grew up. They will respond better when you need to ask for the important stuff—another painkiller, a glass of water, help in shampooing your hair for the first time in four days.

It will always hurt more than your doctor says it will.

He was trying to be encouraging. My doctor at St. Luke's was assessing the fallout of cutting out a piece of tendon, threading it through my left knee and screwing it down to replace the anterior cruciate ligament, and repairing a rip in the medial meniscus cartilage. (One cool thing about surgery is, you get to bandy about terms of anatomy. One bad thing is that nobody wants to hear about it.)

"Let's do it on a Friday; that way you can be back at work on Monday," my doctor said. One patient told how she underwent the same operation and was back tending bar by the next night.

One word on that: Fuhgeddaboudit. Nearly six hours of surgery, of tugging and pushing and cutting and suctioning all masked by a pleasant haze of Valium and narcotics as you lie there awake, turns out to hurt like hell later on. It took me two weeks to get back to work, six weeks on crutches. Maybe my case was an exception. Or maybe I'm just a wuss.

Just say yes.

For some bizarre reason, too many of us have an aversion to painkillers, so we tough it out. Don't be a hero—demand drugs. Nervous the morning of surgery? Get a scrip for Valium ahead of time. Feel a dull ache where the stiletto scalpel cut through layers of muscle? Beep the nurse for another pill. That's what medicine is for.

For sanity's sake, get a private room.

If you can afford the extra $300 or more a day, getting a room of your own is well worth it. I hate to sound unsympathetic, but it avoids the chance that your roommate will tough it out, forgo pain pills and keep you up all night with his moaning (as happened my second night at NYU). Or that he will listen to reruns of "M*A*S*H" at top volume. (First night, first roommate.) This would be bearable normally, but it's a bummer when you've just been cut open and feel alternately miserable and sorry for yourself.

Get a second opinion—not for insurance, but because some doctors are just wrong.

And don't get it from someone the first doctor refers you to; that way, overruling his advice won't be a problem. In trying to detect what might be blocking fluid flow from my left kidney, a doctor at Beekman Hospital wanted to take a look inside by doing an invasive outpatient procedure called a retrograde cystoscopy. Think "Up Periscope" meets "Private Parts."

As noon approached, I waited, hungry and thirsty because you can't consume anything after midnight, and the doctor finally showed up—a half-hour late and eating an ice-cream cone. (Now think "Boston Strangler" meets "Marcus Welby, M.D.")

The procedure found no blockages, and when the chronic pain hadn't eased six months later, Dr. Ice Cream suggested doing it again. This time, to make sure, I checked with a new urologist at a separate hospital. His advice was a jolt: Don't do it, and you shouldn't have done it the first time. The procedure is too painful and invasive on a man in his 30s; it can't show a drainage problem; and whatever snag it had failed to find six months earlier was sure to elude it again. He suggested a "nuclear scan," injecting a radioactive dye into an arm and taking X-ray images of the kidney as it worked or swelled up. It was far less uncomfortable than "Up Periscope," and it pinpointed where the drainpipe had crimped.

Don't hesitate to switch to a better surgeon.

You can get locked into one doctor path: Your regular physician refers you to a specialist at the same hospital, who then refers you to another specialist, and before you know it your fate is set. Yet the third expert may not be the most talented choice.

For back surgery, I started on one path at St. Luke's and then had a chance at a hard-to-get appointment with one of the world's best neurosurgeons at NYU. It was hard not to worry about hurting the first guy's feelings. "Don't you worry about that, he'll live," another doctor told me. "You want somebody just OK, or you want the best?"

Days later, as I lay on a gurney in an NYU operating room, my doctor's team excitedly prepped the operating room, pumped up at assisting this hotshot. When he entered, it felt as if the room would break into applause. It was like waiting for Elvis.

Afterward, try not to whine too much. Especially at home.

Two days after knee surgery, scaling two flights of stairs to enter my apartment was, well, kind of uncomfortable. Within 20 minutes of parking myself in the den, I rattled off requests to my accommodating wife, Kathy. Please get me some water . . . and some ice . . . and something to eat . . . and the ice pack . . . and half a dozen other things, all one at a time.

"He's kind of bossy," a friend whispered sympathetically, but Kathy didn't complain. "It wasn't the whininess as much as it was the order-barking part," she said later. "That was a little trying."

Eventually you may get it right.

One more surgery, at the least, may lie ahead for me: I have been diagnosed with an inguinal hernia. "You should definitely get this fixed, now or in a year or two," the specialist advises. Not to worry; he says it won't hurt at all.

Maybe I'll hold off for a while.

Vital Signs*

ED CASSIDY

Foreword: I thought I was going to die—literally. Until one wonderful nurse looked into my eyes and calmly threatened death if I didn't cut the cheap theatrics.

It must have been about 2 or 3 AM when it hit me. A strange pain shot through the right side of my stomach. What was this? Had the rack of lamb been too spicy? The dessert too rich? I downed about a quart of Pepto-Bismol as I leafed through my home medical dictionary in search of a quick diagnosis.

Within an hour the pain was excruciating. I had finished off both bottles of Pepto-Bismol, tried my personal cure-all of brown rice with ginger ale, chewed every antacid tablet in the house, swallowed handfuls of vitamins B and C (who knows what I was thinking—unbelievable pain makes you do unbelievable things).

As I lay doubled over in the hallway, clutching my side, I made a decision: I had to get to the hospital. In a matter of minutes, my friend Charlie had rushed to my rescue and tossed me in the back of his jeep. We were off to Kaiser Moanalua at double the speed limit. Luckily it was a very early Monday morning and construction hadn't yet begun on Kalaniana'ole.

After a couple of miles of my writhing and screaming, Charlie pulled into the Niu fire station and summoned their ambulance. My "painful" performance was just a bit too much for him to handle.

Inside the ambulance, despite screaming and crying and begging someone—anyone—to shoot me and put me out of my misery, I managed to hear every medical TV show cliché radioed into Kaiser . . . "white caucasian male" (isn't that redundant?), "looks to be early 30s" (thank you, I'm actually 38), "is incoherent" (because it *hurts*, damn it!), "might be appendicitis" (oh no, not the knife!), "or possible stroke victim" (oh great, how will I type my "Foreword" column now?), "vital signs are . . ." What was vital at the moment was pain beyond all imagining.

As we pulled into the emergency entrance at Kaiser, I was amazed by the staff's choreography. Everyone seemed to know exactly what to do, as though the scene had been rehearsed a dozen times. There was none of that silly "but we must know your insurance card number first" that the media love to use when taking potshots at emergency rooms. In an odd way, I was alarmed and yet flattered at the serious attention I was being given.

Several doctors and nurses were trying to get me to explain the pain, describe the symptoms—give any sort of clue as to what was wrong. But the best I could do was scream, "I wanna die, I wanna die," while flopping around the gurney like a fish in an evaporating tidepool.

Then one of the emergency nurses—a handsome hapa woman—grabbed my face in her hands, locked into my rolling eyes and very calmly said, "If you don't tell me what's wrong, you *are* going to die."

I was yanked from my wailing and into reality, explained to her that the pain had begun in the small of my back and shot through to the right side of my stomach. "Kidney stone! No appendicitis, no stroke. It's a kidney stone," she announced. And then, as I launched back into total hysteria, this remarkable nurse held out her very strong arm and let me clutch it, punch it, hang from it, and practically bite it as I was rushed in for x-rays.

By the end of the day I was back home, doped up on painkillers and waiting for that tiny stone to pass. Talk about a watermelon going through the head of a pin! At least women can proudly hold up some cute baby after childbirth—all I had to show for the godawful experience was a piece of sand.

Amidst the chaos of my Oscar-worthy performance (motivated by pain), the ambulance ride and the astounding care and efficiency of the Kaiser emergency room, I never did find out the name of that wonderful nurse. I wish I had, I'd like to thank her. I know I was a real pain in the—butt.

Hawai'i is blessed with some great doctors, and behind every good doctor is a great nurse. Since I will probably never know the name of that Kaiser emergency room nurse (but I'll bet she groans whenever she remembers me), let me just thank every nurse in Hawai'i for your attention, your care, and your patience.

I know your hours are ridiculous, your headaches numerous, and your pay pretty lousy. But from one melodramatic, very difficult patient, thank you.

*Reprinted with permission from Honolulu Magazine, ©1992; 26(12).

Wake up, It's Time to go to Bed*

MAYNARD GOOD STODDARD

At the time I was plighting my troth, or troughing my plight, however that goes, a young man's choices were pretty well limited. There was the homebody skilled in the art of cooking, dusting, and raising kids, or there was the rare career girl whose range of careers ran the gamut from schoolteacher to nurse.

In opting for the nurse, I never stopped to think—honestly—that the schoolteacher works only nine months out of the year as opposed to the nurse's opportunity of working seven days a week year round. Or that some nurses work two shifts year round. Or that until I got on my literary feet, however wobbly, this extra income might come in handy.

It *had* crossed my mind that by joining plights with a nurse, I would be locking in free nursing service for the rest of my life, or until death did us part, whichever came first. I mean, here was a woman who would coddle me at every hangnail, show compassion at every headache, run for a Band-Aid at every razor scratch. And just between us—I wouldn't want this to go any further—I had heard a rumor that for passion, no mammal on earth could hold a candle to the *Homo sapiens* female nurse.

To all of which I now say, "Hogwash!" with a capital "hog."

Taking last things first, the passion theory went down the drain when she came sagging through the door after her first post-marriage eight-hour shift. Turned out that after eight hours of tending to the demands of sick sapiens, she was up to here with sapiens, both feeble and in fine fettle.

And then there was the Hippocratic oath, which commits every nurse to the dumping of a bucket of disinfectant—also known as hospital cologne—over her head before leaving for home. One whiff of that stuff is enough to bank the fire of a man's passion for at least the next 24 hours.

The free nursing service I'd been counting on was shot down the morning a can of Alpo rolled off the kitchen counter and landed across three of the best toes on my naked right foot, already blue from the cold linoleum. I figured that before news of the pain could reach my brain computer terminal, she would have assisted me to the nearest chair, drawn a bucket of warm water, rustled up the Epsom salt, and had her arms around me in case the pain would cause me to begin hopping around and possibly break a leg.

If she had any such fears she managed to mask them behind a facade of ear-splitting laughter. Between shrieks she cried, "You should have seen the fellow we had in traction yesterday . . . Both legs in casts clear to his hips . . . Did you hurt your toes?"

No fooling—I could come into the house with my head hanging by a thread, and she would still leave it up to me to find the Elmer's glue. And while I was applying the glue she would tell me about a guy coming into Emergency that day carrying his head in a Wal-Mart shopping bag.

In the confusion of choosing the appropriate wife, I had failed to consider that a nurse might be bringing her work home with her. Especially at mealtime. Especially when we were having stew. Whereas a schoolteacher would be discussing the proper positioning of a predicate adjective, a nurse says, "I saw my first evisceration today."

With my first slurp of stew poised in midair, I say, "That's nice—what's an evisceration?"

"They took this guy's insides out. Would you please pass the steak sauce?"

I managed to eat a few crackers, but they didn't go down easy.

Even having overlooked these major surprises, I still had to consider the no-small matter of what I choose to call plain old creature comfort. What you choose to call it is your business.

You know how nurses in the movies and on the tube are always showing up in the patient's room to coax him to have a slug of orange juice, fluff his pillows, rub his back, pull up the covers, and coo, "Now you try to get some sleep" and then tippytoe out of the room? All that solicitude, believe me, ends at the patient's door.

*Reprinted with permission from The Saturday Evening Post, ©July/August 1990.

One of the greatest pleasures in the life of a married nurse is catching hubby napping on the sofa at the end of the nine o'clock movie, jerking the pillow out from under his head, and cackling, "Wake up—it's time to go to bed!" If my nurse ever tippytoed when I was sleeping, I'd know I was still dreaming.

Then, however, thanks to a bleeding ulcer, it became my turn to take up residence in the Bloomington (Indiana) hospital. Have you got a minute?

Through exercise and diet, I had managed to reduce my baby fat by ten pounds and was about to receive my reward by stopping at the Spencer Dairy Queen for a Hawaiian Blizzard. Naturally, I was feeling good—God was in heaven, the hillside dew pearled, that sort of thing. But no more had we stepped through the door than I said to my dear wife-nurse, "You'll have to order. I've got to sit down." Which I did, laying my head on the table.

The next thing I knew, the table was covered with blood, blood was running off on my new white shoes, my wife was trying in vain to sop up the torrent with paper napkins, a boy was hurrying with a mop, and patrons right and left were suddenly losing their appetites. My nurse later said I had no pulse; the ambulance people could get no blood pressure. Had I been in the mood for conversation, I would have asked how anyone could register blood pressure when the last of his blood was ruining his new white shoes and the stream was already inching toward the door.

But instead of experiencing the great adventure of death, I wound up in the emergency room with a nurse coaxing me to swallow a plastic garden hose intended to siphon off the last few drops of my vital juice. Another nurse was busily engaged in stripping me down to my shorts.

When my dear wife showed up, I managed to mumble, "This girl took off my pants. Do you want to say anything to her?" To which dear wife replied, "I've taken the pants off a lot of men." This brought all activity in the room to a screeching halt until my red-faced mate explained that she also is a nurse.

I won't bore you with the details—if I haven't already—of how the doctor exposed my innards with a flashlight, how he discovered what he said was a *big* ulcer, leaving me to speculate that it must be about the size of a regulation Frisbee. Turned out to be the size of a quarter. Big enough, anyway, that I spent the next four days languishing in the hospital, surviving mostly on gelatin, and trying to forget that gelatin comes from horses' hoofs. And trying not to think where horses' hoofs have been.

What I'm getting at—and it has certainly taken long enough, I'm sure you are saying—it was during this stay that I would learn why a nurse-wife has eccentricities unlike those of, say, a schoolteacher-wife.

In taking the oath upon graduation, a nurse evidently swears that neither rain nor sleet nor dark of night will keep her from waking a patient at least four times during her eight-hour shift. No matter that sleep might do the patient more good than the pill she is serving in that little plastic cup—the pill must go through. The blood-pressure people cleverly time their intrusions to fall midway between the pill servers. One nurse woke me one night—no kidding—just to ask how I was feeling.

In an effort to outsmart the night owl Nightingales, I tried sleeping during the day. Tried is the definitive word. The parade of doctors, nurses, nurses' aides, candy stripers, flower arrangers, gelatin stewards, custodians, IV replacers, and TV adjusters through my room make a beehive by comparison look about as active as a muskrat house in the Sahara.

How I was allowed to sleep long enough to dream on my last night there is a mystery. But I'm sure heads will roll because of it. Have you got another minute?

In this dream a prospective patient would save money by not routinely accepting admittance to the first hospital where the ambulance people delivered him. If his wits were still intact, he would ask for their price on whatever he had that needed fixing, then have the ambulance driver take him to other hospitals in the area for comparison shopping. So in this dream, I was occupying a bed in the hospital of the lowest bidder.

To keep the prices low, the hospital was on a cost-cutting kick. To save heating costs as well as nurses' time, two patients with the same problem were in the same bed. I was in bed with a fellow ulcer sufferer so both of us could eat from the same gelatin bowl. In the next bed were two men with their legs in traction, one right leg, one left, both hoisted on the same trapeze.

Convalescents got their therapy by helping out around the hospital and cut their hospital bill at the same time. Female patients were cleaning bathrooms, making beds, stirring gelatin, carrying trays, doing the laundry. Their male counterparts flexed their muscles polishing floors, emptying trash, washing windows. I dreamed I had been assigned the windows on the sixth floor, outside, and I was standing on a scaffold and trying to see through my hospital gown, which the wind was whipping over my head.

On one of the windows I saw posted the hospital's business hours: "Open Monday through Friday 8 a.m. to 7 p.m.; Saturday 9 a.m. to 12 noon; closed Sunday. In case of emergency, especially ulcers, try not to bleed until you can get in line on Monday morning."

When the nurse awakened me for my 2 a.m. pill, I might have kissed her except that she had already stuck a thermometer in my mouth.

On my dear wife's daily visit, I reversed tradition and gave *her* a bouquet, one I had spotted in a deserted room on my therapy walk that morning. Dear wife, of course, was overcome with this display of affection, especially when I explained it was my way of apologizing for her nursing nonchalance at home. She was even more overcome when she happened to find a card tucked away in the foliage, a little card that read: "Get well soon, Boss. I miss you." It was signed, "Your friend, Spot."

I'm not sure that a schoolteacher-wife's reaction would have been any kinder or gentler. She very carefully placed the flowers on my chest, then ever-so-gently folded my hands over the stems. It was only a little thing, but the gesture will no doubt influence the rest of my natural as well as unnatural life. Especially on those nights when I am awakened on the sofa and dragged off to bed.

The Wrong Stuff*

MARY ANN WALSH

If you've seen the movie *The Right Stuff,* you may remember the scene involving two would-be astronauts holding enema bags on a crowded elevator. When I first saw the movie, I thought this scene was a scream, but I didn't for a minute think it was based on fact. No way could something like that actually happen. How wrong I was.

Not too long ago, I went to a thoroughly modern, state-of-the-art hospital to have upper and lower gastrointestinal examinations. My physician had recommended the tests because of the high incidence of stomach and colon cancer in my family. The "upper" test was done first and was unremarkable. The "lower" was scheduled for another day.

It was a chill, gray morning in January when I returned to outpatient radiology. It was so early that few people were around, a fact I would later be grateful for. A nurse sitting at a desk in the main waiting area instructed me to select a hospital gown from a nearby cabinet, go into a dressing room, remove my clothes from the waist down, put on the gown (with the opening in the back), and return to the reception area to wait. I did as I was told, clutching the back of the gown to keep it together as best I could. I waited, watching a light snow fly past the sixth-floor window on its way to the sodden ground below. A few more people arrived and went through the routine, returning to the reception area to sit self-consciously and leaf through magazines.

Finally, someone called my name, and I looked up to see a white-uniformed woman (a nurse?) standing in a doorway halfway down the hall and looking our way. I rose, clutching my gown, indicated that I was Mary Walsh, and headed for the examining room. Inside were a tilt-top examining table with a bulky electronic gizmo (a camera, I was soon to discover) suspended above it. At the foot of the table was a metal stand holding a plastic bag filled with a white fluid. A white-coated man, whom I took to be a technician, explained the procedure and showed me how the table worked. Then they helped me up on the table and told me to relax.

After they got me hooked up to the bag at the end of the table, they secured the tube with two or three wide pieces of tape and tilted the head of the table slightly down so the fluid would flow through my bowel. *Then* they checked the camera. Several attempts to take a picture failed. The woman left through a back door to check on something while the man continued to fiddle with the camera and make small talk. The woman came back and said the camera in another room was fine and the room was available.

I lay there listening to the discussion, which concluded with the decision to move to the other room. "Mrs. Walsh," the man said, "I'm really sorry, but this camera isn't working, so we're going to have to go to another room. Is that OK with you?"

"Sure," I replied, uncertain what was expected of

*Reprinted with permission from Health Progress, ©1993; 74(2):72, 71 and the author.

me, but never in my wildest imaginings thinking I would have to walk down the hall in my current condition.

Getting off the table was a delicate process, given the tubes and all in my sitter, but eventually I got to my feet and looked around apprehensively at the stand I was attached to. "You go ahead, slowly," the man said, indicating the open back door through which the woman had apparently fled. "I'll take care of this [the bag]."

Cautiously, I ventured into the blessedly deserted hallway, which must have been a service hallway for staff. "It's the third door on the left," I was told. Acutely aware of my ignominy, I dutifully set off down the hall, with the technician bringing up the rear. He carried my tubal train, clutching the bag like a bridesmaid's bouquet.

"You're a real sport," he said when we reached our destination.

Yeah, but do I get to be an astronaut?

The Other Side of the Bed*

CAROLYN B. STEVENS, L.P.N.

Most nurses would agree that doctors make the worst patients. But many nurses would also agree that other *nurses* run a close second in the worst patient category. After all, who wants to care for a patient who knows the score or one who might be *keeping* score and might judge your nursing care inadequate?

When I was a patient recently, I *did* find my nursing care inadequate. Now, I'm wondering. If I *hadn't* been a nurse, would I have gotten better care, or worse?

When I was admitted, my tentative diagnosis was a dislocated patella. Like most patients, I was apprehensive. How would I handle the pain? The feeling of helplessness? The lack of privacy? I didn't realize that when you're on the other side of the bed, you can't count on anything.

I knew I'd get an identification bracelet, but I hadn't counted on my reaction to the bracelet—I felt like a number. Actually, I felt like *two* numbers, since the bracelet listed my patient identification number and my age.

"Good grief, are you *that* old?" one of the younger nurses said.

Then, my first night in a strange bed, I was restless. My leg ached, my back ached, and I needed an aspirin.

"I'm sorry," the nurse said. "But your doctor didn't order aspirin." When she saw my jaw drop in dismay,

she softened a bit. "I'm awfully busy, but I *could* call the doctor," she said.

"No, no," I said, feeling guilty. So since the doctor had ordered sleeping pills, I took a sleeping pill for pain.

When the day of my surgery came, I was plagued with a new anxiety—body exposure. How could I let the nurses and doctors flop me around naked on the operating table?

"I'm wearing my underpants to the operating room," I said. "Now, Carolyn, you know no one wears underwear during surgery," the nurse cajoled. "My knee's way down there and my underpants are way up here," I pleaded.

The nurse told me that the last nurse-patient who'd worn underpants to surgery had had them removed and hung on an I.V. pole. "Do you want everyone to walk by and say, 'There're Carolyn's pants'?" she asked.

So I went to surgery without my underpants and returned without the meniscus in my left knee. As it turned out, my patella was worse than dislocated—it was torn off, along with the quadriceps of my thigh.

My first postoperative day, I overheard a doctor and nurse discussing a woman patient who hadn't voided since surgery and who might need to be catheterized.

Poor soul, I thought. Then it dawned on me the doctor was *my* doctor, and the patient was *me*. I was almost immobilized by fear, thinking about being catheterized,

*Used with permission from Nursing 80, ©1980; 10(1):104. Edited from the original.

when the doctor walked into my room—the orthopedic specialist who knew $500 words 12 syllables long.

"Why haven't you peed?" he asked.

"Nobody asked me to," I answered.

"Pee," he commanded and left the room.

I could hardly ignore a command so bluntly stated, so since no one offered to help, I put myself on the bedpan.

Carrying out the doctor's orders was easier said than done. Fortunately, I had a lot to think about. Like, whatever happened to all those little tricks we learn to encourage patients to void? Running tap water; warming the bedpan. After an hour, I finally carried out the doctor's order—I "peed."

My leg began to ache badly. My doctor had ordered meperidine (Demerol); but when I asked for the medication, the nurse told me, "You can become addicted to this." I couldn't believe her presumptuousness. *I* knew I could become addicted, but not in the few days I'd be a patient. I wondered what she told her other patients who *didn't* know.

After that episode, I was more hesitant to ask for Demerol. I endured the pain as long as I could, but one night, I went too long without medication. I rang for the nurse three times. An hour later, when I finally got my Demerol, I was clammy, trembling, and crying. And by that time, the Demerol didn't even work.

As far as I'm concerned, my entire 8 days in the hospital were impossible, and I'm sure that my nurses thought I was an impossible patient. I'm convinced that some of the things that happened to me happened *because* I'm a nurse—that my nurses expected me to either take care of myself or patiently go to the end of the line. When I did ask for something, I felt guilty, and my nurses did little to alleviate my guilt. In fact, by their words and actions, they encouraged it.

I don't believe they did this intentionally, but I do believe they didn't give much thought, to how their words or actions might affect me—the patient. But if your nurse doesn't give you any thought, who will?

So I'm still wondering. If I *hadn't* been a nurse, would I have gotten better care, or worse?

AT TIMES LIKE THIS

An exploding health care system seeks seasoned professionals to join our multidisciplinary team. As a key member of the staff, you will be challenged to provide direct patient care, coordinate case management, and conduct independent research. Applicants must demonstrate excellent oral and written communication skills as well as computer literacy. Trilingual ability and proven leadership a plus. Twelve years experience and MS preferred.

Qualified candidates must submit to random drug testing, a polygraph, and a complete background investigation. We offer highly flexible schedules for evenings, nights, shift work, or weekends at per diem rates. Fax resume to 1-800-GET-REAL or visit our website at www.perdiem.org.

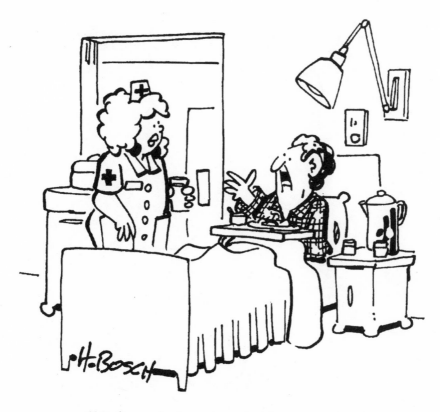

"Two thousand a day and you don't have a wine list?"

Then and Now*

GRACE BUBULKA, R.N., M.S.N.

Of all the changes nursing has undergone recently, the most outwardly obvious is in the "dress code."

As a new graduate back in the 1970s, I remember the feel of wearing my bright white uniform, starched to perfection. While it was always a challenge keeping my shoes neat and clean, the most controversial aspect of our look back then was our nurse's cap.

Caps were an everyday source of frustration to me once I started working in a busy hospital emergency department. My co-workers and I began grumbling at the start of every shift prior to report as we tried to get the darned things right on our heads. Without fail, every time I assisted with a suturing, a spray of local anesthetic and blood would sprinkle across my white cap. Working in codes was particularly difficult. Typically, we would be involved in at least two resuscitations per shift. Every time I performed chest compressions, my cap would get hopelessly entangled in the surrounding intravenous tubing or monitor wires and fall off (bobby pins and all) into a sterile field, infuriating the physicians.

As a group, not many of us felt our caps were particularly attractive. Some of the basic styles were okay, but others were . . . well, different.

Our hospital was preparing for an accreditation site visit. For weeks ahead, we ED nurses were cautioned to wear our caps, per policy, during the survey. Nervous about being noticed by our supervisors or a surveyor for not complying with the rules, we examined our old, stained caps.

The day of survey arrived and we were ready for inspection. Our policy books and charts were perfect, exam rooms were clean and stocked . . . but we still did not have presentable caps. The four of us huddled in the break room when we got the call that the Director of Nurses, our superior, and a surveyor would be coming through the ED in ten minutes. Suddenly one of my buddies had a brilliant flash—and we got to work.

We were ready and waiting in the nursing station for the team to walk through our unit. We heard the rear entrance open and shoes squeaking on the shiny floors. As the examiners approached, we all smiled our professional best, and watched our supervisor's eyes widen at the clean white caps on our heads. Perched on each head was a paper coffee filter from the break room, folded creatively, and pinned in place for the big event.

Our supervisor never discussed this with us, our hospital was accredited . . . and I still won't wear my cap.

*Reprinted with permission from Point of View, ©1995; 32(2):22. Edited from the original.

Top Ten Lists for Doctors— Part 2*

HOWARD J. BENNETT, M.D.

Top Ten Reasons to Work for an HMO

10. You've always wondered what it would be like to see 80 patients a day.
9. The thought of running streptokinase drips at home sounds like fun.
8. Your accountant thinks you should be in a lower tax bracket.
7. You get a free tote bag with the plan's logo on it.
6. It's a good transition job before you make the jump to professional wrestling.
5. You can star in a TV commercial.
4. It gives you something to brag about at high school reunions.
3. It's a challenge to manage patients without any lab work.
2. Big bonuses are earned for reusing tongue depressors.
1. Lawyers rarely belong to HMOs.

Top Ten Rejected Names for Managed Care Plans

10. McHealth Care
9. Suboptimum Choice
8. Sri Lanka Health Plan
7. Equivocare
6. Premiums Plus
5. You'll Get That Procedure Over Our Dead Body Health Plan
4. Cut-Rate Health Care
3. Gatekeepers USA
2. Chapter 11 Health Plan
1. Kevorkian Plus

Answering Service Operators' Top Ten Pet Peeves

10. Patients with multiple personalities who call in six times for the same complaint.
9. New digital headsets that keep picking up *Regis & Kathie Lee*.
8. Grouchy doctors who expect phone numbers to be accurate.
7. Choking patients who garble their phone number.
6. 911 operators who brag about the hunks they work with at the fire station.
5. Working the night shift, but not getting to wake anybody up.
4. People who like *Chicago Hope* more than *E.R.*
3. Tornadoes that knock out power but spare the phone lines.
2. People who call the wrong number and really want *The Friend's Psychic Hotline*.
1. Prank calls from former co-workers who now have really good jobs that *don't* involve working with doctors.

Top Ten Medical Categories Not Seen on *Jeopardy*

10. Rashes that ooze.
9. Health benefits of nicotine.
8. Surgeons General who have been on *Oprah*.
7. Orifices you can reach with one finger.
6. Insurance companies that really care.
5. Diseases you can catch from toilet paper.
4. Famous doctors who cheated in high school.
3. Supreme Court justices who have had liposuction.
2. Organs that have not been dropped in the O.R.
1. What doctors say about patients when they are anesthetized.

*Reprinted from *The Journal of Family Practice,* ©1996; 43(2):110.
Reprinted by permission of Appleton & Lange, and the author.

Nursing Hymns for Every Occasion

AMY Y. YOUNG AND COLLEEN KENEFICK

Administrator	Almost Persuaded
Agency nurse	I'm On My Way To Canaan
Army nurse	Fight the Good Fight With All thy Might!
Camp nurse	Nobody Knows De Trouble I've Seen
Cardiology	From Heart to Heart
Community nurse	I Know Not Where The Road Will Lead
Ear, nose, and throat	Give Ear, O God, to my Loud Cry
Emergency room	We Are Watching, We Are Waiting
Endocrinology	There's a Sweet, Sweet Spirit In This Place
Flight nurse	In Heaven Soaring Up
Geriatrics	Remember, Sinful Youth
Grant applicant	Mysterious Presence! Source of All
Home health nurse	When Shall We All Meet Again?
Hospice nurse	Kind Words Can Never Die
Hospital nurse	A Little Kingdom I Possess
Infertility clinic	For Lo! My Jonah How He Slumped
Labor and delivery	Now From Labor and From Care
Management	Th' Almighty Spoke, and Gabriel Sped
Military nurse	Oh God, Send Men Whose Purpose Will Not Falter
Night shift	For Us No Night Can Be Happier Filled
Nurse anesthetist	Welcome, Sweet Rest
Nurse educator	Trust In Me
Nurse theorist	You That Have Been Often Invited
Nurses aide	Thou Long Disowned, Reviled, Oppressed
Nursing home	We Love the Venerable House
Office nurse	The Voice of God is Calling
Obstetrics and gynecology	Don't You be Like the Foolish Virgin
Occupational health	At Length the Busy Day is Done
Oncology	We Shall Overcome
Ophthalmology	Mine Eyes Have Seen the Glory
Orthopedics	I Spread Out Unto Thee My Hands
Pediatrics	Come, Happy Children
Plastic surgery	O Lord, Turn Not Away Thy Face
Preventive health	Defend Us, Lord, From Every Ill
Proctology	Let the Deep Organ Swell the Lay
Psychiatric	When Wild Confusion Wrecks the Air
Public health	Sinners, Will You Scorn the Message?
Rehabilitation	Be Strong, We Are Not Here to Play
Retiring nurse	Rejoice, Let Alleluias Ring
School nurse	Our School Now Closes Out
Ship nurse	What Ship Is This?
Substance abuse	O For the Happy Hour
Surgical	Lord, At This Closing Hour
Urologic	My Soul Before Thee Prostrate Lies
Vacationing nurse	All Things Bright and Beautiful
Visiting nurse	I've Reached the Land of Corn and Wine

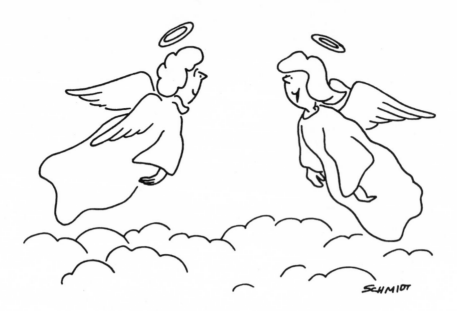

You'll like it here—no nights and no weekends!

Stress and the Single Sybarite*

LEAH L. CURTIN, R.N.

Stress. The dictionary defines it as "strain or pressure." The government studies it. We all wish we had less of it. And I think I've found a cure for it.

Last summer, my sister Patty and I hied ourselves off to Vail—a fancy place in the Colorado Rockies which offers luxury hotels, fancy boutiques and sybaritic spas. Five days of decadent dining, stress reduction classes, and massage. All for a little less than it cost me to put my son through law school.

Despite my general allergy to beaches—infested as they are with women who pose for *Sport's Illustrated's* swimwear edition (I have cooked turkeys bigger than most of them)—Patty convinced me that **spas** are another matter altogether. So I unpacked my 15-year-old

bathing suit—a no-nonsense, one-piece black and pink stripe with industrial strength straps and enough rubber in the bra to support an 18-wheeler—and off we went.

My dears! Feet soaked in an herbal broth. Folks waiting on you hand and foot. After 45 minutes of vigorous massage, you get into a hot tub to soothe your weary body. You've no sooner settled your bones when an athletic looking young man brings you a cool glass of water lest you get too hot in the hot tub. Next you go to the steam room where you *breathe in* (spa people often speak in italics) a wall of steam to purify your vocal cords. Actually, even the soles of my feet were sweating so I figured I must have purified every-

*Used with permission from Nursing Management, ©1993; 24(10):7.

thing. When you get out, **of course** your shower is running to cool you right off. You would be *astounded* at how easy it is to get used to this kind of service.

The personnel in spas are also very big on self-esteem. They have been taught that there is an inverse relationship between self-esteem and stress. So, no matter how much of an uncoordinated blimp you may be, they always find something good to say about you. Patty came back from her pedicure and announced proudly, "The manicurist said that **I** have perfectly shaped toenails."

"Perfect toenails?" I asked.

"**Perfect** toenails," she said.

After my facial, the make-up artist studied my face for a long time. Just as I was mentally preparing myself for the statement, "Only a plastic surgeon can . . .," she came up with my redeeming feature. "My *dear*," she announced triumphantly, "you have a *fabulous patrician* nose."

With a strong sense of superiority, I informed Patty that **I** have a **patrician** nose. She promptly countered with, "My masseuse says I have *beautiful* skin." I topped her, however, when my therapist said, "You have *great* elasticity." Patty can't compete with great elasticity.

Despite the splendid efforts of the spa, Patty and I still suffered from utter flabdom, so we decided that a tougher regime was warranted and headed off to classes on exercise, nutrition and New Age relaxation.

In nutrition classes these days, none of the vegetables are their regular color—red lettuce, yellow bell peppers, green pasta. This is hard to keep up with when you regularly eat pizza, but I did my best. I tried tofu, oat bran and herbal tea. I went to classes on visualization, actualization, meditation and yoga. I like yoga best—exercise without sweat! Patty and I even developed our own mantra. For 20 minutes each day we assumed the lotus position and chanted, "Aoom. I am a slim, trim, healthy human being right noooow. I am . . ." It was hard to keep from laughing.

In every class, the instructors told us that we had to get in touch with our bodies. Mine isn't all that communicative, but I heard from it on Saturday morning when I suggested, "Body, how would you like a nice work out on the Nordictrack?"

Within a heartbeat, my body responded, "Listen, dingbat, do it and you die." Great! I finally get in touch with my body and it turns out to have the personality of Attila the Hun. They told us to listen to our bodies, so we did. Without another word, Patty and I pulled up our one-piece bathing suits and headed for the hot tub again.

On our last day there, I was in my best class—New Age Relaxation—when the instructor said in a soothing voice, "Think of something about yourself that you really like. Take it to your center and hold it there. Believe it. Love it. Our most important task is to learn to love ourselves unconditionally. Each of us must do this for there to be peace in the world."

I thought, "Am I in trouble now. I can **never** find my center, and I have a hard time finding things I like about my body and **world peace** depends on this." Talk about stress! Then it came to me and I took it right to my center. I have a **fabulous** patrician nose.

I laughed. I hope you do, too. It is the only stress reliever that **always** works.

Who Was
That Masked Man?*

MICHAEL ROTH, B.S., R.N., C.N.O.R.

As I arrived at work in the MICU one Saturday night, I was told that I was being pulled to the SICU that shift. It wasn't my turn to be pulled, but I didn't argue. Our one ICU had recently broken up to the three units of MICU, SICU and CCU. All staff members of each unit were cross trained to work on the others. I felt this would be an easy pull and I would skip a turn going to the floors, so I didn't think much about it as I walked down the hall to the SICU.

I opened the door and instead of the usual bustle of a busy unit, all was quiet. Even on the night shift the ICUs are generally well lit, but the SICU was dim. I quickly entered to see what was going on. As soon as the evening nurses, Sue and Cindy, saw me they let out an audible sigh of relief. While most people are eager to go home, this struck me as strange. I asked what was going on, and they laughed. They explained why I was pulled.

Their one and only patient had been shot in the head during a feud between two families. The gunman was still at large and was planning on finishing the job. The patient's family was a little perturbed and they were out hunting for the gunman. Thus, there were two families running around with guns settling scores over one guy. My patient.

Since this hospital was the only trauma center in town, that pretty much narrowed their search to us. I was pulled because I was the only male nurse in the ICUs this shift. Being a new grad, I didn't think of getting suddenly ill. Having judiciously avoided all aspects of military service, including registering for the draft, I bravely and calmly said to Carol, the other nurse with me that shift, "If anyone comes to get him, I'm diving behind this counter."

Everything went smoothly, with Carol and I taking turns caring for our patient. Then, at 4:00 a.m., the nursing supervisor arrived. After we got up from behind the desk, she told us she was just making rounds.

We updated her on our patient. As she was leaving, she said there was no truth to the rumor that a couple of men had been seen in the hospital with shotguns. There was nothing to worry about, and besides, security was making frequent rounds here in the SICU. As she left, Carol and I looked at each other and simultaneously said, "Great, I feel safe now." Carol felt that if security was making frequent rounds we should have seen someone by now. I, having thought they were all graduates from the Barney Fife School of Security, said that I hoped they had their bullet with them tonight.

The night slowly dragged on as Carol and I watched the clock's hands inch forward. Suddenly, at 6:00 a.m., the door opened and in strolled a man in blue jeans and a flannel shirt, about six-foot-two, weighing two hundred plus. He walked purposefully toward our patient. Carol and I looked at each other. She grabbed the phone and called security. She gestured for me to confront that man. I bravely volunteered to hold the phone while she went forth, but she shoved me toward the patient's room.

I arrived at the door, allowing myself plenty of room to escape, and in a deep voice squeaked out, "Can I help you?"

He turned and fixed me with a glare and asked about vital signs, ICP readings, swan readings, and cardiac output. Quick as ever, I responded, "What? Who are you?"

He said, "I'm Dr. J., the new neurosurgeon. I was out and about and decided to check on my patient." He then held out his hand and said, "Nice to meet you." Thirty minutes later, as he was leaving, our crack security team arrived with their hands on their guns. They were finally responding to Carol's STAT call. When Carol and I finished laughing, we cleared Dr. J. with security, and they left. We explained to Dr. J. what happened. He laughed and said that he had better make himself more well known.

*Reprinted with permission from Journal of Nursing Jocularity, ©1997; 7(1):28–29. Edited from the original.

AT TIMES LIKE THIS

What Would Nightingale Say?*

BERNITA DECKER, B.S., G.N.

Dear Ms. Nightingale,

I was so glad to hear that the news of your demise was slightly exaggerated. As a nursing student nearing the end of my first quarter, some things have come to light which disturb and confuse me. Perhaps you can help me, since formal nursing education gained its impetus and respectability largely because of your efforts.

I have looked at my schedule for the next 2 years and can not find a course that teaches what I am struggling to read between the lines. One of my instructors is teaching nursing diagnosis, which includes some aggressive interventions. She has constantly stressed the independent portion of nursing. Good grief, in the space of 9 weeks, I have learned to treat and diagnose everything from urge incontinence to sexual dysfunction, using interventions like dance therapy and therapeutic touch. (I wonder if guided imagery would work for constipation?) Anyway, now my instructor is saying that the only way to function effectively as a nurse is to pretend ignorance and somehow magically let the physician know what to do—sort of like developing an affect of independent subservience. I think that I am missing something, somewhere. Is there a course offered that will tell me how to apply upper-level information without anyone knowing?

As a class, we are told of the evils of paternalism and how this cultural attitude has oppressed nurses. We are also encouraged to welcome men into our profession because they will be instrumental in gaining respect and equal pay for us. Why will it take the very group who oppressed us to unoppress us? (Isn't that rather like encouraging the fox to become a hen? He may pretend for a while, but will eventually take control of the coop.)

Another thing that confuses me is the learning system. If I am soon going to have the responsibility for an individual's mental, spiritual, and physical responses to illness or health, why is the current focus on learning to pass a test? Since passing a test is the prevailing concern, why doesn't the Dean just institute an applicable course and save all of the instructors from having to subtly impart this information in a hodge-podge manner?

I am also supposed to figure out how to incorporate intuition, probably the most abstract of concepts, into the very specific NANDA-approved nursing diagnosis and structured care plans.

There is another thing I can not figure—the instructors say that holism is of prime importance, yet everyone else evaluates and respects a nurse according to her ability to perform tasks. In fact, I am told that an RN barely has time to complete necessary tasks, much less do anything holistic. How did you do it?

Well, those are just a few of the things I am supposed to learn by reading between the lines. I am being taught holism, management skills, and research, but I wish there was a class called N473: Application of Polar Inconsistencies in Nursing.

Sincerely yours,

B. Decker

Bernita Decker,
a very confused nursing student

*Reprinted with permission from Nurse Educator, ©1991; 16(3):12. Edited from the original.

Deck the Wards*

BRIAN BOOTH, R.G.N.

Traditionally, much effort has gone into making Christmas in the wards special.

Over recent years, however, the task has been made more difficult because of the effects of tighter financial constraints. Ward decorations long past their prime are having to be used and reused, because there is no money available for replacements. Even trust funds may have been exhausted by some irresponsible nurses' profligate spending on luxury items such as soap and shampoo for patients or training courses for staff.

Christmas cards

One little-marked effect of the NHS reforms' money-saving programme has been the increase in numbers of senior administrators to whom Christmas cards must be sent. Failure to remember such important personages as the business manager or executive planning officer can have disastrous results in the following year, should you (for example) run out of coffee before the monthly delivery is due or if a window in the bathroom gets stuck open.

Even worse than forgetting these eminent members of the hospital team would be to send a 3in × 4in card bought from the local market in a bargain box of 200 for 49p. This signals an apparent failure to have embraced the values of the internal market, showing that you are unable to prioritise resource allocation.

But do not despair. Unless you have the misfortune to work for one of the Luddite hospitals that has not applied for trust status, there will exist, somewhere, a stack of thousands of glossy brochures extolling the virtues of your provider services. A friendly porter should be able to obtain as many of these as you need.

The cover of each brochure will be constructed from the highest-quality glossy paper, bearing an extremely flattering picture of the, freshly painted, main hospital buildings. By carefully removing the contents, and judiciously trimming the edges, you have the makings of a personalised Christmas card.

A quick poll of patients, particularly the older ones, will undoubtedly turn up someone who was taught to write legibly at school, and that person will be happy to write in the details in return for an extra digestive biscuit with his or her morning tea.

Consultants

Christmas presents for your consultants can be problematic and expensive. However, with a little forward planning, you can come up with a delightful surprise at very little cost.

In early December, you will need to establish at what time they propose to drop in on Christmas Day (if they are always around to carve the turkey, this will be much easier for you). However, it is essential that they all arrive within five minutes of each other.

When the first one enters the ward, he or she will hand you the gift-wrapped traditional bottle of sherry. You must take this with the usual thanks and protestations, at which point a member of staff will, according to a pre-arranged signal, call you away to take an urgent telephone call. As you move away, carefully remove the gift tag and replace it with one of your own.

Timing is crucial at this point. You should now be moving to greet the next consultant and as he or she hands you a bottle, you in turn give them the one that you are holding, murmuring something about 'a small token of our esteem.' The tag replacement gambit is then repeated with each person, not forgetting the first.

Note: it is unwise to try this technique on nurse managers, as they are likely to wrap gifts themselves and may well recognise the paper.

Decorations

These are a major drain on resources, but Christmas decorations can be obtained at minimal cost, providing a little ingenuity and imagination is used.

• *Artificial snow for windows:* apart from the effect on the ozone layer, aerosol snow sprays are prohibitively expensive for the cash-strapped ward. A perfect substitute is available, though, thanks to the cutbacks in domestic services.

*Reprinted from Nursing Times, ©1993; 89(50):42–43 with permission from Macmillan Magazines, Ltd.

In the run-up to Christmas, a monthly check under the beds should yield large amounts of fluff. By dabbing this on locker tops, sticky with accumulated Lucozade spillages, you have a self-adherent product, ready to be applied where needed.

Note: bed fluff can also be utilised to make a cost-effective and realistic beard for Santa.

• *Paper chains:* your ward clerk will have large supplies of audit forms, special requisition documentation and so on that have been superseded by new improved ones. If you have achieved trust status, the amounts will be larger, not least because of outdated forms bearing the old hospital name, which will all have been removed from circulation. If your application was turned down, there should be an unlimited supply of headed notepaper bearing the proposed new name.

These forms, which often come in a variety of colours, make handsome decorations.

Crêpe paper is extremely expensive nowadays, but have you considered the use of crêpe bandages? Ones that have been used and laundered several times can be given a slight twist and run from corner to corner of the dayroom. If you have access to bandages that have been used on heavily exudating wounds—for example, leg ulcers—you will see that unique patterns have been created, adding that missing touch of colour.

• *Tree decorations:* every ward has a wealth of material that cries out to be used.

Tinsel: by carefully stripping the backs from blister packs of tablets, you can amass large amounts of high-quality silver paper in no time.

Candles: the barrels of used syringes are a perfect shape; but if the tree is a small one, catheter spigots may be more suitable.

Fairy lights: in today's high-tech medical world, there is a plethora of machinery equipped with warning lights, many of which flash attractively.

Artificial snow: if all the saved bed fluff has been used up on the windows, the interiors of continence pads can be shredded and used to gently powder the branches.

Baubles: multi-dose drug vials, being made of glass, catch the light charmingly, while the inside of adhesive tape rolls spin in an intriguing way.

Streamers: draping catheters and intravenous-giving sets across branches creates an unusual effect.

We hope this guide has helped set off some ideas of your own and trust that forward-thinking management will reward staff who brighten up their places of work in such a cost-effective manner.

New Year's Resolutions— and All That Jazz!*

GLORIA ROSENTHAL

I'm not fooling around anymore. I made my New Year's resolutions this year, like I do every year, but I'm sticking to them this time. I even wrote them down in a nice, neat, numbered list. So you can see how serious I am about this entire business.

Actually, the first one practically wrote itself right after the holidays. I was sitting around thinking about not having to stuff another turkey until next November, and I started thinking about how lucky a turkey is. I mean, look at it this way. A turkey gets stuffed, and before you know it, there's nothing left but skin and bones. I get stuffed at just about the same time, and before you know it, I'm . . . well, never mind what I am, but you can be sure it's not skin and bones. That's why the first resolution had to be:

1. Lose 10 pounds.

I took the advice of a magazine article and stood naked in front of a full length mirror (without holding in my stomach, for heaven's sakes!) They promised this would point up my major figure flaws.

They were right.

2. My second resolution was to never stand naked in front of a full length mirror.

Before I go on with the rest of the list, there's something I want to explain about number one. You know, the one about losing 10 pounds? It seems that Larry and I had this bet. He said I wouldn't stick to my resolutions again this year, and I, knowing my determination and strength of character, said of course I would and ha! ha! what did he want to bet? We bet a hot fudge sundae. And as soon as he saw I was winning, he paid off.

So I lost.

I'm still trying to figure out what happened there. No matter. It pushed me into being more reasonable and realistic about my goals. To wit:

3. Serve something really different for dinner at least one night a week.

I'm starting tonight. Won't they be surprised to get oatmeal for dinner!

4. Don't spread gossip.

Of course, it isn't always easy to tell the difference between spreading gossip and imparting information.

5. Don't listen to gossip.

And I suppose you think it's easy to tell the difference between listening to gossip and my inalienable "right to know"?

6. Cut phone conversations short.

7. Don't insult friends.

Cutting phone conversations short might insult friends.

8. Keep a record of expenses to help cut down unnecessary spending.

For example: if I leave the house, like I did this morning, with $23.57, and I have $2.87 left when I return home, I will immediately write down that I bought . . . I bought . . . er . . . I spent it on. . .

9. Eliminate sources of irritation.

Keeping expense records is irritating.

10. Stop nagging.

When I want the kids to do something, I will ignore them and talk directly to the wall.

11. Check how words are spelt when not sure.

You might not believe this, but I freqwently make mistakes.

12. Look up the meanings of new words and use them if they fit naturally into conversations without sounding forced.

I'd say this resolution is sui generis; and it should prove to be efficacious.

12a. Get over that superstition about the number thirteen.

14. Always finish what you start.

In other words, I won't leave something in the middle of . . .

*Reprinted with permission from American Journal of Nursing, ©1977; 77(1):174.

The Harmonics of Nursing*

RUTH E. MALONE, R.N.

According to mystical tradition, we're just beginning a New Age. The celebration of this Harmonic Convergence began one Sunday last August.

"Wouldn't you know it?" I remarked to a friend. "One Harmonic Convergence every 5,000 years, and *I* have to work."

We all know how it is when you're a nurse—and why there's a shortage. Actually, it's more of an outage than a shortage. Almost everyone knows someone who used to be a nurse and now makes 65 grand a year selling cosmetics. You can't make a lot of money in everyday life-and-death work, but peddle something that covers the tracks life makes and just watch your income balloon.

Our profession requires a certain ducklike ability to immerse ourselves in reality, yet shed it off naturally, just swimming on through. Not everyone can do this. "Oh, I could never be a nurse!" rates number one of the three phrases nurses hear most. This phrase is usually followed by a brief explanation, such as "I could never stand all that blood" or "I can't stand sick people."

Why do people feel the need to say this to us? Have I ever blurted out, "Oh, I could never stand to be an accountant!" when getting my taxes done? This phrase always gives me a vaguely backhanded feeling, as if someone had remarked, "Gee, you are courageous for someone with bad breath."

Then there's the heartfelt exclamation, "I think what you do is just wonderful!" This remark is well intentioned, yet few people actually know what nurses do. Good nursing care is often invisible: we often step in and work our magic before the problem becomes apparent to anyone else.

But the phrase that makes me want to throw up my hands is, "Are you going to go on and become a doctor?" I always make a point of explaining how nursing is *very* different from medicine, yet people are still skeptical (even after I flash such a winner as "carecure

dichotomy"). They don't understand it. Eyes narrowing, they silently consider other explanations:

- *Doesn't want the responsibility?* (But the doctor isn't even here—the nurse is in charge right now!)
- *Too dumb to get into medical school?* (But I heard this nurse explaining my ECG to a doctor earlier!)
- *Too lazy to go to medical school?* (Unlikely. Everyone knows how hard nurses work—on their feet all day—or all night.)
- *Too crazy to go to medical school?* (Hmmmm. . .)

I guess it's easy to understand why people think that nursing is a stepping-stone to doctoring. After all, aren't the main "ingredients" of our work the same: people who are patients, injured or sick (or at least not well) and treatment?

But I like to think the differences bear some relationship to why a person chooses to become a musician rather than a mathematician, or a sculptor instead of an engineer. For me, nursing seems a little closer to the nerve and the bone, a little more personal than medicine.

In the middle of the night, when fears throng thick and fast, the nurse helps the patient wrestle with whatever demons he must face. These struggles are the ones every human being faces at one time or another. At dark moments, we all search desperately for meaning, reevaluating all priorities, questioning all values.

Physicians are taught to find the right answers—and that's important in what doctors do. Nurses learn there aren't any right answers—except the ones their patients discover for themselves. When we help patients make those discoveries, our rhythms fall into step with theirs. Now that's convergence. And to think we celebrate it once every 5,000 years.

My head nurse promised me that since I worked this time, I get the next Harmonic Convergence off. Unless somebody calls in sick . . .

*Reprinted with permission from American Journal of Nursing, ©1988; 88(1):144.

Sick of the Sick*

BARBARA EHRENREICH

The insurance industry would be perfectly healthy if sick people would just quit their bellyaching.

Once again we are being deafened by complaints that the U.S. medical system "doesn't work." We spend $500 billion a year on medical care, the complainers allege, for no tangible benefits beyond what could easily be achieved through sorcery, environmental cleanup, or the free distribution of prescription drugs to all comers, regardless of ailment.

But let us look beyond the facile charges of the chronic malcontents. Who's doing the complaining, anyway? Is it the people who are in a position to *know* whether the medical system is working or not, i.e., the real experts—the doctors, hospital executives and hardworking CEOs of the companies that make silicon breast inserts and lifelike hair transplants? No, from them comes only the profound silence of the recently and abundantly fed. The complaining comes almost entirely from—let us be honest—the *sick.*

And no wonder the sick are complaining! The medical system was not designed for people who have declined from the full bloom of health. Doctors don't like them, because sickness, along with injury and death, is a reliable source of malpractice suits. Hospitals don't like them, because sickness, especially the more painful and flamboyant varieties, is deeply disruptive to the hospital routine and disorienting to the personnel. Insurance companies positively hate them, which is why an exhaustive physical exam is required for those seeking insurance—to rule out anyone who is now, has ever been, or may someday become, sick.

And let us be really honest. *We* don't like them either. Consider their appearance: the hideous rashes, the open sores, the feverish ravings, the ghastly neglect of personal grooming. We don't let sick people be president. We don't want to see them playing the romantic lead next to Kim Basinger. Why should we let them tell us how to run our medical system?

Another thing about sick people: they'll complain about *anything.* Put a tasty meal in front of them, attractively arranged on a tray—say, mashed potatoes, army-green vegetables, color-coordinated meat, and a savory lime jello—and what do you get? Complaints! Because that is almost the definition of sickness, the one universal symptom underlying the myriad varieties of disease—kvetching!

The truth is, we have the finest medical technology in the world. What other country offers in-vitro fertilization, with its fabulous success rate of over 5 percent, not only to the landed aristocracy, but to the average possessor of $10,000? What other nation can guarantee that no infant need fight its way out of the birth canal as long as there are scalpels around, and thousands of debt-ridden anesthesiologists?

I scarcely need mention our staggering diagnostic capabilities, which leave those poor socialistic types—the English, the Canadians, the Swedes, and their ilk—gasping in envy. There's a brand-new, multimillion-dollar infrasonic-magneto detonator for the detection of earwax, for example. Or the temple-sized ultra-quark-powered graviton for the visualization of intestinal gas. And so forth. Of course the sick feel left out. The rigors of our burgeoning diagnostic technology can be safely survived only by the most robust and able-bodied.

Take the sick out of the system and, I tell you, the system works just fine. So long, of course, as you understand what it's trying to *do.*

Hospitals, for example, are best appreciated as an extractive industry, on a par with the more familiar forms of mining. In a hospital, human parts—blood, urine, kidneys, limbs, uteruses, etc.—are removed, thus leaving the general population lighter and sleeker. Some of these parts are recycled to people who are themselves in need of kidneys, blood, or, for that matter, urine. It is true, a few parts cannot adequately be accounted for. The fat removed in liposuction, for example, may have something to do with the texture of the french fries served at McDonald's, though that is only conjecture.

The rest of the human tissue removed is essential to

*Reprinted with permission from *Mother Jones* Magazine, ©1989; 14(9):7,10. Foundation for National Progress.

the production of medical waste. Some analysts believe that the syringes washing up in our surf represent a unique laissez-faire approach to socialized medicine: load up the syringes and trust that each swimmer gets the medication appropriate to his or her condition! Who knows? But it cannot be denied that medical waste, inhaled as air pollution, contributes to the painless removal of the aged, infirm, and asthmatic.

Moving on to the medical profession. It is easily faulted, of course, if its mission is confused with mercy. Sociologists have long regarded the medical profession as a guild, but more recently they have decided it is more accurately described as a gang. Hence the characteristic white jackets, and the wearing of masks for undertakings of unusual violence or questionable legality.

The initiation rite—which clearly distinguishes medicine from rival gangs like the Crips or the Bloods—is organic chemistry, in which the competition for grades is so fierce that premeds are led to steal the reference books and smash the lab apparatus of their fellow students. Such rituals assure that our medical profession continues to select for the criminal element.

Like the aforementioned rivals, the medical profession has two main preoccupations: the protection of turf, especially from upstarts in the nursing or midwifery professions, and, naturally, the distribution of drugs. Current laws put penicillin, for example, in much the same category as cocaine: it cannot be freely purchased over the counter, but obtained only through specialized salespersons, and then only by the wealthy, the wily, or the unusually desperate.

But the *sick*, you say. Where do they fit in amid all this grasping, grabbing, hustling, hacking, and feverishly rapid metabolism of money and body parts? Is there no place for them?

Yes, indeed, there's a place. It's called Canada, or Sweden, or even England. So get out and get better! And leave our medical system for those who really need it—the insurance execs, the hospital directors, and, of course, the gang in white coats.

BOOK BIBLIOGRAPHY

Adams, Patch: Gesundheit! Bringing Good Health to You, the Medical System, and Society through Physician Service, Complementary Therapies, Humor, and Joy. Rochester, VT, Healing Arts Press, 1993.

Allan, Robert, and Scheidt, Stephen. Heart and Mind: The Practice of Cardiac Psychology. Washington, D.C., American Psychological Association, 1996.

Andrus Volunteers: Humor: The Tonic You Can Afford, A Handbook on Ways of Using Humor in Long Term Care. Los Angeles, Ethel Percy Andrus Gerontology Center, 1983.

Blumenfeld, Esther, and Alpern, Lynne: The Smile Connection: How to Use Humor in Dealing with People. Englewood Cliffs, N.J., Prentice-Hall, 1986.

Bokun, Branko: Humour Therapy in Cancer, Psychosomatic Diseases, Mental Disorders, Crime, Interpersonal and Sexual Relationships. London, Vita Books, 1986.

Buxman, Karyn, LeMoine, Anne (eds): Nursing Perpectives on Humor. New York, Power Publications, 1995.

Cousins, Norman: Anatomy of an Illness as Perceived by the Patient. New York, W.W. Norton, 1979.

Cousins, Norman: Head First: The Biology of Hope. New York, E.P. Dutton, 1989.

Cousins, Norman: The Healing Heart: Antidotes to Panic and Helplessness. New York, W.W. Norton, 1983.

Felson, Benjamin: Humor in Medicine . . . And Other Topics. Cincinnati, RHA, Inc., 1989.

Fry, William F., Salameh, Waleed A. (eds): Advances in Humor & Psychotherapy. Sarasota, Professional Resource Exchange, Inc., 1993.

Fry, William F., Salameh, Waleed A. (eds): Handbook of Humor and Psychotherapy: Advances in the Clinical Use of Humor. Sarasota, Professional Resource Exchange, Inc., 1987.

Goodheart A: Laughter Therapy: How to Laugh about Everything in Your Life that Isn't Really Funny. Santa Barbara, Less Stress Press, 1994.

Haig, Robin Andrew: The Anatomy of Humor: Biopsychosocial and Therapeutic Perspectives. Springfield, CC Thomas, 1988.

Hay, Louise L: You Can Heal Your Life. Carson, CA, Hay House, Inc., 1987.

Holland, Norman N: Laughing: A Psychology of Humor. Ithaca, Cornell University Press, 1982.

Keller, Dan: Humor As Therapy. Wauwatosa, WI, Med-Psych Publications, 1984.

Klein, Allen: The Healing Power of Humor. Los Angeles, J.P. Tarcher, 1989.

Kuhlman, Thomas L: Humor and Psychotherapy. Homewood, IL., Dow Jones-Irwin, 1984.

LeDoux, Joseph: The Emotional Brain: The Mysterious Underpinnings of Emotional Life. New York, Simon & Schuster, 1996.

Lefcourt, Herbert M., Martin, Rod A: Humor and Life Stress: Antidote to Adversity. New York, Springer-Verlag, 1986.

McGhee, Paul E., Goldstein, Paul E (eds): Handbook of Humor Research, volume II Applied Studies. New York, Springer-Verlag, 1983.

McGuire, Francis A., Boyd, Rosangela K., James, Ann: Therapeutic Humor with the Elderly. New York, Haworth Press, 1992.

Mallett, Jane: Humor and Laughter Therapy. In: Slater, VE, Rankin-Box, DF (eds): The Nurses' Handbook of Complementary Therapies. New York, Churchill Livingstone, 1996.

Metcalf, C.W., Felible, Roma: Lighten Up: Survival Skills for People Under Pressure. Reading, MA, Addison-Wesley Publishing Co., 1992.

Morreall, John: The Philosophy of Laughter and Humor. Albany, State University of New York Press, 1987.

Morreall, John: Taking Laughter Seriously. Albany, State University of New York Press, 1983.

Moyers, Bill D., Flowers, Betty Sue (eds): Healing and the Mind. New York, Doubleday, 1993.

Nahemow, Lucille, McCluskey-Fawcett, Kathleen A, McGhee, Paul E. (eds): Humor and Aging. Orlando, Academic Press, Inc., 1986.

Oring, Elliott: Jokes and Their Relations. Lexington, University Press of Kentucky, 1992.

Pennebaker, James W: Emotion, Disclosure, and Health. Washington, D.C., American Psychological Association, 1995.

Peter, Laurence J., Dana, Bill: The Laughter Prescription. New York, Ballantine Books, 1982.

Robinson, Vera M: Humor and the Health Professions: The Therapeutic Use of Humor in Health Care, 2nd ed. Thorofare, NJ, Slack Incorporated, 1991.

Schaeffer, Neil: The Art of Laughter. New York, Columbia University Press, 1981.

Shea, Ursula: The Perceptions of Faculty and Students Concerning the Use of Humor in Nursing Education. Doctoral Dissertation, University of Massachusetts, 1991.

Sherman, James R: The Magic of Humor in Caregiving. Golden Valley, MN, Pathway Books, 1995.

Siegel, Bernie S: Love, Medicine, & Miracles: Lessons Learned About Self-Healing from a Surgeon's Experience with Exceptional Patients. New York, Harper & Row, 1986.

Sochen, June: Women's Comic Visions. Detroit, Wayne State University Press, 1991.

Strean, Herbert S. (ed): The Use of Humor in Psychotherapy. Northvale, NJ, J. Aronson, 1994.

Walker, Nancy A: A Very Serious Thing: Women's Humor and American Culture. Minneapolis, University of Minnesota Press, 1988.

Wooten, Patty: Compassionate Laughter: Jest for Your Health. Salt Lake City, Commune-A-Key Pub., 1996.

Wooten, Patty (ed): Heart, Humor & Healing. Mt. Shasta, CA, Commune-A-Key Publishing, Inc., 1994.

Ziv, Avner: Personality and Sense of Humor. New York, Springer Publishing Company, 1984.

JOURNAL BIBLIOGRAPHY

ADMINISTRATION

Executives ought to be funnier. Journal of Nursing Administration 1984 Oct;14(10):7,22,31.

Having fun being a manager. Hospital Food and Nutrition Focus 1991 Oct;8(2):7–8.

Balzer JW. Humor adds the creative touch to CQI teams. Journal of Nursing Care Quality 1994 Jul;8(4):13–19.

Balzer JW. Humor—a missing ingredient in collaborative practice. Holistic Nursing Practice 1993 Jul;7(4):28–35.

Bennett AC. It's no joke—healthcare exec needs sense of humor to be good manager. Modern Healthcare 1981 Aug;11(8):146,150.

Brown BL. Improving communication: the use of management parables. Health Care Supervisor 1988 Jan;6(2):13–26.

Brown RE. Brownisms: words of wisdom on management style. Hospitals 1989 Dec 5;63(23):88.

Copp LA. In-box humor. Journal of Professional Nursing 1990 Mar–Apr;6(2):65–67.

Davidhizar R. Humor—no nurse manager should be without it! Today's OR Nurse 1988 Jan;10(1):18–21.

Davidhizar RE. Enjoying management: the positive benefits of liking the job. AORN Journal 1989 Feb;49(2):576–578.

Eaton B. Career management. Humour's potential as a management tool. Leadership in Health Services 1995 Nov–Dec;4(6):30–31.

England D. Leadership: as my father used to say. Seminars for Nurse Managers 1996 Dec;4(4):196–199.

Fry PS. Perfectionism, humor, and optimism as moderators of health outcomes and determinants of coping styles of women executives. Genetic, Social, and General Psychology Monographs 1995 May;121(2):213–245.

Greene GJ. The practical unit administrator's toolkit. Hospital and Health Services Review 1982 Sep;78(8):227.

Harmon S. How to become changehardy. MLO: Medical Laboratory Observer 1993 Aug;25(8):41–5,48.

Henry BM, Moody LE. Energize with laughter. Nursing Success Today 1985 Jan;2(1):4–8,36.

Hilbert KL. Starting a humor board or how to make that crack in the wall look better cheaply. Journal of Nursing Jocularity 1997 Sum;7(2):26–27.

Kennedy MM. Was that really funny? The politics of humor. Physician Executive 1995 Jul;21(7):44–45.

Klein A. Humor: how to use it. Health Confidential 1995 Jul;9(7):13–14.

Lee BS. Humor relations for nurse managers. Nursing Management 1990 May;21(5):86–92.

McCloskey JC. Creating an environment for success with fun, hope and trouble. Journal of Nursing Administration 1991 Apr;21(4):5–6.

Marquand B. Laughter is the best medicine. RDH 1993 Mar;13(3):12–13.

Miller DA. Laughter in leadership: bringing out your lighter side. Creative Nursing: a Journal of Values, Issues, Experience & Collaboration 1997;3(2):6–7.

Popka BG. Humor for hospital public relations; prescription for prn use. Profiles in Hospital Marketing 1983 Apr;10:50–55.

Robinson VM. Humor is a serious business. Dimensions of Critical Care Nursing 1986 May–Jun;5(3):132–133.

Rodgers JA. An invitation to laugh. Journal of Professional Nursing 1988 Sep–Oct;4(5):314.

Schroeder P. Making fun a part of quality. Nursing Quality Connection 1992 Sep–Oct;2(2):1,4.

Schwab P. Those who laugh . . . last! PMA 1993 Mar–Apr; 26(2):8–10.

Sleeter MR. Are you humoring your employees? Management World 1981 May;10(5):25–27.

Strickland D. Coping with chaos and change. AORN Journal 1996 Nov;64(5):804–807.

Strickland D. How to use humor as a management tool. Kansas Nurse 1994 Mar;69(3):1–2.

Thomas KW, Iannone JM. Humor as a retention strategy for nurses. Hospital Topics 1989 Sep–Oct;67(5):26–27.

Weishaus G. Humor in the home care office. Home Healthcare Nurse 1997 Apr;15(4):276–278.

Whaley C. Humor: prescription for the work place. Journal of Diagnostic Medical Sonography 1993 Mar/Apr;9:88–89.

Wilson CN. Fun at work, work at fun. Hospital Pharmacy 1989 Jul;24(7):543–544.

CLOWNING

Carlisle D. Comic relief. Nursing Times 1990 Sep 19;86(38): 50–51.

D'Anna BA. Nurse clowns in the OR. An interview with Barbara Ann D'Anna. Today's OR Nurse 1993 Nov–Dec;15(6):25–27.

Deutsch N. Double duty. Canadian Nurse 1994 Dec;90(11): 60,59.

Finnerty A. Send in the clowns. American Health 1995 Sep; 14(7):68–69,105.

Gustafson MB. The newest member on the healthcare team: clowns. Creative Nursing 1996;2(3):14.

Jackson MM. The nurse who laughs, lasts: the comic spirit in nursing. Michigan Nurse 1980 Apr;53(4):12–14.

Killeen ME. Clinical clowning: humor in hospice care. American Journal of Hospice and Palliative Care 1991 May–Jun;8(3):23–27.

Kluny R. From Russia with love. Beginnings: The Official Newsletter of the American Holistic Nurses Association 1995 Jun/Jul;15(6):1,9.

Maddry L. He helps cure'em with laughter. Executive Housekeeping Today 1985 May;6(5):12–13.

Mancke RB, Maloney S, West M. Clowning: a healing process. Health Education 1984 Oct–Nov;15(6):16–18.

Manning E. Does clowning help the medicine go down? New Scientist 1996 Feb 10;149(2016):10.

Montague J. Clowning for comfort. Hospitals & Health Networks 1995 Jul 5;69(13):45.

Paquet JB. Nurse clowns in the OR: an interview with Barbara Ann D'Anna. Today's O.R. Nurse 1993 Nov–Dec; 15(6):25–27.

Rotton J. Trait humor and longevity: do comics have the last laugh? Health Psychology 1992;11(4):262–266.

COLLEAGUES

A funny thing happened on the way to recovery. Journal of the American Medical Association 1992 Apr 1;267(13):1856, 1861.

Akinwunmi P, Hulatt I. Legend has it. Nursing Standard 1994 Jun 1;8(36):46–47.

Banning MR, Nelson DL. The effects of activity-elicited humor and group structure on group cohesion and affective responses. American Journal of Occupational Therapy 1987 Aug;41(8):510–514.

Barnes RH. You have a good sense of humor. You should be a doctor. Pharos 1991 Fall;54(4):27–29.

Bennett HJ. Humor in the medical literature. Journal of Family Practice 1995 Apr;40(4):334–336.

Boyd EF. Use, don't lose, the wind. American Journal of Obstetrics and Gynecology 1996 Jun;174(6):1675–1677.

Brown L. Laughter: the best medicine. RNABC News 1990 Nov–Dec;22(6):11–13.

Bruce H, Cumming B. Surely you jest: bringing humour to the workplace. Canadian Nurse 1997 Aug;93(7):51–52.

Catanzaro TE. Keys to coping: a healthy life-style and a healthy sense of humor. Journal of the American Veterinary Medical Association 1992 Feb 15;200(4):441–442.

Chaney JA, Folk P. A profession in caricature: changing attitudes towards nursing in the American Medical News, 1960–1989. Nursing History Review 1993:1(1):181–202.

Chrisp DR. The lighter side. Nursing 1997 May;27(5):61.

Coombs RH, Chopra S, Schenk DR, Yutan E. Medical slang and its functions. Social Science and Medicine 1993 Apr; 36(8):987–998.

Cushner FD, Friedman RJ. Humor and the physician. Southern Medical Journal 1989 Jan;82(1):51–52.

Davidhizar R, Wysong PR. Positive and negative criticism: strategies for professional growth. Critical Care Nurse 1992 Aug;12(6):94–99.

Devereaux EB. Occupational therapy's challenge: the caring relationship. American Journal of Occupational Therapy 1984 Dec;38(12):791–798.

Dirckx JH. Doctor, I'm [sic]. American Journal of Dermatopathology 1992 Aug;14(4):369–371.

Duncan WJ. The superiority theory of humor at work. Small Group Behavior 1985 Nov;16(4):556–564.

Fay MF. Special focus on humor in the OR. Today's O.R. Nurse 1993 Nov–Dec;15(6):5.

Goodman JB. Laughing matters: taking your job seriously and yourself lightly. Journal of the American Medical Association 1992 Apr 1;267(13):1858.

Goodman JB. Laughing matters: taking your job seriously and yourself lightly. Orthopaedic Nursing 1989 May–Jun;8(3): 11–13.

Haig R. Some sociocultural aspects of humour. Australian and New Zealand Journal of Psychiatry 1988 Dec; 22(4):418–422.

Hammond P. Sick with laughter. Nursing Times 1993 Mar 24;89(12):24.

Hill MJ. Laughter really is the best medicine. Dermatology Nursing 1995 Oct;7(5):280,282.

Hott JR. To see ourselves as others see us. Imprint 1984 Feb–Mar;31(1):45–48.

Huckaby C. Take time to laugh. Nursing 1987 Apr;17(4):81.

Hulatt I. Just a laugh? Nursing Times 1993 Sep 8;89(36):41.

Klass P. Sick jokes. Discover 1987 Nov;8(11):30,34–35.

Kuhlman TL. Gallows humor for a scaffold setting: managing aggressive patients on a maximum-security forensic unit. Hospital and Community Psychiatry 1988 Oct;39(10):1 085–1090.

Liechty RD. Humor and the surgeon. Archives of Surgery 1987 May;122(5):519–522.

Madden T. Joking relationships. Journal of the Royal College of General Practitioners 1986 May;36(286):197.

Mandell HN. Frivolity in medicine—is there a place for it? Postgraduate Medicine 1988 Jun;83(8):24–28.

Nordberg M. Laughing with Loretta. Emergency Medical Services 1996 Jan;25(1):27.

Peace BL. President's message. Journal of the American Medical Record Association 1990 Sep;61(9):29–30.

Russett C. Sense of humor in the workplace adds perspective. Oncology Nursing Forum 1993 Jul;20(6):963.

Schaefer KM, Peterson K. Effectiveness of coping strategies among critical care nurses. Dimensions of Critical Care Nursing 1992 Jan–Feb;11(1):28–34.

Scogin FR, Pollio HR. Targeting and the humorous episode in group process. Human Relations 1980 Nov;33(11):831–852.

Shea ME, Buxa B. The best prescription—humor in the workplace. Prairie Rose 1994 Dec;63(4):7a.

Sumners AD. Professional nurses' attitudes towards humour. Journal of Advanced Nursing 1990 Feb;15(2):196–200.

Thomas P. The anatomy of coping: medicine's funny bone. Medical World News 1986 Jul 14;27(13):42–66.

Tooper VO. Humor as an adjunct to occupational therapy interactions. Occupational Therapy in Health Care 1984;1:49–57.

Tooper VO. Improving your laugh life. Nursing Life 1985 Mar–Apr;5(2):58–61.

Van Wormer K, Boes M. Humor in the emergency room: a social work perspective. Health & Social Work 1997 May; 22(2):87–92.

Vergeer G, MacRae A. Therapeutic use of humor in occupational therapy. American Journal of Occupational Therapy 1993 Aug;47(8):678–683.

Wender RC. Humor in medicine. Primary Care 1996 Mar; 23(1):141–154.

Wooten P. Jest for the health of it! Making humor work. Journal of Nursing Jocularity 1993;3(4):40–42.

DEATH AND DYING

Barnum B. Losses and laughter. Nursing and Health Care 1989 Feb;10(2):59.

Bottorff JL, Gogag M, Engelberg-Lotzkar M. Comforting: exploring the work of cancer nurses. Journal of Advanced Nursing 1995 Dec;22(6):1077–1084.

Huggins R. The get-away room. Oncology Nursing Forum 1990 Sep–Oct;17(5):764.

Klein A. Humor and death: you've got to be kidding. American Journal of Hospice Care 1986 Jul–Aug;3(4):42–45.

Knight J. The need to laugh. Nursing 1990 Aug;20(8):20.

Mager M, Cabe PA. Effect of death anxiety on perception of death-related humor. Psychological Reports 1990 Jun;66(3 pt 2):1311–1314.

Metcalf CW. Humor, life, and death. Oncology Nursing Forum 1987 Jul–Aug;14(4):19–21.

Radziewicz RM, Schneider SM. Using diversional activity to enchance coping. Cancer Nursing 1992 Aug;15(4):293–298.

Redman M, Guarnieri C. Daily activities relieve stress of patients and staff members. Oncology Nursing Forum 1993 Jul;20(6):964–965.

Simon JM. Humor techniques for oncology nurses. Oncology Nursing Forum 1989 Sep–Oct;16(5):667–670.

Stevenson RG. We laugh to keep from crying: coping through humor. Loss, Grief and Care: a Journal of Professional Practice 1993; 7(1–2):173–179.

Thorson JA, Powell FC. Relationships of death anxiety and sense of humor. Psychological Reports 1993 Jun;72(3 pt 2):1364–1366.

GERIATRICS

Barrick AL, Hutchinson RL, Deckers LH. Humor, aggression, and aging. Gerontologist 1990 Oct;30(5):675–678.

Buckwalter KC, Gerdner LA, Hall GR, Stolley JM, Kudart P, Ridgeway, S. Shining through: the humor and individuality of person's with Alzheimer's disease. Journal of Gerontological Nursing 1995 Mar;21(3):11–16.

Buckwalter KC. What is the impact of the use of humor as a coping strategy by nurses working in geropsychiatric settings? Journal of Psychosocial Nursing 1991 Jul;29(7): 41–42.

Dawson P. Humour and cognitive impairment. Perspectives 1992 Spr;16(1):2–6.

Demos V, Jache A. When you care enough: an analysis of attitudes toward aging in humorous birthday cards. Gerontologist 1981 Apr;21(2):209–215.

Dillon KM, Jones BS. Attitudes toward aging portrayed by birthday cards. International Journal of Aging and Human Development 1981;13(1):79–84.

Drummond G. Laughter is better than medicine—a support group for caring relatives. Health Visitor 1984 Jul;57(7): 201–202.

Herth KA. Humor and the older adult. Applied Nursing Research 1993 Nov;6(4):146–153.

Hulse JR. Humor: a nursing intervention for the elderly. Geriatric Nursing 1994 Mar–Apr;15(2):88–90.

Isola A, Astedt-Kurki P. Humour as experienced by patients and nurses in aged nursing in Finland. International Journal of Nursing Practice 1997 Mar;3(1):29–33.

Kavanaugh K. Residents benefit from use of humor as a therapeutic tool. Brown University Long Term Care Quality Letter 1995 Nov 27;7(22):6.

Kehl DG. Thalia meets tithonus: gerontological wit and humor in literature. Gerontologist 1985 Oct;25(5):539–544.

Labott SM, Martin RB. Emotional coping, age, and physical disorder. Behavioral Medicine 1990 Sum;16(2):53–61.

Parse RR. The experience of laughter: a phenomenological study. Nursing Science Quarterly 1993 Spr;6(1):39–43.

Parse RR. Laughing and health: a study using Parse's research method. Nursing Science Quarterly 1994 Sum;7(2):55–64.

Peck R. A little nursing home humor. Nursing Homes 1995 Nov–Dec;44(9):4.

Prerost FJ. A strategy to enhance humor production among elderly persons: assisting in the management of stress. Activities, Adaptation and Aging 1993;17(4):17–24.

Richman J. The lifesaving function of humor with the depressed and suicidal elderly. The Gerontologist 1995 Apr;35(2):271–273.

Rodvik B. Life too important to take seriously, says humor advocate Lila Green. Nursing Homes and Senior Citizen Care 1988 Nov–Dec;37(6).

Ruch W, McGhee PE, Hehl FJ. Age differences in the enjoyment of incongruity—resolution and nonsense humor during adulthood. Psychology and Aging 1990 Sep;5(3): 348–355.

Ruxton JP, Hester MP. Humor: assessment and interventions. Clinical Gerontologist 1987 Fal;7(1):13–21.

Seltzer MM. Speculative gerontology revisited: the herd instinct. International Journal of Aging and Human Development 1992;34(3):199–208.

Simon JM. Humor and its relationship to perceived health, life satisfaction, and morale in older adults. Issues in Mental Health Nursing 1990;11(1):17–31.

Simon JM. Humour and the older adult: implications for nursing. Journal of Advanced Nursing 1988 Jul;13(4):441–446.

Simon JM. The therapeutic value of humor in aging adults. Journal of Gerontological Nursing 1988 Aug;14(8):9–13.

Solomon JC. Humor and aging well. American Behavioral Scientist 1996 Jan;39(3):249–271.

Sullivan JL, Deane DM. Humor and health. Journal of Gerontological Nursing 1988 Jan;14(1):20–24.

Tennant KF. Laugh it off, the effect of humor on the well-being of the older adult. Journal of Gerontological Nursing 1990 Dec;16(12):11–17.

Townsend CH. Humor and elderly caregivers. Home Healthcare Nurse 1994 Nov/Dec;12(6):35–41.

Weisberg J, Haberman MR. Drama, humor, and music to reduce family anxiety in a nursing home. Geriatric Nursing 1992 Jan–Feb;13(1):22–24.

Wooten P. What is the impact of the use of humor as a coping strategy by nurses working in geropsychiatric settings? Journal of Psychosocial Nursing 1991 Jul;29(7):42–43.

Yoder MA, Haude RH. Sense of humor and longevity: older adults' self-ratings compared with ratings for deceased siblings. Psychological Reports 1995 Jun;76(3 pt 1):945–946.

HEALING

A humor test. Ardell Wellness Report 1994 Fall:1.

Adams P, Mylander M. Good health is a laughing matter. Caring 1992 Dec;11(12):16–20.

Audette IM. The use of humor in intravenous nursing. Journal of Intravenous Nursing 1994 Jan/Feb;17(1):25–27.

Cohen M. Caring for ourselves can be funny business. Holistic Nursing Practice 1990 Jul;4(4):1–11.

Collins HL. How well do nurses nurture themselves? RN 1989 May:39–41.

Coulehan J. The incredible lightness: antidote for the heaviness of illness. Pharos 1990 Fall;53(4):15–17.

Cousins N. The laughter prescription. Saturday Evening Post 1990 Sep;262(6):32–37.

Cousins N. The laughter prescription. Saturday Evening Post 1990 Oct;262(7):34–39.

Cousins N. Proving the power of laughter. Psychology Today 1989 Oct;23(10):22–25.

Cousins N. Therapeutic value of laughter. Integrative Psychiatry 1985;3:112–114.

Crawford PR. A national laughter day: are you serious? Canadian Dental Association Journal 1993 Jul;59(7):569.

Dolan MB. A drug you can't overuse. RN 1985 Nov;48(11):47–48.

Elgee NJ. Norman Cousins' sick laughter redux. Archives of Internal Medicine 1990 Aug;150(8):1588.

Ferguson S, Campinha-Bacote J. Humor in nursing. Journal of Psychosocial Nursing and Mental Health Services 1989 Apr;27(4):29–35.

Gibson L. Healing with humor. Nursing 1994 Sep;24(9):56–57.

Granick S. The therapeutic value of laughter. USA Today Magazine 1995 Sep;124(2604):72–74.

Groves DF. A merry heart doeth good like a medicine. Holistic Nursing Practice 1991 Jul;5(4):49–56.

Herring ME. Humor in the management of serious medical disorders. Trends in Health Care, Law and Ethics 1993 Win;8(1):80–82.

Hillman S. The healing power of humour at work. Nursing Standard 1994 Jul 13;8(42):31–34.

Kohn A. Aspects of laughter. Omni 1990 Sep;12(12):25.

Laura R, Ashton J. Laugh your way to health. Good Health 1993 May–Jun;23:16–20.

McNutt K. Let's lighten up. Nutrition Today 1994 Jun;29:36–39.

Macaluso MC. Humor, health and healing. ANNA Journal 1993 Feb;20(1):14–16.

May C. Moruya Hospital laughter room: an experiment. Lamp 1996 Mar;53(2):6.

Rawnsley MM. H-e-a-l-t-h: A Rogerian perspective. Journal of Holistic Nursing 1985;3(1):25–29.

Rodning CB. Humor and healing: a creative process. Pharos 1988 Sum;51(3):38–40.

Samra C. A time to laugh. Journal of Christian Nursing 1985 Fall;2(4):15–19.

Saper B. Humor in psychiatric healing. Psychiatric Quarterly 1988 Win;59(4):306–319.

Seaward BL. Humor's healing potential. Health Progress 1992 Apr;73(3):66–70.

Silberman IN. Humor and health, an epidemiological study. American Behavioral Scientist 1987 Jan/Feb;30(1):100–112.

Slater S. Health professionals learn healing power of humor. Health Care 1986 Jun;28(5):10–12.

Strickland D. Seriously, laughter matters. Today's O.R. Nurse 1993 Nov–Dec;15(6):19–24.

Sumners AD. Humor: coping in recovery from addiction. Issues in Mental Health Nursing 1988;9(2):169–179.

Van Zandt S, LaFont C. Can a laugh a day keep the doctor away? Journal of Practical Nursing 1985 Sep;35(3):32–35.

Warner SL. Humor & self-disclosure within the milieu. Journal of Psychosocial Nursing 1984 Apr;22(4):16–21.

Weiss R. Healing through humor. Health Progress 1993 Jul–Aug;74(6):84–85,92.

Williams H. Humor and healing, therapeutic effects in geriatrics. Gerontion 1986 May–Jun;1(3):14–17.

Yonge O. Humour: more than Ho! Ho! Ho! AARN Newsletter 1985 Dec;41(11):1,4.

ONCOLOGY/PAIN

How humor can help when you hurt. Coping 1989;3:14–15.

Adams ER, McGuire FA. Is laughter the best medicine? A study of the effects of humor on perceived pain and affect. Activities, Adaptation and Aging 1986;8(3–4):157–175.

Bellert JL. Humor: a therapeutic approach in oncology nursing. Cancer Nursing 1989 Apr;12(2):65–70.

Dant D. The effects of humor on self-reported mood and pain levels in the oncology patient population. Kentucky Nurse 1993 Jul–Aug;41(4):21.

Davies D. Special motto enforces the importance of humor and hugs. Oncology Nursing Forum 1993 Jul;20(6):964.

Dean RA. Humor and laughter in palliative care. Journal of Palliative Care 1997 Spr;13(1):34–39.

Erdman L. Laughter therapy for patients with cancer. Oncology Nursing Forum 1991 Nov–Dec;18(8):1359–1363.

Frankenfield PK. The power of humor and play as nursing interventions for a child with cancer: a case report. Journal of Pediatric Oncology Nursing 1996 Jan;13(1):15–20.

Gilligan B. A positive coping strategy; humour in the oncology setting. Professional Nurse 1993 Jan;8(4):231–233.

Graham LL, Cates JA. Responding to the needs of the terminally ill through laughter and play. American Journal of Hospice Care 1989 Jan/Feb;6:29–30.

Gullo SM. Props and jokes provide patients with healing hugs. Oncology Nursing Forum 1993 Jul;20(6):964.

Herth K. Contributions of humor as perceived by the terminally ill. American Journal of Hospice Care 1990 Jan–Feb; 7(1):36–40.

Huggins R. The get-away room. Oncology Nursing Forum 1990 Sep–Oct;17(5):764.

Hunt AH. Humor as a nursing intervention. Cancer Nursing 1993 Feb;16(1):34–39.

Leise CM. The correlation between humor and the chronic pain of arthritis. Journal of Holistic Nursing 1993 Mar;11(1):82–95.

Lipsyte R. Roc the docs. American Health 1992 Sep;11(7): 92–93.

Lipsyte R. Tumor humor. American Health 1992 Mar;11(2): 28,30.

Ljungdahl L. Laugh if this is a joke. Journal of the American Medical Association 1989 Jan 27;261(4):558.

Menke C. Humor book provides release for nurses. Oncology Nursing Forum 1993 Jul;20(6):964.

Michaud M. Humour: an approach to brief episodes of pain. AARN Newsletter 1992 Jul–Aug;48(7):37.

Nowak K. Pain beneath the humor. Nursing 1991 Oct:21(10) 168.

Ruxton JP. Humor intervention deserves our attention. Holistic Nursing Practice 1988 May;2(3):54–62.

Schultes LS. Humor with hospice clients: you're putting me on! Home Healthcare Nurse 1997 Aug;15(8):561–566.

Schunior C. Nursing and the comic mask. Holistic Nursing Practice 1989 May;3(3):7–17.

Scott C. Go ahead, laugh. It's good for you. Nursing Success Today 1985 Jan;2(1):8.

Smolenski SC. Unit offers unique and fun approaches to therapy. Oncology Nursing Forum 1993 Jul;20(6):964.

Southam M, Cummings M. The use of humor as a technique for modulating pain. Occupational Therapy Practice 1990;1(3):77–84.

Trent B. Ottawa lodges add humour to armamentarium in fight against cancer. Canadian Medical Association Journal 1990 Jan 15;142(2):163–166.

Weaver J, Zillman D. Effect of humor and tragedy on discomfort tolerance. Perceptual and Motor Skills 1994 Apr; 78(2):632–634.

Weisenberg M, Tepper I, Schwarzwald J. Humor as a cognitive technique for increasing pain tolerance. Pain 1995 Nov;63(2):207–212.

Whaley AP. Humor comes in many forms. Oncology Nursing Forum 1993 Jul;20(6):963.

PATIENTS

Aoki C. If the humor fits, use it to ease a patient's exam fears. Asrt Scanner 1997 Jun;29(9):6.

Astedt-Kurki P, Liukkonen A. Humour in nursing care. Journal of Advanced Nursing 1994 Jul;20(1):183–188.

Bakerman HM. Humour as a nursing intervention. Axone 1997 Mar;18(3):56–61.

Bagdanovich JB. Humor . . . the best medicine, or is it? Imprint 1993 Apr–May;40(3):123,127.

Barra JM. High kicks in the ICU. RN 1986 Apr;45–46.

Baum N. Medicine, marketing and the worth of mirth. American Medical News 1993 Sep 13;36(34):30.

Behi R. Using humor as therapy in clinical practice. British Journal of Nursing 1992 Sep 2–Oct 7;1(10):484.

Bennett HJ. Using humor in the office setting: a pediatric perspective. Journal of Family Practice 1996 May;42(5): 462–464.

Bigelow AE. President's perspective. Journal: Society of Otorhinolaryngology Head and Neck Nurses 1988;6(3):3.

Blackburn W. Laughter and humor may be the best medicine. Axon 1992 Mar;13(3):inside front cover.

Broccolo-Philbin A. Laughing & crying. Current Health 1995 Dec;22(4):26–27.

Buxman K. Make room for laughter. American Journal of Nursing 1991 Dec;91(12):46–51.

Campbell C. Laughter on the ward. Nursing Mirror 1982 Nov 24;155(21):41–44.

Campinha-Bacote J. Soul therapy: humor and music with African-American clients. Journal of Christian Nursing 1993 Spr;10(2):23–26.

Carpenter A. Humor brings a new perspective. Oncology Nursing Forum 1992 Sep;19(8):1261.

Crane AL. Why sickness can be a laughing matter. RN 1987 Feb;50(2):41–42.

Creech S. Kate's comeback. Nursing 1990 Oct;20(10):200.

Davidhizar R, Shearer R. Using humor to cope with stress in home care. Home Healthcare Nurse 1996 Oct;14(10):825–830.

Davison M, O'Brien D. Humour in midwifery. Modern Midwife 1997 Apr;7(4):11–14.

Demott B. Inside joke: humor is one antidote to insensitivity. American Health 1992 May;11(4):30–31.

Dolan MB. Rx: laughter, 15 min/day. RN 1994 Dec;57(12):80.

Draheim MD. Humor: a powerful tool for health-care professionals and patients. Diabetes Spectrum 1995 May;8(3):137.

Dunn B. Use of therapeutic humour by psychiatric nurses. British Journal of Nursing 1993 May 13–26;2(9):468–473.

Elliott-Binns CP. Laughter and medicine. Journal of the Royal College of General Practitioners 1985 Aug;35(277):364–365.

Fogel M. The humorous side. Journal-American Health Care Association 1981 Jan;7(1):18–21.

Gaberson KB. The effect of humorous distraction on preoperative anxiety. AORN Journal 1991 Dec;54(6):1258–1264.

Gaberson KB. The effect of humorous and musical distraction on preoperative anxiety. AORN Journal 1995 Nov;62(5):784–791.

Harries G. Use of humour in patient care. British Journal of Nursing 1995 Sep;4(17):984–986.

Henn MB. Intervening with humor. Free Association: A Newsletter for Psychiatric Nurses 1983 Mar–Apr;10(2):5–6.

Herth KA. Laughter, a nursing Rx. American Journal of Nursing 1984 Aug;84(8):991–992.

Johnson CAS. The humor basket project. Nursing News 1988 Dec;38(6):4–5.

Johnston W. To the ones left behind. American Journal of Nursing 1985 Aug;85(8):936.

Kelly D. Three tips for closer caring. Nursing 1995 May;25(5):72.

Lee M. AJN interview: Sandy Ritz. American Journal of Nursing 1995 Aug;95(8):39–41.

Linn LS, DiMatteo MR. Humor and other communication preferences in physician-patient encounters. Medical Care 1983 Dec;21(12):1223–1231.

McCallum J. Don't laugh—this is serious. Australian Nurses Journal 1981 May;10(10):39–40.

Mallett J, A'Hern R. Comparative distribution and use of humour within nurse-patient communication. International Journal of Nursing Studies 1996 Oct;33(5):530–550.

Mallett J. Humour and laughter therapy. Complementary Therapies in Nursing & Midwifery 1995 Jun;1(3):73–76.

Mallett J. Use of humour and laughter in patient care. British Journal of Nursing 1993 Feb 11;2(3):172–175.

Moore JL. A smile for Jenny. Health Progress 1992 Apr;73(3):88,87.

Osterlund H. Humor, a serious approach to patient care. Nursing 1983 Dec;13(12):46–47.

Parish AB. It only hurts when I don't laugh. American Journal of Nursing 1994 Aug;94(8):46–47.

Pedersen KA. Another language. Nursing 1987 Jul;17(7):19.

Raber WC. The caring role of the nurse in the application of humor therapy to the patient experiencing helplessness. Clinical Gerontologist 1987 Fal;7(1):3–11.

Schmitt N. Patients' perceptions of laughter in a rehabilitation hospital. Rehabilitation Nursing 1990 May–Jun;15(3):143–146.

Sheldon LM. An analysis of the concept of humour and its application to one aspect of children's nursing. Journal of Advanced Nursing 1996 Dec;24(6):1175–1183.

Warner SL. Appropriate uses of humor in critical care. Dimensions of Critical Care Nursing 1986 May–Jun;5(3):168–170.

Warner U. The serious import of humour in health visiting. Journal of Advanced Nursing 1984 Jan;9(1):83–87.

Worth A. Humor used to cope with difficult camp experience. Pediatric Nursing 1991 Jul–Aug;17(4):395.

PHYSIOLOGY

Have a belly laugh. Canadian Nurse 1993 May;89(5):14.

Laughter . . . the best medicine. Canadian Operating Room Nursing Journal 1984 Sep;2(4):25.

Laughter: can it keep you healthy? Mayo Clinic Health Letter 1993 Mar;11(3):5.

Why laughter is good for the body and soul. Addiction Letter 1996 Feb;12(2):4.

Arnold MK. Why laughter is good for the body and soul. Psychotherapy Letter 1996 Mar;8(3):8–9.

Askenasy JJM. The functions and dysfunctions of laughter. Journal of General Psychology 1987 Oct;114(4):317–334.

Berk LS. Neuroendocrine and stress hormone changes during mirthful laughter. American Journal of Medical Sciences 1989 Dec;298(6):390–396.

Berk LS, Tan SA, Napier BJ, Eby WC. Eustress of mirthful laughter modifies natural killer cell activity. Clinical Research 1989 Jan;37(1):115A.

Berk LS, Tan SA, Nehlsen-Cannarella SL, Napier BJ, Lewis JE, Lee JW, Eby WC, Fry WF. Humor associated laughter decreases cortisol and increases spontaneous lymphocyte blastogenesis. Clinical Research 1988 Apr;36(3):435A.

Brody R. Anatomy of a laugh. American Health 1983 Nov–Dec;11(2):43–47.

Callahan P. Watch some Monty Python and call me in the morning. Omni 1994 Feb;16(5):30–31.

Cogan R. Effects of laughter and relaxation on discomfort thresholds. Journal of Behavioral Medicine 1987 Apr;10(2):139–144.

Deaner SL, McConatha JT. The relation of humor to depression and personality. Psychological Reports 1993 Jun;72(3 pt 1):755–763.

Dillon KM, Minchoff B, Baker KH. Positive emotional states and enhancement of the immune system. International Journal of Psychiatry in Medicine 1985–86;15(1):13–18.

Dillon KM, Totten MC. Psychological factors, immunocompetence, and health of breast-feeding mothers and their infants. Journal of Genetic Psychology 1989 Jun;150(2):155–162.

Doskoch P. Happily ever laughter. Psychology Today 1996 Jul;29(4):32–35.

Fry WF, Savin WM. Mirthful laughter and blood pressure. Humor: International Journal of Humor Research 1988;1(1):49–62.

Fry WF. The physiologic effects of humor, mirth, and laughter. Journal of the American Medical Association 1992 Apr 1;267(13):1857–1858.

Goodman S. Jest for the health of it. Current Health 1989 Jan;15(5):18–19.

Griffiths J. The mirthful brain: where the belly laugh begins. Omni 1992 Aug;14(11):18.

Halley FM. Self-regulation of the immune system through biobehavioral strategies. Biofeedback and Self-Regulation 1991 Mar;16(1):55–74.

Hubert W, Moller M, de Jong-Meyer R. Film-induced amusement changes in saliva cortisol levels. Psychoneuroendocrinology 1993;18(4):265–272.

Hudak DA, Dale JA, Hudak MA, DeGood DE. Effects of humorous stimuli and sense of humor on discomfort. Psychological Reports 1991 Dec;69(3 pt 1):779–786.

Johnson AM. A study of humor and the right hemisphere. Perceptual and Motor Skills 1990 Jun;70(3 pt 1):995–1002.

Kamei T, Kumano H, Masumura S. Changes of immunoregulatory cells associated with psychological stress and humor. Perceptual & Motor Skills 1997 Jun;84(3 Pt 2):1296–1298.

Labott SM, Ahleman S, Wolever ME, Martin RB. The physiological and psychological effects of the expression and inhibition of emotion. Behavioral Medicine 1990 Win;16(4):182–189.

Lambert RB, Lambert NK. The effects of humor on secretory immunoglobin A levels in school-aged children. Pediatric Nursing 1995 Jan–Feb;21(1):16–19.

Lippert L. Humor and health. Kansas Nurse 1994 Mar;69(3):5.

Lowe G, Taylor SB. Effects of alcohol on responsive laughter and amusement. Psychological Reports 1997 Jun;80(3 Pt 2):1149–1150.

McClelland DC, Cheriff AD. The immunoenhancing effects of humor on secretory IgA and resistance to respiratory infections. Psychology & Health 1997;12(3):329–344.

Martin RA, Dobbin JP. Sense of humor, hassles, and immunoglobulin A: evidence for a stress-moderating effect of humor. International Journal of Psychiatry in Medicine 1988;18(2):93–105.

Newman MG, Stone AA. Does humor moderate the effects of experimentally-induced stress? Annals of Behavioral Medicine 1996;18(2):101–109.

Prerost FJ, Ruma C. Exposure to humorous stimuli as an adjunct to muscle relaxation training. Psychology: A Quarterly Journal of Human Behavior 1987;24(4):70–74.

Rynk P. Laughter and good health: a positive connection. Let's Live 1993 Feb;61(2):34–37.

Stone AA, Cox DS, Valdimarsdottir, Jandorf L, Neale JM. Evidence that secretory IgA antibody is associated with daily mood. Journal of Personality and Social Psychology 1987 May;52(5):988–993.

Svebak S. The effect of mirthfulness upon amount of discordant right-left occipital EEG Alpha. Motivation and Emotion 1982 Jun;6(2):133–147.

Ziegler J. Immune system may benefit from the ability to laugh. Journal of the National Cancer Institute 1995 Mar 1;87(5):342–343.

PSYCHOLOGY

Berger AA. Humor: an introduction. American Behavioral Scientist 1987 Jan–Feb;30(3):6–15.

Biermann J, Toohey B. Part III: the role of a positive attitude. Diabetes in the News 1995 Jan–Feb;14:22–23.

Black DW. Laughter. Journal of the American Medical Association 1984 Dec 7;252(21):2995–2998.

Blank AM, Tweedale M, Cappelli M, Ryback D. Influence of trait anxiety on perception of humor. Perceptual and Motor Skills 1983 Aug;57(1):103–106.

Burbach HJ, Babbitt CE. An exploration of the social functions of humor among college students in wheelchairs. Journal of Rehabilitation 1993 Jan/Feb/Mar;59(1):6–9.

Carroll JL. The relationship between humor appreciation and preceived physical health. Psychology: A Journal of Human Behavior 1990;27(2):34–37.

Carroll JL, Shmidt JL. Correlation between humorous coping style and health. Psychological Reports 1992 Apr;70(2):402.

Clabby JF. The wit: a personality analysis. Journal of Personality Assessment 1980 Jun;44(3):307–310.

Clark HH. On the pretense theory of irony. Journal of Experimental Psychology 1984 Mar;113(1):121–126.

Davies C. Ethnic jokes, moral values and social boundaries. British Journal of Sociology 1982 Sep;33(3):383–403.

Dundes A. At ease, disease—AIDS jokes as sick humor. American Behavioral Scientist 1987 Jan–Feb;30(3):72–81.

Fry WF. Humor and chaos. Humor: International Journal of Humor Research 1992;5(3):219–232.

Fry WF. Humor and paradox. American Behavioral Scientist 1987 Jan–Feb;30(3):42–71.

Fry WF. Misconception of humor: part one of a three part series. Journal of Nursing Jocularity 1997 Sum;7(2):38–40.

Gelkopf M, Kreitler S, Sigal M. Laughter in a psychiatric ward; somatic, emotional, social and clinical influences on schizophrenic patients. Journal of Nervous and Mental Disease 1993 May;181(5):283–289.

Gelkopf M, Sigal M, Kramer R. Therapeutic use of humor to improve social support in an institutionalized schizophrenic inpatient community. Journal of Social Psychology 1994 Apr;134(2):175–182.

Johnston RA. Humor: a preventive health strategy. International Journal for the Advancement of Counselling 1990 Jul;13(3):257–265.

Kennedy P, Marsh NJ. Effectiveness of the use of humor in the rehabilitation of people with SCI: a pilot study. Journal of the American Paraplegia Society 1993 Oct;16(4):215–218.

Kuiper NA, Martin RA. Humor and self-concept. Humor: International Journal of Humor Research 1993;6(3):251–270.

Lowe G, Taylor SB. Relationship between laughter and weekly alcohol consumption. Psychological Reports 1993 Jun;72(3 pt 2):1210.

Lowis MJ, Nieuwoudt JM. The use of a cartoon rating scale as a measure for the humor construct. The Journal of Psychology 1995 Mar;129(2):133–144.

McCauley C, Woods K, Coolidge C, Kulick W. More aggressive cartoons are funnier. Journal of Personality and Social Psychology 1983 Apr;44(4):817–823.

McCullough LS. A cross-cultural test of the two-part typology of humor. Perceptual and Motor Skills 1993 Jun;76(3 pt 2):1275–1281.

Mannell RC, McMahon L. Humor as play: its relationship to psychological well-being during the course of a day. Leisure Sciences 1982;5(2):143–155.

Martin RA, Kuiper NA, Olinger LJ, Dance KA. Humor, coping with stress, self-concept, and psychological well-being. Humor: International Journal of Humor Research 1993; 6(1):89–104.

Molitor D. HaHa: measuring a sense of humor. Journal of Irreproducible Results 1988 Jan–Feb;33(3):13–15.

Moran CC. Short-term mood change, perceived funniness, and the effect of humor stimuli. Behavioral Medicine 1996 Spr;22(1):32–38.

Pettifor JL. A touch of ethics and humor. Canadian Psychology 1982 Oct;23(4):261–263.

Porterfield AL. Does sense of humor moderate the impact of life stress on psychological and physical well-being? Journal of Research in Personality 1987 Sep;21(3):306–317.

Saper B. The therapeutic use of humor for psychiatric disturbances of adolescents and adults. Psychiatric Quarterly 1990 Win;61(4):261–272.

Schimel JL. The role of humor as an integrating factor in adolescent development. Adolescent Psychiatry 1992;18:118–126.

Shaw E. What's so funny? Today's O.R. Nurse 1984 Jul;6(7):36.

Thorson JA, Powell FC. Depression and sense of humor. Psychological Reports 1994 Dec;75(3 pt 2):1473–1474.

Thorson JA, Powell FC. Development and validation of a multidimensional sense of humor scale. Journal of Clinical Psychology 1993 Jan;49(1):13–23.

Thorson JA, Powell FC. Measurement of sense of humor. Psychological Reports 1991 Oct;69(2):691–702.

Thorson JA, Powell FC. Sense of humor and dimensions of personality. Journal of Clinical Psychology 1993 Nov; 49(6):799–809.

Turner RG. Self-monitoring and humor production. Journal of Personality 1980 Jun;48(2):163–172.

Wyer RS, Collins JE. A theory of humor elicitation. Psychological Review 1992 Oct;99(4):663–688.

Yoon CK. Anatomy of a tickle is serious business at the research lab. New York Times 1997 Jun 3;B10.

PSYCHOTHERAPY

Bader MJ. The analyst's use of humor. Psychoanalytic Quarterly 1993 Jan;62(1):23–51.

Banmen J. The use of humour in psychotherapy. International Journal for the Advancement of Counseling 1982; 5(2):81–86.

Bernet W. Humor in evaluating and treating children and adolescents. Journal of Psychotherapy Practice and Research 1993 Fall;2(4):307–317.

Bloch S, Browning S, McGrath G. Humour in group psychotherapy. British Journal of Medical Psychology 1983 Mar;56(1):89–97.

Bloomfield I. Humour in psychotherapy and analysis. International Journal of Social Psychiatry 1980 Sum;26(2):135–141.

Buxman K. Humor in therapy for the mentally ill. Journal of Psychosocial Nursing 1991 Dec;29(12):15.

Campinha-Bacote J. Humor therapy for culturally diverse psychiatric patients. Journal of Nursing Jocularity 1997 Spr;7(1):38–40.

Coale H. Use of humor in stepfamily therapy. Stepfamilies 1992 Win;12(4):10–11.

Dimmer SA, Carroll JL, Wyatt GK. Uses of humor in psychotherapy. Psychological Reports 1990 Jun;66(3 pt 1):795–801.

Ehrenberg, DB. Playfulness and humor in the psychoanalytic relationship. Group 1991 Win;15(4):225–233.

Eisenman R. Using humor in psychotherapy with a sex offender. Psychological Reports 1992 Dec;71(3 pt 1):994.

Falk DR, Hill CE. Counselor interventions preceding client laughter in brief therapy. Journal of Counseling Psychology 1992;39(1):39–45.

Forsyth AS. Humour and the psychotherapeutic process. British Journal of Nursing 1993 Oct 28–Nov 10;2(19):957–961.

Gelkopf M, Kreitler S. Is humor only fun, an alternative cure or magic? The cognitive therapeutic potential of humor. Journal of Cognitive Psychotherapy 1996;10(4):235–254.

Gervaize PA, Mahrer AR, Markow R. Therapeutic laughter: what therapists do to promote strong laugher in patients. Psychotherapy in Private Practice 1985 Sum;3(2):65–74.

Haig RA. Therapeutic uses of humor. American Journal of Psychotherapy 1986 Oct;40(4):543–553.

Harman RL. Humor and gestalt therapy. Voices: The Art and Science of Psychotherapy 1981 Win;16(4):62–64.

Kennedy LR. Humor in group psychotherapy. Group 1991 Win;15(4):234–241.

Korb LJ. Humor: a tool for the psychoanalyst. Issues in Ego Psychology 1988;11(2):45–54.

Kruger A. The nature of humor in human nature: cross-cultural commonalities. Counselling Psychology Quarterly 1996 Sep;9(3):235–241.

Lederman S. Discussion of "Humor: a tool for the psychoanalyst" by Linda Korb. Issues in Ego Psychology 1988;11(2):55–59.

Lusterman DD. Humor as metaphor. Psychotherapy in Private Practice 1992;10(1–2):167–172.

McHale M. Getting the joke: interpreting humor in group

therapy. Journal of Psychosocial Nursing 1989 Sep;27(9): 24–28.

MacHovec F. Humor in therapy. Psychotherapy in Private Practice 1991;9(1):25–33.

Mahrer AR, Gervaize PA. An integrative review of strong laughter in psychotherapy: what it is and how it works. Psychotherapy 1984 Win;21(4):510–516.

Malamud DI. The laughing game: an exercise for sharpening awareness of self-responsibility. Psychotherapy: Theory, Research and Practice 1980 Spr;17(1):69–73.

Megdell JI. Relationship between counselor-initiated humor and client's self-perceived attraction in the counseling interview. Psychotherapy 1984 Win;21(4):517–523.

Odell M. The silliness factor: breaking up repetitive and unproductive conflict patterns with couples and families. Journal of Family Psychotherapy 1996;7(3):69–75.

Pasquali EA. Learning to laugh: humor as therapy. Journal of Psychosocial Nursing 1990 Mar;28(3):31–35.

Pasquali G. Some notes on humour in psychoanalysis. International Review of Psycho-Analysis 1987;14(2):231–236.

Poland WS. The gift of laughter: on the development of a sense of humor in clinical analysis. Psychoanalytic Quarterly 1990 Apr;59(2):197–225.

Pollio DE. Use of humor in crisis intervention. Families in Society 1995 Jun;76(6):376–384.

Prerost FJ. Evaluating the systematic use of humor in psychotherapy with adolescents. Journal of Adolescence 1984 Sep;7(3):267–276.

Prerost FJ. Humor as an intervention strategy during psychological treatment: imagery and incongruity. Psychology: A Journal of Human Behavior 1989;26(4):34–40.

Prerost FJ. A procedure using imagery and humor in psychotherapy: case applicaton with longitudinal assessment. Journal of Mental Imagery 1985 Fal;9(3):67–76.

Reynes RL, Allen A. Humor in psychotherapy: a view. American Journal of Psychotherapy 1987 Apr;41(2):260–270.

Richman J. Points of correspondence between humor and psychotherapy. Psychotherapy 1996;33(4):560–566.

Rogers FB. Myth, mirth, and madness. Transactions and Studies of the College of Physicians of Philadelphia 1990;Ser 5. 12(1):103–106.

Rosenheim E, Golan G. Patients' reactions to humorous interventions in psychotherapy. American Journal of Psychotherapy 1986 Jan;40(1):110–124.

Rutherford K. Humor in Psychotherapy. Individual Psychology 1994 Jun;50:207–22.

Ruvelson L. The empathic use of sarcasm: humor in psychotherapy from a self psychological perspective. Clinical Social Work Journal 1988 Fal;16(3):297–305.

Sands S. The use of humor in psychotherapy. Psychoanalytic Review 1984 Nov;71(3):441–460.

Saper B. Humor in psychotherapy: is it good or bad for the client? Professional Psychology: Research and Practice 1987;18(4):360–367.

Schnarch DM. Therapeutic uses of humor in psychotherapy. Journal of Family Psychotherapy 1990;1(1):75–86.

Shaughnessy MF, Wadsworth TM. Humor in counseling and psychotherapy: a 20-year perspective. Psychological Reports 1992 Jun;70(3 pt 1):755–762.

Thomson BR. Appropriate and inappropriate uses of humor in psychotherapy as perceived by certified reality therapists: a Delphi study. Journal of Reality Therapy 1990 Fal;10(1):59–65.

Tuttman S. On utilizing humor in group psychotherapy. Group 1991 Win;15(4):246–256.

SEX DIFFERENCES

Crawford M, Gressley D. Creativity, caring, and context. Psychology of Women Quarterly 1991 Jun;15(2):217–231.

Gruner CR, Gruner MW, Travillion LJ. Another quasi-experimental study of understanding/appreciation of editorial satire. Psychological Reports 1991 Dec;69(3 pt 1): 731–734.

Hampes WP. Relation between humor and generativity. Psychological Reports 1993 Aug;73(1):131–136.

Hampes WP. Relation between intimacy and humor. Psychological Reports 1992 Aug;71(1):127–130.

Janus SS. Humor, sex, and power in American society. American Journal of Psychoanalysis 1981 Sum;41(2):161–167.

Jeffress JE. Sexual jokes. Medical Aspects of Human Sexuality 1985 May;19(5):178,184.

Johnson AM. Language ability and sex affect humor appreciation. Perceptual and Motor Skills 1992 Oct;75(2):571–581.

Kuhlman TL. A study of salience and motivational theories of humor. Journal of Personality and Social Psychology 1985 Jul;49(1):281–286.

Martin RA, Lefcourt HM. Situational humor response questionnaire: quantitative measure of sense of humor. Journal of Personality and Social Psychology 1984 Jul;47(1): 145–155.

Neitz MJ. Humor, hierarchy, and the changing status of women. Psychiatry 1980 Aug;43(3):211–223.

O'Quin, K, Aronoff J. Humor as a technique of social influence. Social Psychology Quarterly 1981 Dec;44(4):349–357.

Prerost FJ. Developmental aspects of adolescent sexuality as reflected in reactions to sexually explicit humor. Psychological Reports 1980 Apr;46(2):543–548.

Prerost FJ. The effects of high spatial density on humor appreciation: age and sex differences. Social Behavior and Personality 1980;8(2):239–244.

Prerost FJ. Humor preferences among angered males and females: associations with humor content and sexual desire. Psychological Reports 1995 Aug;77(1):227–234.

Prerost FJ. Reactions to humorous sexual stimuli as a function of sexual activeness and satisfaction. Psychology: A Quarterly Journal of Human Behavior 1984;21(1):23–27.

Richman J. Sexual jokes. Medical Aspects of Human Sexuality 1985 Feb;19(2):196,201.

Rose JF. Psychologic health of women: a phenomenologic study of women's inner strength. Advances in Nursing Science 1990 Jan;12(2):56–70.

Scott EM. Humor and the alcoholic patient: a beginning study. Alcoholism Treatment Quarterly 1989;6(2):29–39.

Shibles W. Feminism and the cognitive theory of emotion: anger, blame and humor. Women and Health 1991;17(1):57–69.

Wahl CW. Sexual jokes. Medical Aspects of Human Sexuality 1985 Apr;19(4):150,152.

Wilson DW, Molleston JL. Effects of sex and type of humor on humor appreciation. Journal of Personality Assessment 1981 Feb;45(1):90–96.

STRESS REDUCTION

Ackerman MA. Humor won, humor too: a model to incorporate humor into the healthcare setting (revised). Nursing Forum 1994 April–June;29(2):15–21.

Anderson CA. An examination of perceived control, humor, irrational beliefs, and positive stress as moderators of the relation between negative stress and health. Basic and Applied Social Psychology 1989 Jun;10(2):101–117.

Bowen M, Davidhizar R. Tension reduction in the operating room. Today's O.R. Nurse 1990 Nov;12(11):32–34.

Buchwald A. On laughter. Journal of the American Medical Association 1984 Dec 7;252(21):3014.

Carroll JL, Dimmer S. Humor for the health of it. Michigan Hospitals 1989 May;25(5):22–25.

Chipman D. Did you hear the one about. Revolution: The Journal of Nurse Empowerment 1993 Fal;3(3):54–58, 105.

Cohen S. Humor beats stress. Training & Development 1996 Apr;50(4):66.

Darwish M. So you thought the Internet was only serious: humor resources to keep us balanced. Beginnings 1997 Mar;17(3):8.

Davidhizar R, Bowen M. The dynamics of laughter. Archives of Psychiatric Nursing 1992 Apr;6(2):132–137.

DesCamp KD, Thomas CC. Buffering nursing stress through play at work. Western Journal of Nursing Research 1993; 15(5);619–627.

Ditlow F. Humor is a serious remedy for stress. Imprint 1989 Apr–May;36(2):80.

Ditlow F. The missing element in health care. Humor as a form of creativity. Journal of Holistic Nursing 1993 Mar; 11(1):66–79.

Dixon NF. Humor: a cognitive alternative to stress? In: Sarason IG, Spielberger CD (eds), Stress and Anxiety 7, Washington D.C., Hemisphere Publishing Corp., 1980:281–289.

Donnelly GF. How do I know I'm on the right track? RN 1980 Sep;43(9):44,46.

Dugan DO. Laughter and tears: best medicine for stress. Nursing Forum 1989;24(1):18–26.

Eccles AM. Using humor to relieve stress. Point of View 1990 Jan 1;27(1):8–9.

Goldstein JH, Mantell M, Pope B, Derks, P. Humor and the coronary-prone behavior pattern. Current Psychology: Research and Reviews 1988 Sum;7(2):115–121.

Goodwin S. He who laughs, lasts. Nursing Times 1986 Jun 4;82(23):24.

Grumet GW. Laughter: nature's epileptoid catharsis. Psychological Reports 1989 Dec;65(3 pt 2):1059–1078.

Gullickson C. Laughter jest for the health of it. Healthcare Trends and Transition 1992 Nov–Dec;4(2):28–35.

Hutchinson S. Self-care and job stress. Image: Journal of Nursing Scholarship 1987 Win;19(4):192–196.

James DH. Humor: a holistic nursing intervention. Journal of Holistic Nursing 1995 Sep;13(3):239–247.

Kennedy KD. Invest in yourself: have a laugh! have a health laugh! Nursing Forum 1995 Jan–Mar;30(1):25–30.

Labott SM, Martin RB. The stress-moderating effects of weeping and humor. Journal of Human Stress 1987 Win;13(4):159–164.

Leff N. Ten ways nurses can change their lives with laffter and play. Revolution: The Journal of Nurse Empowerment 1993 Win;3(4):62–63,94.

Leiber DB. Laughter and humor in critical care. Dimensions of Critical Care Nursing 1986 May–Jun;5(3):162–170.

McGhee PE. How humor helps nurses manage job stress. Journal of Practical Nursing 1993 Sep;43(3):37–40.

McGhee PE. Laughter is the cure for terminal seriousness. Addiction Letter 1996 Feb;12(2):3.

McFadden B. Laughter can make your day. Neonatal Network 1997 Jun;16(4):54.

Martin RA, Lefcourt HM. Sense of humor as a moderator of the relation between stressors and moods. Journal of Personality and Social Psychology 1983 Dec;45(6):1313–1324.

Mattera MD. Relax! RN 1997 Aug;60(8):7.

Nelson DS. Humor in the pediatric emergency department: a 20-year perspective. Pediatrics 1992 Jun;89(6 pt 1):1089–1090.

Nezu AM, Nezu CM, Blissett SE. Sense of humor as moderator of the relation between stressful events and psychological distress: a prospective analysis. Journal of Personality and Social Psychology 1988 Mar;54(3):520–525.

Paquet JB. Laughter and stress management in the OR. Today's O.R. Nurse 1993 Nov–Dec;15(6):13–17.

Pasquali EA. Humor: preventive therapy for family caregivers. Home Healthcare Nurse 1991 May–Jun;9(3);13–17.

Prerost FJ. Health locus of control, humor, and reduction in aggression. Psychological Reports 1987 Dec;61(3):887–896.

Prerost FJ. Intervening during crises of life transitions: promoting a sense of humor as a stress moderator. Counselling Psychology Quarterly 1989;2(4):475–480.

Prerost FJ. Use of humor and guided imagery in therapy to

alleviate stress. Journal of Mental Health Counseling 1988 Jan;10(1):16–22.

Roach M. Can you laugh your stress away? Health 1996 Sep; 10(5):92–96.

Robinson VM. The purpose and function of humor in OR nursing. Today's O.R. Nurse 1993 Nov–Dec;15(6):7–12.

Rosenberg L. A qualitative investigation of the use of humor by emergency personnel as a strategy for coping with stress. Journal of Emergency Nursing 1991 Aug;17(4) 197–202.

Safranek R, Schill T. Coping with stress: does humor help. Psychological Reports 1982 Aug;51(1):222.

Schill T, O'Laughlin S. Humor preference and coping with stress. Psychological Reports 1984 Aug;55(1):309–310.

Shoss B. Smile if you're feeling stressed. Family Safety & Health 1993 Spr;52:24–25.

Simon JM. Therapeutic humor, who's fooling who? Journal of Psychosocial Nursing and Mental Health Services 1988 Apr;26(4):8–12.

Smail N, Lynch M. The best medicine. Journal of Practical Nursing 1996 Mar;46(1):24–25.

Vinton KL. Humor in the workplace: is it more than telling jokes. Small Group Behavior 1989 May;20(2):151–166.

Weishaus G. Share the laughter. Home Healthcare Nurse 1996 Nov;14(11):903–904.

White C, Howse E. Managing humor: when is it funny-and when is it not? Nursing Management 1993 Apr;24(4): 80–92.

Woodhouse DK. The aspects of humor in dealing with stress. Nursing Administration Quarterly 1993 Fall;18(1): 80–89.

Wooten P. Humor: an antidote for stress. Holistic Nursing Practice 1996 Jan;10(2):49–56.

Yovetich NA, Dale JA, Hudak MA. Benefits of humor in reduction of threat-induced anxiety. Psychological Reports 1990 Feb;66(1):51–58.

TEACHING

Austin L, Fry C. Mandatory education: a successful, creative approach. Journal of Nursing Staff Development 1993 Jul/Aug;9(4):200–201.

Bennett HJ. Keeping up with the literature. Journal of the American Medical Association 1992 Feb 19;267(7):920.

Bonheur BB. Creating a new learning experience: "The story of Art" and "Prudent Art". Journal of Continuing Education in Nursing 1994 Sep/Oct;25(5):237–240.

Chan B. Does humour have a place in nursing education? Hong Kong Nursing Journal 1993 Mar;61:15–16.

Christy NP. The passive voice is deemed to be bad. Hospital Practice 1984 May;19(5):155,158–159.

Clarridge A, Couchman WA, Holloway IM. Interaction in the classroom: district nurse students and their teachers. Nurse Education Today 1992 Jun;12(3):200–206.

Endlich E. Teaching the psychology of humor. Teaching of Psychology 1993 Oct;20(3):181–183.

Felson B. Humor in medicine. Seminars in Roentgenology 1987 Jul;22(3):141–143.

Fennell R. Using humor to teach responsible sexual health decision making and condom comfort. Journal of American College Health Association 1993 Jul;42(1):37–39.

Flavier JM. The lessons of laughter. World Health Forum 1990;11(4):412–415.

Gigliotti E. Let me entertain..er..teach you: gaining attention through the use of slide shows. Journal of Continuing Education in Nursing 1995 Jan/Feb;26(1):31–34.

Glass E. Humor helps to "break the ice" during patient education. Oncology Nursing Forum 1993 Jul;20(6):965.

Grahame C. Frontline revolt. Nursing Times 1987 Apr 22; 83(16):60.

Harrison N. Using humour as an educational technique. Professional Nurse 1995 Dec;11(3):198–199.

Jones L. Consultant's corner. Journal of Shared Governance 1996 Apr;2(2):7–8.

Karrei I. Fun & games. Canadian Nurse 1992 Jun;88(6):28–30.

Kuhrik M, Kuhrik N, Berry PA. Facilitating learning with humor. Journal of Nursing Education 1997 Sep;36(7):332–334.

Lamp JM. Humor in postpartum education: depicting a new mother's worst nightmare. MCN 1992 Mar–Apr;17(2): 82–85.

Leidy K. Enjoyable learning experiences—an aid to retention? Journal of Continuing Education in Nursing 1992 Sep–Oct;23(5):206–208.

Lorensi EA. Humor in the testing situation. Nurse Educator 1996 Jan–Feb;21(1):12,14.

McDermott TJ. Cartooning: a humorous approach to medical and health education. Journal of Biocommunication 1989;16(4):20–27.

Maher MF, Smith D. I could have died laughing. Journal of Humanistic Education and Development 1993 Mar;31(3): 123–129.

Modic MB. A reinforcement technique: the goody bag. Journal of Continuing Education in Nursing 1994 May/Jun; 25(3):143–144.

Mooney NE. Juggling performance checklist. Journal of Continuing Education in Nursing 1993 Jan/Feb;24(1):43–44.

Moses NW, Friedman MM. Using humor in evaluating student performance. Journal of Nursing Education 1986 Oct; 25(8):328–333.

Parfitt JM. Humorous preoperative teaching; effect on recall of postoperative exercise routines. AORN Journal 1990 Jul;52(1):114–120.

Parkin CJ. Humor, health, and higher education: laughing matters. Journal of Nursing Education 1989 May;28(5):229–230.

Parrott TE. Humor as a teaching strategy. Nurse Educator 1994 May–Jun;19(3):36–38.

Pease RA. Cartoon humor in nursing education. Nursing Outlook 1991 Nov–Dec;39(6):262–267.

Robbins J. Using humor to enhance learning in the skills laboratory. Nurse Educator 1994 May/Jun;19(3):39–41.

Rosenberg L. A delicate dose of humor. Nursing Forum 1989;24(2):3–7.

Schmidt SR. Effects of humor on sentence memory. Journal of Experimental Psychology: Learning, Memory, and Cognition 1994 Jul;20(4):953–967.

Schmitz K. Surviving nursing school with humor. Imprint 1989 Nov;36(4):105–109.

Schoenknecht H. How to use humor to help educate physicians in necessary PPS skills. Hospital Topics 1985 Nov–Dec;63(6):30–39.

Shiffner JM. The family medicine game: using humor to teach residents about endings. Family Medicine 1991 Feb;23(2):156–158.

Struthers J. An exploration into the role of humour in the nursing student-nurse teacher relationship. Journal of Advanced Nursing 1994 Mar;19(3):486–491.

Tupler J. Humor, learning & labor: laughter is a life skill. Childbirth Instructor 1993 Win;3(1):18–20.

Warner SL. Humor: a coping response for student nurses. Archives of Psychiatric Nursing 1991 Feb;5(1);10–16.

Watson MJ, Emerson S. Facilitate learning with humor. Journal of Nursing Education 1988 Feb;27(2):89–90.

White LA, Lewis DJ. Humor: a teaching strategy to promote learning. Journal of Nursing Staff Development 1990 Mar–Apr;6(2):60–64.

Williams BL, Hubbard B. Teaching theory through cartoons. Journal of Health Education 1994 May/Jun;25(3):179–180.

Wise PSY. Maintaining the perspective. Journal of Continuing Education in Nursing 1997 May/Jun;28(3):101.

Wright D. The princess and the chemo spill—a policy magically turned into a fairy tale. Journal of Continuing Education in Nursing 1993 Jan/Feb;24(1):37–38.

Wylie MA. This nurse educator is hooked on humor. Journal of Emergency Nursing 1997 Jun;23(3):272–273.

Ziv A. The effect of humor on aggression catharsis in the classroom. The Journal of Psychology 1987 Jul;12(4):359–364.

AUTHOR INDEX

DATE DUE

JA 08 '01			
MR 8 '04			

DEMCO 38-297